The Folate Fix

Exploring the Role of Folate in Autism and Neurodevelopmental Disorders

By Dr. Richard E. Frye, MD, PhD

The Folate Fix

Exploring the Role of Folate in Autism and Neurodevelopmental Disorders

By Dr. Richard E. Frye, MD, PhD

©2025 Richard E. Frye
ISBN: 979-8-99-28893-0-7
Published by The Metabolic Learning Resource, LLC

Dedication

This book is dedicated to all the parents that have worked tirelessly to fight for their children to have the best life despite being faced with medical science that could not provide answers. These heroes will be the ones to move the world forward and create a better place for their children, their families, and the others who come behind them.

Acknowledgements

I would like to thank my colleagues that have helped me along the journey to better understand central folate abnormalities, especially for their encouragement and assistance in completing and publishing the science in order to prove the importance of folate in neurodevelopmental disorders such as autism spectrum disorder.

I would like to thank the parents of children affected by this disorder for their faith that a treatment could be found. Their trust in my work was a clear motivating force which propelled the research forward.

I thank my friends, wife and children for their support though this long journey. I need to especially thank Shana Anderson for her incredible assistance with making the idea of a book a reality.

Disclosures

The publisher and the author provide this book and its contents on an "as is" basis and make no representations or warranties of any kind, express or implied, with respect to the accuracy, applicability, fitness, or completeness of the contents. The publisher and the author expressly disclaim all warranties, including but not limited to any warranties of medical efficacy, merchantability, or fitness for a particular purpose.

The content presented in this book is for informational purposes only and is not intended to diagnose, treat, cure, or prevent any medical condition or disease. This book is not a substitute for professional medical advice, diagnosis, or treatment. Readers should consult their own licensed healthcare providers regarding any medical condition and before implementing any health-related recommendations described in this book.

By using this book, you acknowledge and accept that the authors and publisher are not responsible for any adverse effects or consequences resulting from the use of the information herein. Individual results may vary. The testimonials and examples provided are not intended to represent or guarantee that any individual will achieve the same or similar outcomes.

Financial and Professional Disclosures

Dr. Frye serves in an uncompensated advisory role for ReligenDX, a diagnostic testing company. He also has a patent pending for the development of a folate biomarker test. Portions of the research discussed in this book were supported by grants from Arizona Biomedical Research Centre, Autism Speaks, the National Institutes of Health (NIH), the Department of Defense (DoD), and the BRAIN Foundation.

Table of Contents

Acronyms Used in This Book — xiv

Part I. Vitamins — 1

Chapter 1. The Importance of Vitamins — 3
What are Vitamins? — 3
Essential Versus Non-Essential Vitamins — 4
Vitamins are Precursors to Important Molecules — 4
Vitamins are Carriers of Important Compounds — 5
Vitamins are Important Cofactors — 6
Vitamins Send Important Messages — 7
Vitamins Offer Protection — 8
Fat Soluble vs. Water Soluble Vitamins — 10

Chapter 2. Folate: The Most Essential Vitamin — 11
The Discovery of Folate — 11
Nutritional Sources of Folate — 13
Recommended Dietary Allowance of Folate — 13
The Importance of the Microbiome — 15
Folate Absorption & Transportation in the GI Tract — 19
Liver Metabolism — 19
Understanding Oxidation and Reduction — 23

Chapter 3. Folate: The Workhorse Vitamin — 25
Brain Development and Nutrition — 26
Folic Acid versus Folinic Acid — 28
Folinic Acid (Leucovorin) – The Chemistry — 29
The Folate Cycle — 31
Purine Metabolism — 33
Purine Production — 35
Methylation Metabolism — 36
Redox Metabolism — 37

Part II. If the Brain Lacks Folate — 41

Chapter 4. Cerebral Folate Deficiency (CFD) — 43
Background — 43
CFD as a Syndrome — 45
The Scientific Evidence — 46
Folate Receptor Autoantibodies (FRAAs) — 48
Other Causes of CFD — 50
CFD Treatment — 50
Caroline's Story — 52
A Physician's Perspective — 57
Marley's Story — 59
A Physician's Perspective — 63

Chapter 5. Autism Spectrum Disorder	67
Background	67
The Scientific Evidence	71
Evan's Story	79
Kai's Story	87
Mason's Story	91
CFD and Autism Spectrum Disorder	94
A Physician's Perspective	94
Chapter 6. Down Syndrome	103
Background	103
The Scientific Evidence	105
Brooklyn's Story	107
Reeve's Story	112
Bella's Story	118
CFD and Down Syndrome	124
A Physician's Perspective	127
Chapter 7. Epilepsy	129
Background	129
The Scientific Evidence	136
Folinic Acid Responsive Seizures	137
CFD and Epilepsy	139
Victor's Story	140
Patrick's Story	144
A Physician's Perspective	151
Chapter 8. Neuroinflammation	155
Background	155
Daniel's Story	158
How Leucovorin Helped Me - Daniel in His Own Words	162
A Physician's Perspective	164
Daniel's Complicated Story Comes Together	165
CFD and Neuroinflammation	169
Chapter 9. Genetic Disorders	173
Background	173
From Genetic Code to Useful Protein	175
The Scientific Evidence	176
Leland's Story	180
A Physician's Perspective	184
Chapter 10. So What About Vaccines?	187
Horror Vacui	187
"We Know Autism is Genetic"	188
"Vaccines are Absolutely Safe"	189
"The Debate is Finally Over"	190
Then Came COVID	191
Compassion as a Subversive Activity	192

Part III. Folate in Psychiatric Conditions — 193

Chapter 11. Psychiatric Disorders — 195
Background — 195
CFD and Psychiatric Disorders — 197
Implications — 199

Chapter 12. Neurocognitive Disorders of Older Age — 201
Background — 201
CFD and Neurocognitive Disorders — 202
Implications — 204

Part IV. Working Your Way Through CFD — 205

Chapter 13. Who Should Be Tested? — 207

Chapter 14. The Symptoms of CFD — 211
CFD Checklist — 212
Microcephaly — 213
Ataxia — 214
Pyramidal Signs — 214
Movement Disorders — 215
Neurodevelopmental Regression — 216
Electrical Status Epilepticus in Sleep (ESES) — 216
Enlarged Ventricles — 217
Intellectual Disability — 218
Communication Disorder — 218
Repetitive and Restrictive Behavior — 219
Irritability — 219
Self-Injurious Behavior — 220
Obsessive Compulsive Disorder — 220
Catatonia — 220
Vision Changes — 221
Hearing Loss — 221

Chapter 15. Diagnosing CFD — 223
To Lumbar Puncture or Not to Lumbar Puncture: That is the Question — 223
What is a Normal CSF Folate Level? — 225
Non-Invasive Testing for Cerebral Folate Deficiency — 227
Specific Genetic Testing — 227
Folate Receptor Autoantibodies — 230
Beyond the Folate Autoantibody — 231
Mitochondrial Disorders — 232
Other Testing — 234
CFD or CFD-like: What is the Diagnosis? — 235

Chapter 16. Milk and CFD	237
Milk: It Does the Body Good?	237
Breastmilk: A Bioactive, Adaptive Fluid	238
The History of Human Milk Drinking Practices	239
Milk Allergies and Intolerances	239
How Milk Differs from Other Dairy Products	240
Biological Components of Milk	241
Milk and Folate Receptor Autoantibodies	242
The Role of Milk in CFD	244

Chapter 17. Treating CFD	245
Why Leucovorin	246
Dosing	247
Brands	250
Coincidence or True Effect of Brands?	251
Alternate Routes of Administration	252
Intravenous (IV) Administration	253
Subcutaneous (SC) Administration	255
Intramuscular (IM) Administration	256
Intrathecal	257
Use of 5-methyltetrahydrofolate (5-MTHF)	257
Use of Deplin® to Treat CFD	258
What About Folic Acid?	259
Adjunctive Treatments	259

Chapter 18. Following Outcomes	263
Parent Rated Autism Symptomatic Change Scale (PRASC)	265

Part V. Frequently Asked Questions

Chapter 19 Frequently Asked Questions (FAQs)	269
FAQs: Diagnosis	269
FAQs: Treatment	277
FAQs: Other Questions	287

References	296
About the Autism Discovery & Treatment Foundation (ADTF)	313
About the Metabolic Learning Resource (MLR)	314
About the Author	315

Acroynms Used in This Book

5-HTP	5-Hydroxytryptophan
5-MTHF	5-Methyltetrahydrafolate
ABC	Aberrant Behavior Checklist
AD	Alzheimer's Disease
ADOS	Autism Diagnostic Observation Schedule
AED	Antiepileptic Drug
ASD	Autism Spectrum Disorder
ATP	Adenosine Triphosphate
BBB	Blood Brain Barrier
BCSFB	Blood Cerebrospinal Fluid Barrier
BH_4	Tetrahydrobiopterin
CFD	Cerebral Folate Disorder
CSF	Cerebrospinal Fluid
CNS	Central Nervous System
CNV	Copy Number Variation
DFE	Dietary Folate Equivalents
DNA	Deoxyribonucleic Acid
DHPR	Dihydropteridine Reductase
DHF	Dihydrofolate
DHFR	Dihydrofolate Reductase
DS	Down Syndrome
DSRD	Down Syndrome Regression Disorder
EEG	Electroencephalogram
ESES	Electrical Status Epilepticus in Sleep
FAD	Flavin Adenine Dinucleotide
FBP	Folate Binding Protein
FDH	Folate-dependent Hydroxymethyltransferase
FRAA	Folate Receptor Alpha Autoantibody
FRAT	Folate Receptor Autoantibody Test
FRα	Folate Receptor Alpha
FOLR1	Gene Encoding the Folate Receptor Alpha Protein
GALT	Gut-Associated Lymphoid Tissue
GGH	Gamma Glutamyl Hydrolase
HPLC	High-performance liquid chromatography
LP	Lumbar Puncture

MCI	Mild Cognitive Impairment
MRI	Magnetic Resonance Imaging
MRP3	Multidrug-Resistance-Associated Protein 3
MS	Methionine Synthase (as used in Chapter 3)
MS	Multiple Sclerosis (as used in Chapter 8)
NAD	Nicotinamide Adenine Dinucleotide
NDR	Neurodevelopmental Regression
NNT	Number Needed to Treat
NTD	Neural Tube Defects
OCD	Obsessive-Compulsive Disorder
PANDAS	Pediatric Autoimmune Neuropsychiatric Disorder Associated with Streptococcal Infections
PANS	Pediatric Acute-onset Neuropsychiatric Syndrome
PCFT	Proton-Coupled Folate Transporter
PD	Parkinson's Disease
PKU	Phenylketonuria
PPI	Proton Pump Inhibitor
RDA	Recommended Dietary Allowance
sFBP	Soluble Folate Binding Protein
SRS	Social Responsiveness Scale
SUDEP	Sudden Unexplained Death in Epilepsy
UMFA	Unmetabolized Folic Acid
VNS	Vagus Nerve Stimulator

Part I.
Vitamins

In 1820, medical physician Dr. Usher Parsons, MD, vividly summarized a harrowing disease that led to a dreadful and agonizing death.

The doctor wrote:

> *It commences with unusual weariness – dejection of spirits – sluggishness, and offensive breath. The gums become soft, livid, and swollen, are apt to bleed from the slightest cause, and separate from the teeth, leaving them loose. About the same time the legs swell, are glossy, and soon exhibit foul ulcers.*
>
> *At first the ulcers resemble black blisters, which spread and discharge a dark-coloured matter...these ulcers increase...bleedings occur at the nose and mouth, all evacuations from the body become intolerably fetid, and death closes the scene.*

One might assume that this 200-year-old ailment was an inescapable death sentence, particularly in an era when medicine had yet to uncover cures for such complex and devastating diseases. However, this assumption would be wrong.

Immediately after detailing the grim progression of the disease, Dr. Parsons outlined a surprisingly simple, safe, and effective cure:

> *Treatment: Medicine is almost unnecessary. Among the most celebrated and infallible remedies are succulent fruits, of which oranges, lemons, limes, and apples, are the best.*

This excerpt is from a medical textbook titled Sailor's Physician.[1] The disease Dr. Parsons, a navy surgeon, described is scurvy—a Vitamin C deficiency that often crippled ship crews from the 16th to 18th centuries.

Though Vitamin C itself would not be officially discovered until more than a century later, Dr. Parsons' account reflects an almost intuitive understanding among early physicians: certain components of food contain substances vital to human health. This historical recognition laid the groundwork for our modern understanding of vitamins and their indispensable role in preventing disease.

Even today, these insights have profound and far-reaching implications. They highlight how nutrient deficiencies can often mimic or exacerbate complex health conditions. From metabolic disorders to immune dysfunction, understanding the role of vitamins in maintaining health remains one of the most critical—and often overlooked—approaches to reducing disease burden. By addressing underlying deficiencies through proper nutrition and supplementation, we have the opportunity to prevent a range of conditions, emphasizing that the simplest solutions can sometimes yield the most significant health outcomes.

---

1. Parsons, Usher. Sailor's Physician – Exhibiting the Symptoms, Causes and Treatment of Diseases Incident to Seamen and Passengers in Merchant Vessels with Directions for Preserving their Health in Sickly Climates. Cambridge. Hiliard and Metcalf. 1820.

CHAPTER 1.
The Importance of Vitamins

What are Vitamins?

Doctors advocate for the regular intake of daily multivitamins, emphasizing their significance in supporting bodily functions. But what are vitamins and what do they do?

Vitamins are organic compounds that keep the body functioning normally. Categorized as either "essential" or "non-essential," vitamins fulfill a multitude of roles within the body, underscoring their indispensable value.

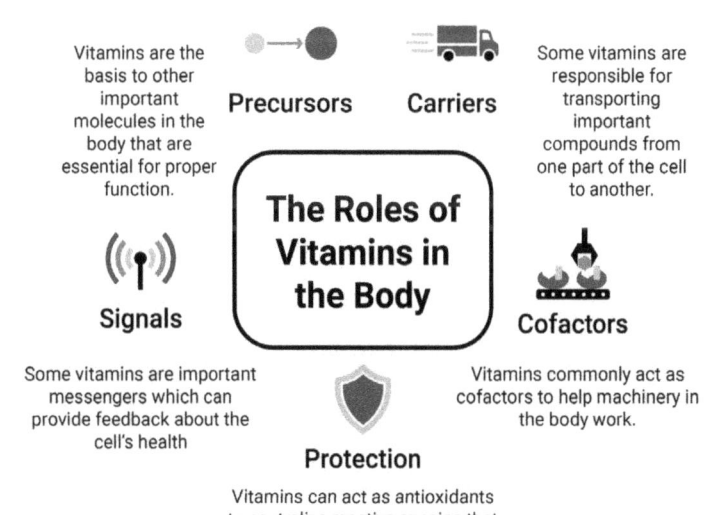

Figure 1.1 Vitamins are involved in many important processes in the body.

Essential Vitamins	Non-Essential Vitamins
Must be obtained through diet - body cannot synthesize.	Body can produce on its own through metabolic processes.

 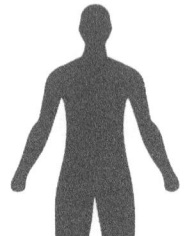

Figure 1.2 Essential vs Non-Essential Vitamins

Essential Versus Non-Essential Vitamins

Essential vitamins are specific nutrients that the body cannot produce in sufficient amounts to maintain proper function; hence, they must be sourced from dietary intake. The diversity and quantity of vitamins available to the body are directly influenced by an individual's dietary choices. This is very important, particularly for people adhering to specialized diets or facing restricted eating patterns, as these individuals are at risk of developing specific vitamin deficiencies.

In contrast, non-essential vitamins are those that the body can synthesize internally. While some may also be obtained from food sources, the body generally manufactures them. Storage capabilities vary: some vitamins are stored for future use, while others necessitate regular consumption to maintain optimal levels.

Vitamin requirements are different for each person due to their genetic make-up. An individual must be able to absorb and activate vitamins to use them. Consequently, certain individuals may require higher quantities or specific forms of vitamins for optimal function. Notably, this is especially pertinent in the case of folate, an essential vitamin, which is the focus of this book.

Vitamins are Precursors to Important Molecules

Many vitamins serve as precursors to essential biomolecules. For instance, riboflavin (Vitamin B2) and niacin (Vitamin B3) form the foundation of flavin adenine dinucleotide (FAD) and nicotinamide adenine dinucleotide (NAD), both of which are crucial for cellular function. Similarly, adenine (Vitamin B4) is a key precursor for several vital cellular compounds. It is a fundamental component of deoxyribonucleic acid (DNA), the blueprint of our genetic code, and a building block of adenosine triphosphate (ATP), the primary energy currency of the cell.

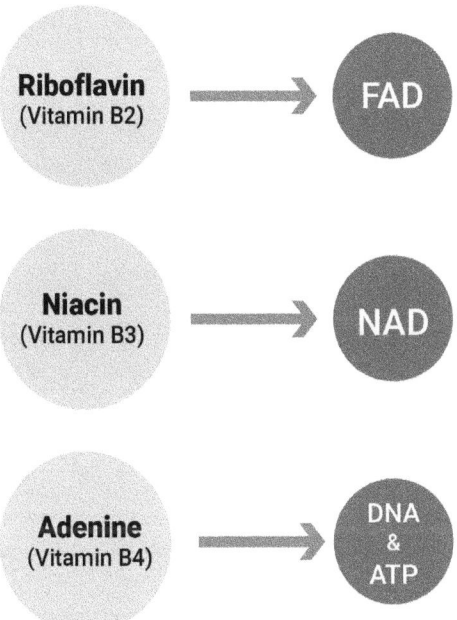

Figure 1.3 Vitamins act as precursors to important molecules.

Vitamins are Carriers of Important Compounds

Many vitamins function as carriers of essential molecules, playing a critical role in cellular processes. For instance, several vitamins are vital for the mitochondria, the energy-producing organelles often referred to as the "powerhouses of the cell." Mitochondria generate energy by converting nutrients from food into a usable form.

Sugars and fats undergo initial processing in the mitochondria through the citric acid cycle, which extracts electrons from molecules to release energy. These electrons are then transported by FAD and NAD to the electron transport chain, where they drive the production of cellular energy (See Figure 1.4).

Cells require energy to function efficiently and can contain anywhere from hundreds to tens of thousands of mitochondria, depending on their energy demands. Mitochondria are uniquely complex structures that contain their own genetic material, which is inherited exclusively from the mother.

Remarkably, mitochondria can produce energy from carbohydrates, fats, and proteins. However, protein utilization is typically conserved due to its essential role in growth and repair.

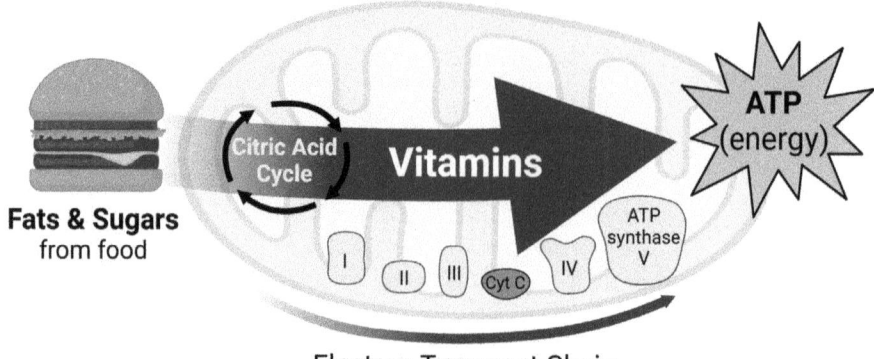

Figure 1.4. Vitamins act as electron carriers in the mitochondria. Electrons generated from the citric acid cycle are carried by vitamin-derived cofactors (NAD and FAD) and transferred through the electron transport chain—from Complex I to Complex II, then to Complex III and IV—culminating in ATP production at Complex V. Image created with BioRender.

Mitochondria represent a complex aspect of cellular biology, featuring numerous pathways dedicated to breaking down nutrients into metabolites for energy production. One of the most well-known pathways is the citric acid cycle, which generates energy carriers that fuel the electron transport chain. This chain consists of five distinct protein complexes that sequentially process energy, ultimately leading to the synthesis of ATP, the cell's primary energy currency. Notably, Complex IV of the electron transport chain relies on oxygen to catalyze energy production, highlighting oxygen's critical role in cellular function.

When NAD and FAD work in the mitochondria, they are known as electron carriers. NAD (in the form of NADH) and FAD (in the form of FADH$_2$) transport the electrons from the citric acid cycle to the complexes. NADH feeds Complex I, and FADH$_2$ feeds Complex II. Complex I and II both use another vitamin called CoQ$_{10}$ (also known as Ubiquinol) to transport the electrons to Complex III. Complex III uses a compound called cytochrome c to transport electrons to Complex IV. In cytochrome c, Iron (Fe) holds the electrons, which is why iron is another important nutrient. Lastly, inside Complex IV, copper (Cu), another vital element, holds the electrons. As this example illustrates, each vitamin plays a vital role, working in harmony to ensure the body functions properly. Without the necessary vitamins for the mitochondria, cells cannot produce energy, and the body's systems fail to operate as they should.

One of the most important carriers for our body is folate. Folate is known as the basis for one-carbon metabolism because it provides the source of methyl (one-carbon) groups. Methyl is essential for many important functions in the cell that will be discussed in the next chapter.

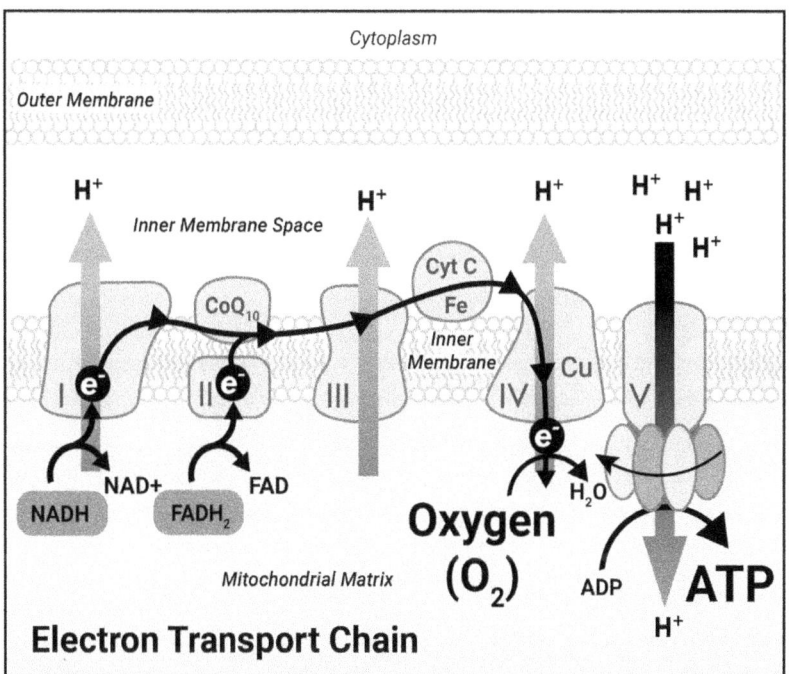

Figure 1.5 The electron transport chain is in the space between the inner and outer membrane of the mitochondria.

Vitamins are Important Cofactors

Vitamins also act as cofactors to help enzymes work. Enzymes can be thought of as small machines in our body that transform one chemical into another. These machines often need assistance from special molecules. In this way, vitamins act as coenzymes to work alongside the main enzymes. This is particularly important for B vitamins which act as cofactors for hundreds of enzymes.

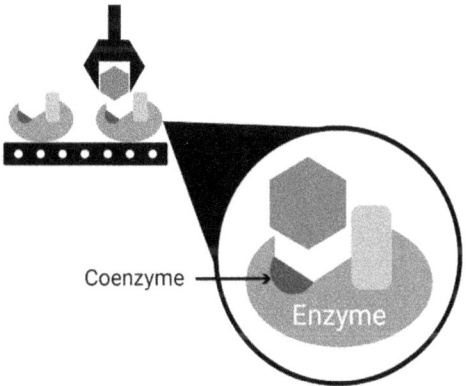

Figure 1.6 Vitamins act as coenzymes during chemical reactions.

Vitamins Send Important Messages

Vitamins also act as signals that send important messages to different cells. Because vitamins are used by various processes in the body, the amount of free-floating vitamins provides important information about the body's metabolic state.

As previously mentioned, NAD (Nicotinamide Adenine Dinucleotide) derives from niacin, also known as Vitamin B3. NAD serves as both a cofactor and an electron carrier in numerous vital reactions within the body. Its pivotal role in energy metabolism makes NAD levels a significant indicator of metabolic activity. Elevated NAD levels typically signify heightened energy production, while low levels suggest a slower metabolic rate. A diminished amount is often associated with aging and neurodegenerative conditions.[1]

Supplementation with NAD is believed to mitigate the aging process and enhance metabolism. This is achieved through the activation of the sirtuin pathway, a specialized mechanism that stimulates cellular activity and facilitates the repair of damaged cells. Consequently, NAD compounds have gained popularity as anti-aging supplements.

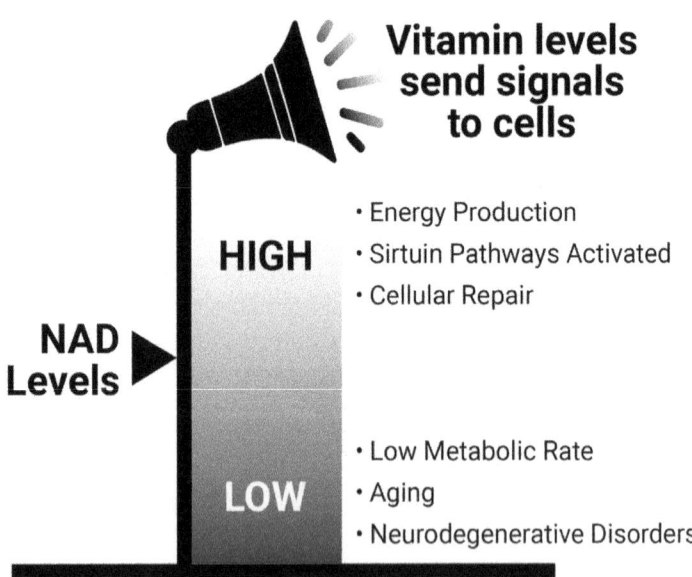

Figure 1.7 NAD levels act as signals, providing important information about cellular function.

Vitamins Offer Protection

Reactive species are small molecules characterized by their unstable electrons, which have the propensity to transfer to other substances, leading to damage. This electron transfer can adversely affect proteins, lipids (integral components of cell membranes), and genetic material.

Numerous vitamins, including Vitamins C, E, and CoQ_{10}, serve as antioxidants, playing a pivotal role in shielding the body by counteracting these reactive species. While the body inherently produces antioxidants and possesses repair mechanisms to rectify damage caused by reactive species, an overwhelming presence of these molecules can overpower the body's defenses, resulting in impaired cells. Hence, the availability of vitamins as antioxidants is of paramount importance.

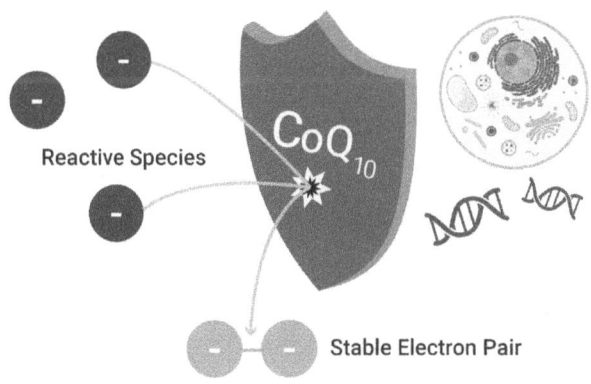

Figure 1.8 CoQ_{10} acts as an antioxidant to neutralize a reactive species. Image created with BioRender.

Antioxidants mitigate the impact of reactive species by donating an electron to them, forming a more stable electron pair configuration that prevents molecular damage. Upon depletion, antioxidants require replenishment or elimination from the body.

CoQ_{10} stands out as a multifaceted antioxidant, undertaking three distinct roles. Aside from neutralizing reactive species, it also replenishes Vitamins C and E, while facilitating electron transport within mitochondria for energy production. Should the demands of any of these functions become excessive, insufficient CoQ_{10} availability may result.

As we delve into subsequent chapters, it becomes evident that other vitamins such as B12 and folate play integral roles in the body's antioxidant system, aiding in the production of glutathione, another key antioxidant.

Fat-Soluble vs Water-Soluble Vitamins

Vitamins can be classified as either fat-soluble or water-soluble. Fat-soluble vitamins, as the name suggests, are stored in fat deposits and accumulate over time. Deficiencies in these vitamins may not manifest until these storage reserves are depleted. Supplementing fat-soluble vitamins requires caution, as blood concentrations may not rise until the fat stores are replenished. Consequently, once replenished, blood concentrations of these vitamins may significantly increase with supplementation.

Conversely, some individuals may struggle to maintain adequate levels of water-soluble vitamins in their bloodstream. This is because water-soluble vitamins dissolve in water and are rapidly eliminated from the body. Unlike fat-soluble vitamins, water-soluble vitamins are not stored. Examples include the nine B vitamins and Vitamin C, which require frequent replenishment. The following chapter will provide an in-depth exploration of folate, a water-soluble vitamin that serves numerous essential functions in the body.

FAT-SOLUABLE	WATER-SOLUABLE
Vitamin A	Thiamin (B1)
Vitamin E	Riboflavin (B2)
Vitamin D	Niacin (B3)
Vitamin K	Adenine (B4)
	Pantothenic Acid (B5)
	Pyridoxine (B6)
	Biotin (B7)
	Folate (B9)
	Cobalamin (B12)
	Vitamin C

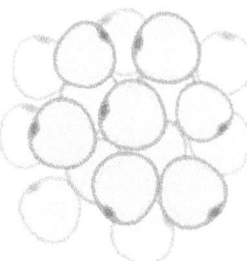
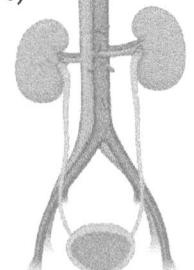

- Stored in fat
- Stores deplete slowly
- Daily dosing not needed

- Not stored
- Depleted in urine
- Daily dosing needed

Figure 1.9 The differences between fat-soluble and water-soluble vitamins. Created with BioRender.

CHAPTER 2.
FOLATE: THE MOST ESSENTIAL VITAMIN

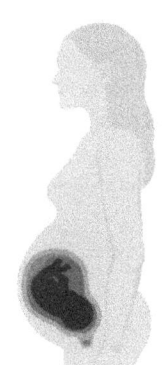

Most people know that folate is an important water-soluble vitamin. They may be familiar with the recommendation for pregnant women to take folate supplements to prevent birth defects. Likewise, many people are aware that everyday foods, such as breads and cereals, are fortified with folate, meaning folate has been added to them. But why is folate so important?

The Discovery of Folate

It was not until the 1800s that scientists began understanding the role of dietary factors in the prevention and onset of diseases. In the late 1800s, doctors realized that certain foods, particularly liver, were effective in treating and preventing anemia. Anemia was prevalent in poorer populations where people had deficient diets. In the early 1900s, an English physician, Lucy Wills, went to Bombay to investigate macrocytic anemia in pregnancy. She found that anemia could similarly be induced in rats by feeding them a deficient diet. When yeast was added to the diet, anemia was prevented, leading to Dr. Wills' discovery that brewer's yeast extracts cured megaloblastic anemia during pregnancy.[2]

In the early days, what is now called "folate" went by many different names, including: Vitamin M, Vitamin Bc and Norit eluate factor. In the mid-1900s, the substance in brewer's yeast was identified and isolated from spinach leaves by Herschel K. Mitchell, Esmond E. Snell, and Roger J. Williams.[3] The derivation of this substance from spinach leaves led to its name "folic acid" as this term is derived from the Latin *folium*, which means "leaf." At the same time, the "folic acid boys," led by the American biochemist Yellapragada Subbarow, extracted the pure crystalline form of folate. Shortly thereafter, Bob Stokstad and Robert Angier synthesized folate and determined its chemical structure.[4] Through these experiments and others, scientists learned that natural folates differed from folic acid in several biochemical ways. These differences will be discussed in further detail later in this chapter.

In the 1950-60s, the biochemical reactions involving folate and folate's importance in one-carbon metabolism and DNA synthesis were discovered. Several important observations helped to illuminate the role of folate in the body. Firstly, doctors observed that folate enhanced the growth of tumors. This led to the development of anti-folate compounds for cancer treatment.[5]

Subsequently, doctors observed that women receiving anti-folate compounds during pregnancy delivered babies with neural tube defects, such as spina bifida. Other physicians noticed that women with folate deficiency anemia also had high incidences of neural tube defects in their offspring. Scientists then realized that folate was needed for cell division and essential for normal growth and development.[6]

It was not until many years later that these findings were definitively confirmed. In 1991, the Medical Research Council Vitamin Study Research Group showed that folate supplementation could protect women from having babies with a neural tube defects.[7] This confirmation of folate's importance led to many of the recommendations seen today, such as the high intake of folate-rich foods and folic acid supplementation for pregnant women, as well as the fortification of grain products in the United States and other countries.

THE HISTORY OF FOLATE

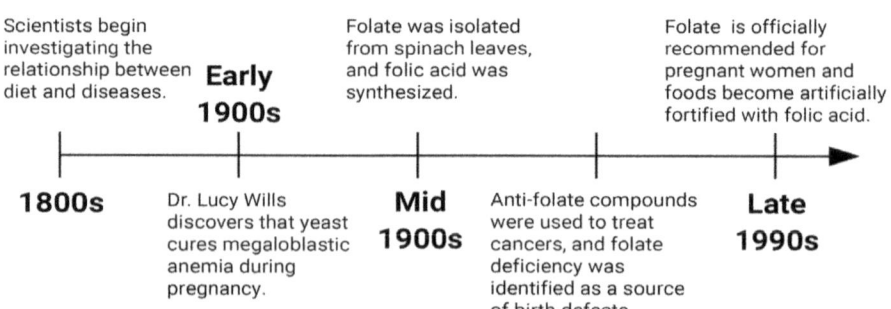

Figure 2.1 Summary of key events in the scientific history of folate.

Nutritional Sources of Folate

People typically consume natural forms of folate through their diets from foods like broccoli, eggs, legumes, and leafy greens; or they receive folate from supplements or fortified foods. While there are many sources of folate, it is important to know that these sources of folate are not equivalent. Only about 50% of folate in food is bioavailable, and the bioavailability of folate taken as a supplement is dependent on whether or not it is consumed with food. Because of these variations, a method for equating the amount of folate from different sources was developed. This is called dietary folate equivalents (DFEs).

Dietary Folate Equivalents (DFE)

1 mcg DFE =

- 1 mcg folate derived from food
- 0.6 mcg supplement consumed with food
- 0.6 mcg folate dervied from fortified foods
- 0.5 mcg supplement taken on an empty stomach

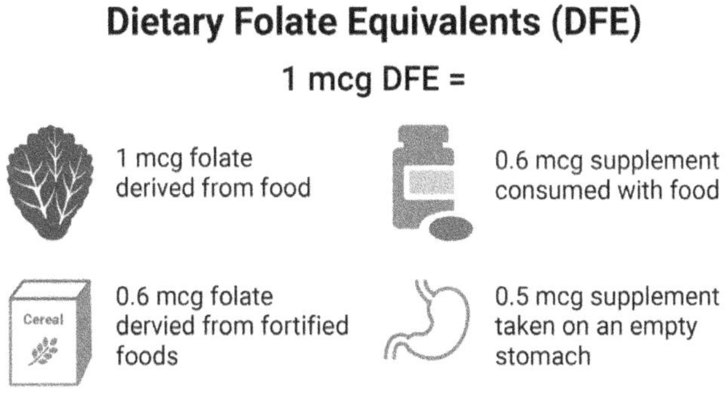

Figure 2.2 Explanation of Dietary Folate Equivalent (DFE).

Another way to interpret DFE is to complete the following statement: "If a person wants to consume the equivalent of 1.0 mcg of folate from food, they could intake (amount) from (source) in (manner)." For example: If a person wants to consume 1.0 DFE, they will need to take 0.5 mcg of folic acid on an empty stomach. Generally, folate taken from supplements yields more folate than what is derived from foods.

Recommended Dietary Allowance of Folate

The recommended dietary allowance (RDA), which represents the average daily intake sufficient for most people, is given in dietary folate equivalents (DFEs). The amount is rather modest, typically less than 1 milligram (mg). This requirement varies depending on age. Generally speaking, older individuals with larger bodies require more folate. For women, the requirement depends on pregnancy and/or lactation status.

During pregnancy and lactation, a woman's body is metabolically active and must supply folate, either through the blood or through milk, to the fetus or infant.

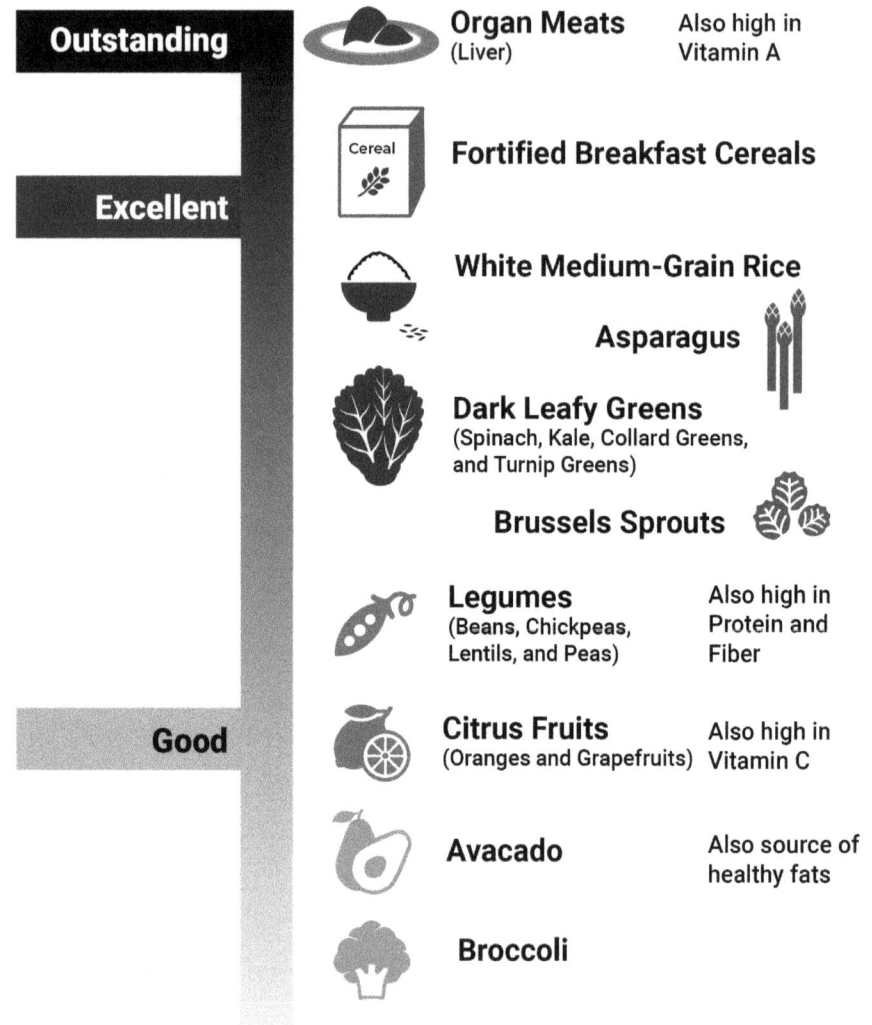

Figure 2.3 Different nutritional sources of folate, ranked by quality from good to outstanding. Folate is sensitive to heat, so cooking methods that minimize heat and use short cooking times can help preserve the folate content in foods.

Folate protects the fetus in multiple ways. As mentioned previously, folate intake during pregnancy has been shown to prevent birth defects.

Additionally, folate supplementation during pregnancy may protect the fetus against the damaging effects of some prescription drugs.[8] Newer research shows that taking folate during pregnancy, or even in the preconception period, may also prevent autism spectrum disorder (ASD) in the offspring.[9]

Folate is a water-soluble vitamin that is exceedingly safe, which is why so many national food fortification programs have been implemented around the world. Despite folate's benefits and safety, and even though folate has not been associated with adverse effects after short- or long-term exposure, some scientists worry that excessive folate intake may lead to negative outcomes. Because of this, the Institute of Medicine recommends an upper limit to folate intake. These limits are listed in Figure 2.4.

Recommended Dietary Allowance (RDA) and Upper Limits of Folate

Age	RDA	Upper Limit
0-6 Months	65 mcg	
7-12 Months	80 mcg	
1-3 Years	150 mcg	300 mcg
4-8 Years	200 mcg	400 mcg
9-13 Years	300 mcg	600 mcg
14-18 Years	400 mcg	800 mcg
Typical Adult	400 mcg	1000 mcg
Pregnant (14-18 Years)	600 mcg	800 mcg
Pregnant (>18 Years)	600 mcg	1000 mcg
Lactating (14-18 Years)	500 mcg	800 mcg
Lactating (>18 Years)	500 mcg	1000 mcg

Figure 2.4 Folate Recommendations Based on Age and Status.

Because folate is an important nutrient for rapidly replicating cells, some researchers hypothesized that folate may accelerate existing cancers. Consequently, many studies have been designed to investigate the relationship between folate intake and cancer. Surprisingly, research is showing the opposite of what was hypothesized—it is now believed that folate deficiency, rather than folate intake, is associated with an increased risk of some cancers. While study results have varied, overall, folate intake appears to have a protective effect on many cancers including breast,[10] pancreatic,[11] esophageal,[12] lung,[13] endometrial,[14] and colorectal.[15]

The Importance of the Microbiome

The gastrointestinal (GI) tract is not sterile but rather contains a diverse ecosystem of bacteria, fungi, and viruses called the enteric microbiome. While people often assume bacteria are bad, most of the bacteria present in the GI tract are helpful, not harmful. This microbiome has a multifaceted relationship with folate. Not only does it help breakdown and process dietary folate, but it also helps to produce folate. There are not just a few foreign organisms in the enteric microbiome, but rather up to 1,000 different species, and the number of bacteria in the gut outnumbers the number of cells in the human body by a factor of ten. Furthermore, since each species of bacteria has its own genome and a human only has one genome, the number of genes in the microbiome outnumbers those of a person by a factor of 100!

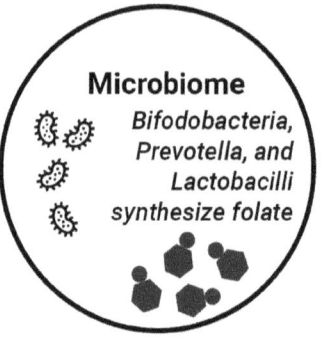

Figure 2.5 Enteric Microbiome.

A person's microbiome is thought to originate from their mother. Specifically, it is believed that bacteria are picked up when a baby goes through the birth canal. Emerging research suggests that the amniotic fluid surrounding a developing baby may not be sterile, as previously believed. Instead, the mother's womb appears to provide a microbiome that the baby inherits. These findings raise important considerations about events surrounding birth. For instance, studies reveal that newborns delivered by cesarean section have distinct microbiomes compared to those delivered vaginally.[16] Similarly, antibiotics administered to the mother during or shortly after delivery can significantly alter the newborn's microbiome.[17]

While these interventions are often essential to safeguard the health of both mother and child and cannot always be avoided, they do raise concerns. Changes in the microbiome have been linked to various health conditions, including diseases of infancy such as necrotizing enterocolitis and infantile colic, childhood atopic conditions like asthma, metabolic disorders such as diabetes, psychiatric conditions including mood and anxiety disorders, and ASD. Therefore, establishing a healthy microbiome from birth is crucial for long-term health.

In cases where microbiome transfer may be compromised, some have proposed "seeding" the newborn with vaginal fluids to replicate microbiome transfer, though this approach remains unproven. Conversely, research suggests that introducing probiotics early in life, either to the mother during pregnancy or directly to the newborn, shows the most evidence for reducing the risk of childhood diseases, particularly allergic conditions.[18] Notably, the microbiome is most malleable within the first two years of life, after which it becomes difficult to modify.

This highlights the importance of breastfeeding, which facilitates the transfer of the mother's microbiome to the infant, and emphasizes the role of proper nutrition and gut health in the first years of life.

Another emerging concern is the "disappearing microbiome," attributed to the Western diet. Compared to non-Western populations, the Western microbiome has 15-30% fewer species and lacks key bacteria such as *Firmicutes* and *Proteobacteria*.

What can be done to maximize a healthy microbiome? Figure 2.6 demonstrates some simple precautions that can be taken to minimize detrimental changes in the microbiome in the mother and child early in life.

Remediation Plan for Microbiome

Avoid	Promote
+ Possible Remediation Plan	+ Healthy Practices
Antibiotics Remediation: Prebiotics and/or Probiotics. Supplement with canitine if using β-Lactams antibiotics.	**Folate Metabolism & Absorption** Use reduced folates (see explanation later in this chapter). Avoid folic acid.
Acetaminophen Remediation: Pretreat with N-acetyl-cysteine if unavoidable.	**Psychological Stress Management** Practice meditation, yoga, and relaxation.
Bovine Milk Products Eliminate or minimize use.	**Good Diet** Eat foods high in microbiota accessible carbohydrates along with fruits and vegetables.
Maternal Infection Minimize exposure, avoid treatments that affect development.	**Breastfeeding** Breastfeed for at least 6 months and/or supply breastmilk from donors over formula feeding or pasturized milk.
Maternal Autoimmune Reaction Remediation: Prebiotics and/or Probiotics. Immune supporting agents.	
Pre/Postnatal Toxins Avoid air pollution, solvents, polychlorinated biphenyls (PCBs), phthalates, bisphenol A, and mercury exposure, cigarette smoking, illicit drug use, and alcohol exposure.	**Adequate Vitamin D** Supplement Vitamin D if needed. **Good Maternal Sleep Hygiene** Introduction of sleep protocols to improve sleep quality.
C-Sections Avoid elective C-Sections and reserve for emergency situations only.	

Figure 2.6 Ways to protect and improve the microbiome.

Gut bacteria keep people healthy in these ways:

- Good bacteria in the gut help prevent the growth of harmful bacteria simply by establishing themselves first. These beneficial bacteria occupy space and consume available nutrients, leaving no room or resources for bad bacteria to thrive. Additionally, some beneficial bacteria produce natural antibiotics, further inhibiting the growth of harmful microbes.
- The GI tract contains gut-associated lymphoid tissue, which significantly influences the body's immune system by regulating responses to various substances. This regulation impacts antibody production and immune cells, controlling the immune system and preventing inflammation. Consequently, the gut's immune system can affect the entire body. The gut bacteria help program and modulate the immune system, making a healthy microbiome essential for proper immune function.
- Gut bacteria ferment carbohydrates to make short chain fatty acids, particularly propionate, butyrate, and acetate. These fatty acids have important effects on the gut and the body. Butyrate has been shown to be protective of cancer and can be used as a fuel by the cells that line the intestine. In fact, in mice, butyrate is the only fuel that the intestinal lining can use. In contrast, propionic acid can be inflammatory to the gut and the brain. Thus, it is important to have an adequate balance of various gut bacteria to produce the correct amounts of these short-chain fatty acids.
- The microbiome is significantly involved in drug metabolism. It can both activate and inactivate medications that are ingested, and even modify drugs so they can become more or less toxic.
- The microbiome can also consume, modify, or produce vitamins such as folate. Certain enteric bacterial species, particularly *Bifidobacteria, Prevotella* and *Lactobacilli* synthesize folate. Interestingly, breastfeeding is the primary source of *Bifidobacteria* in infancy.

Folate Absorption & Transportation in the GI Tract

Dietary folate is a very complex molecule that needs to be simplified. In the upper GI tract, an enzyme called gamma glutamyl hydrolase (GGH) simplifies folates from their polyglutamated form to monoglutamated form that are easier to absorb. Likewise, folic acid, the oxidized form of folate, is reduced by dihydrofolate reductase (DHFR) so that it can be utilized by the body.

Folate is transported from the GI tract into the body using three transporters. The first is in the upper part of the small intestine, the jejunum. In this part of the GI tract, the environment is acidic because of the stomach juices (acidity measures the number of protons present). The proton-coupled folate transporter (PCFT) transports folate from the space inside the gut into the enterocytes, the cells that line the gut, by using available protons to drive the transporter.

In the lower GI tract, the reduced folate carrier transports folate from the space inside the GI tract to inside the enterocyte cells that line the ileum. For this transporter to work, folate needs to be in a reduced form. That is why DHFR in the upper gut is so important. In both the upper and lower gut, folate is transported out of the enterocytes to the blood by the third transporter called the multidrug-resistance-associated protein 3 (MRP3). Unlike the other two transporters, the MRP3 is not specific to folate.

Blood is drained from the gut using a special part of the circulation system which connects the GI tract directly to the liver. This pathway is known as the portal vein. Everything absorbed in the gut must be filtered through the liver. The liver can convert one type of folate into another and uses folate for several metabolic processes. Some folate is stored in the liver, and the remaining folate is transported out of the liver and into the bloodstream for other parts of the body to use. (See the 2-page spread on the next page).

GI disease, diet, and certain medications can affect the absorption of folate. Proton pump inhibitors (PPIs), which are prescribed for stomach inflammation, can decrease acidity in the upper gut, potentially leading to decreased function of the PCFT. However, studies in adults suggest that PPIs do not significantly change blood folate levels.[19]

Liver Metabolism

As previously described, various forms of folate are absorbed into the cells of the intestinal lining, enter the bloodstream through a network of blood vessels called capillaries, and travel to the liver via the portal vein. In the liver, 5-methyltetrahydrofolate (5-MTHF) is involved in metabolic processes, including the synthesis of other important compounds. Some 5-MTHF is stored in the liver, some is

Absorption of Folate

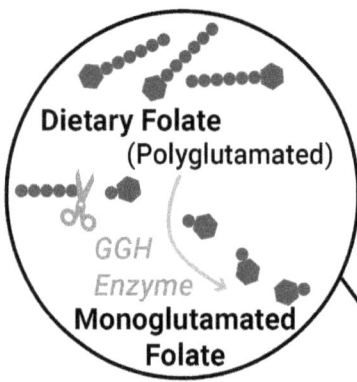

Breakdown of Dietary Folate
In the upper GI tract, an enzyme called gamma glutamyl hydrolase (GGH) simplifies dietary folates from their polyglutamated form to a monoglutamated form which is easier to absorb.

Upper Small Intestine
In the jejunum, the upper part of the small intestine, the environment is acidic, meaning there are many protons. The proton-coupled folate transporter (PCFT) transports folate from the space inside the gut into enterocytes, the cells that line the gut.

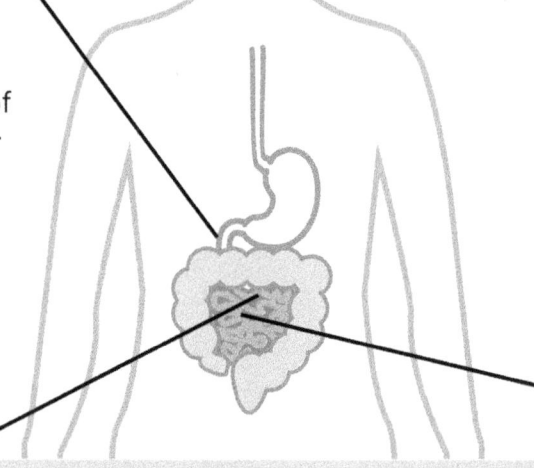

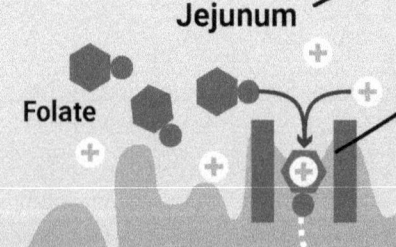

The Folate Fix - 20

Reduction of Folic Acid

Folic acid, the oxidized form of folate, can be more easily absorbed if it is transformed into a reduced form. Dihydrofolate reductase (DHFR) in the upper gut changes folic acid into a reduced form which can be better absorbed.

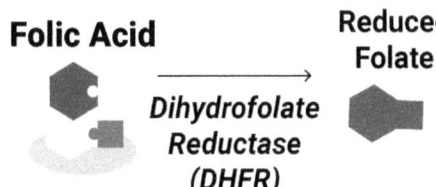

Folate in the Liver

Blood is drained from the gut using a special part of the circulation system which connects the GI tract directly to the liver. This pathway is known as the portal vein.

Lower Small Intestine

In the ileum, the lower part of the small intestine, the reduced folate carrier (RFC) transports reduced folate from the space inside the GI tract to inside enterocytes. In both the upper and lower gut, folate is transported out of the enterocytes to the blood by a special transporter that is not specific for folate called the multidrug resistance-associated protein 3 (MRP3).

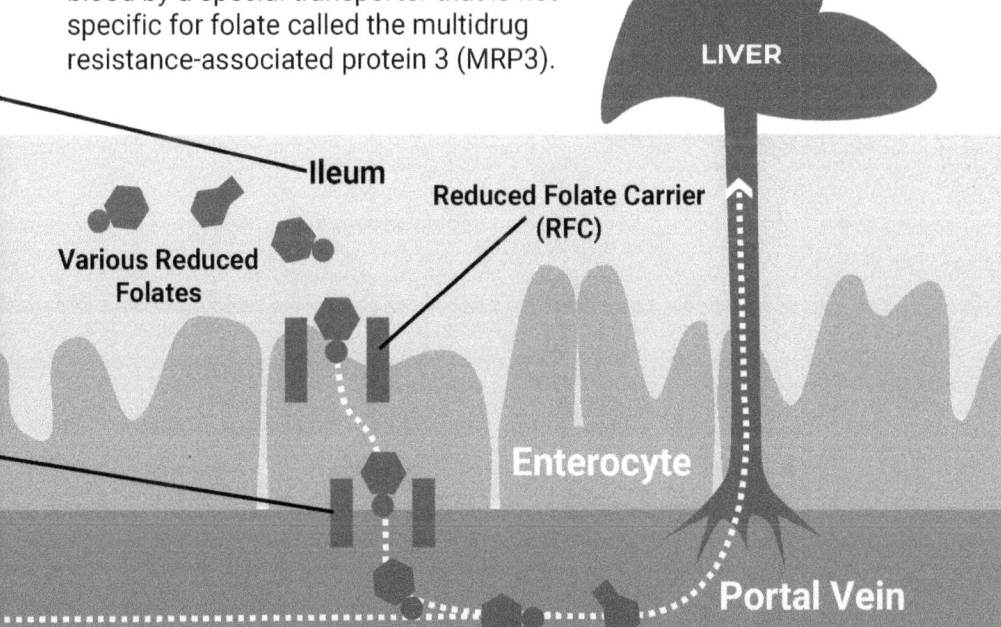

Chapter 2. - Folate: The Most Essential Vitamin

transported throughout the body via the bloodstream where it is used in various tissues for functions such as DNA synthesis, cell division, and the methylation of molecules. Unused 5-MTHF moves through the kidneys where it is excreted in urine.

Folic acid can also be absorbed into the blood stream. It can be reduced by DHFR to a usable folate or eliminated by the kidneys. However, recent research has found that unmetabolized folic acid (that portion which is not reduced by DHFR) can inhibit folate metabolism when it is at high concentrations.[20] Thus, folic acid can build up in people whose DHFR enzyme works slowly or in people who take excess folic acid, overwhelming the DHFR enzyme. This is one of the important nuances of the use of folate supplementation since everyone has a unique folate metabolism. The next chapter will explore folate's biochemical pathways in more detail.

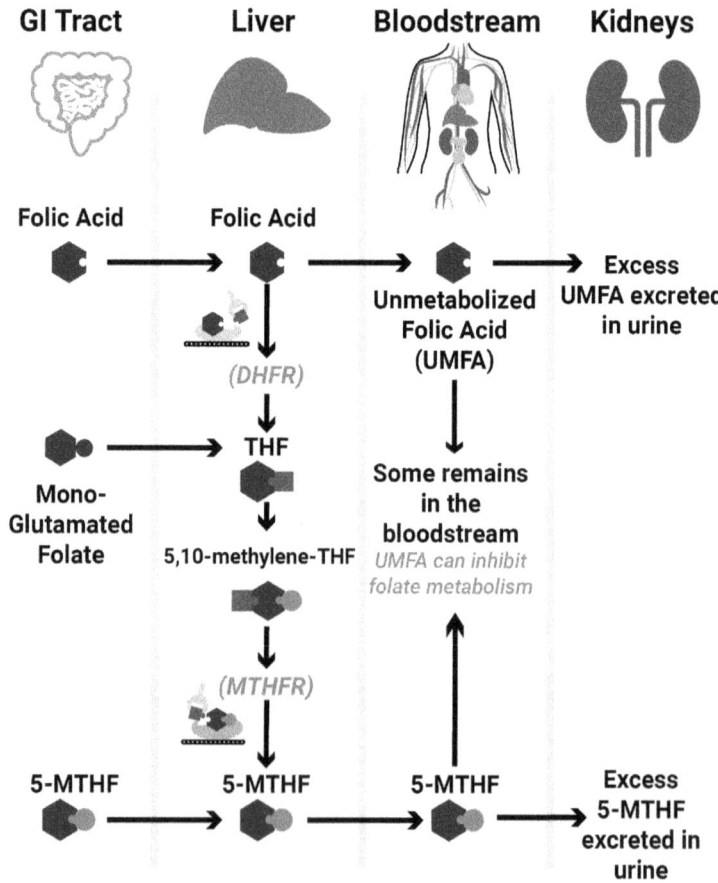

Figure 2.7 How folates move through the body.

Understanding Oxidation and Reduction

Throughout this book, terms such as "oxidized" and "reduced" will be used to describe various compounds and reactions, but what do those terms mean? A simplified explanation is that oxidation-reduction chemical reactions are those in which two molecules exchange electrons. When these reactions occur, scientists often refer to the molecule that lost electrons as "oxidized" and the molecule that gained electrons as "reduced." Combined, these reactions are called by their shortened name, "redox" reactions. It is important to note that redox reactions do not necessarily involve oxygen.

Likewise, reduction may be confusing at first because "being reduced" usually means losing something, not gaining something. But it is helpful to think of the reduction in terms of charge. Electrons are negatively charged subatomic particles; therefore, the more electrons gained, the more the charge is reduced.

In biological processes involving carbon-based molecules, oxidized molecules are often those that lose a hydrogen, and reduced species are those that gain a hydrogen. Hydrogen holds its electrons very weakly, so when it binds to another atom, that other atom generally assumes its electrons. Consequently, when a molecule loses a hydrogen, it is oxidized and loses the hydrogen's electron.

As various biochemical processes are described in this book, it may be helpful to remember the acronym "OIL RIG."

O.I.L. = Oxidized Is Lost Electron (Hydrogen)

R.I.G. = Reduced Is Gained Electron (Hydrogen)

Folic Acid

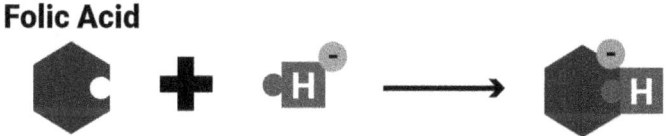

This shows Folic Acid being reduced because an electron is gained (R.I.G.).

CHAPTER 3.
Folate: The Workhorse Vitamin

Folate is an essential nutrient that plays a critical role in maintaining proper bodily function. Since the body cannot produce sufficient folate on its own, individuals must regularly obtain it from food or supplements. This is especially important for women during pregnancy, as they need to meet the increased folate demands of a growing fetus. Because folate is a water-soluble vitamin, it is continuously excreted through urine and cannot be stored like fat-soluble vitamins. As a result, regular replenishment of folate is necessary to support optimal health.

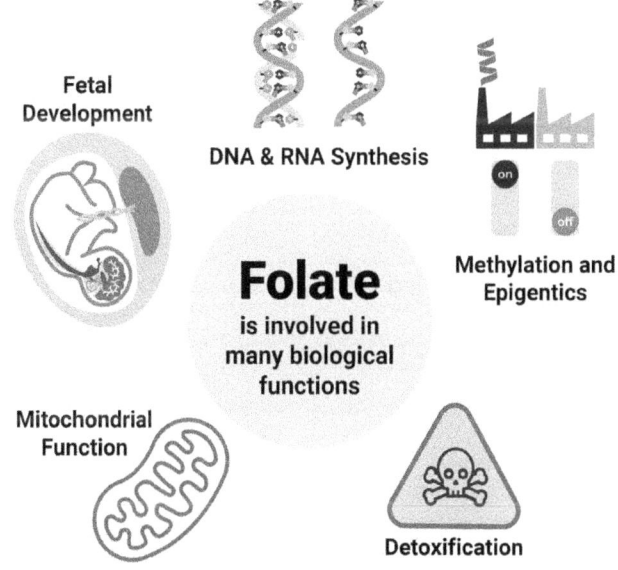

Figure 3.1 The many roles of folate in the body.

Folate can be consumed in various forms and is processed through different pathways within the folate cycle—a key metabolic process involved in numerous biochemical functions, including development and detoxification.

From the earliest stages of embryonic development, folate is vital for forming the nervous system, including the brain and spinal cord. Another primary role of folate is in the synthesis of genetic material, which begins shortly after conception and remains crucial throughout a person's life. Folate is also essential for two critical processes: methylation, which regulates gene activity, and redox metabolism, which protects cells from stress and toxins. Additionally, folate aids brain function by facilitating the production of neurotransmitters, the brain's chemical messengers, and is crucial for the mitochondria, the energy-producing powerhouses of cells.

This chapter will explore the numerous biological functions of folate and delve into why it is often referred to as the "workhorse of the body."

Brain Development and Nutrition

The brain undergoes rapid and critical development during the prenatal period, laying the foundation for future cognitive and physical growth. Once a human egg is fertilized by a sperm, the resulting zygote—the first cell of new human life—begins a process of rapid cell division. This process forms a cluster of cells called a morula (a solid ball of cells), which then progresses into a blastocyst—a fluid-filled structure with an inner cell mass that will develop into the embryo and an outer layer that will form the placenta.

This early phase of prenatal development, particularly the first four weeks, often occurs before many women realize they are pregnant. As these critical stages happen so early, proper nutrition and healthy habits before conception are essential. Research consistently highlights the importance of folate before and during early pregnancy. Around the third week post-fertilization, the blastocyst implants into the uterine lining, initiating gastrulation. During this phase, cells differentiate into three primary layers: the ectoderm (which forms the nervous system and skin), the mesoderm (which becomes muscles and organs), and the endoderm (which develops into the digestive and respiratory systems). At this time, another pivotal event begins—the formation of the nervous system.

The neural tube, the precursor to the brain and spinal cord, forms during this stage. Initially a flat sheet called the neural plate folds into a tube. Adequate folate is essential during this phase, as its deficiency can lead to neural tube defects (NTDs). NTDs occur when the neural tube fails to close completely, leaving parts of it exposed. One of the most recognized disorders this results in is spina bifida, where incomplete closure of the lower neural tube affects the development of the spinal

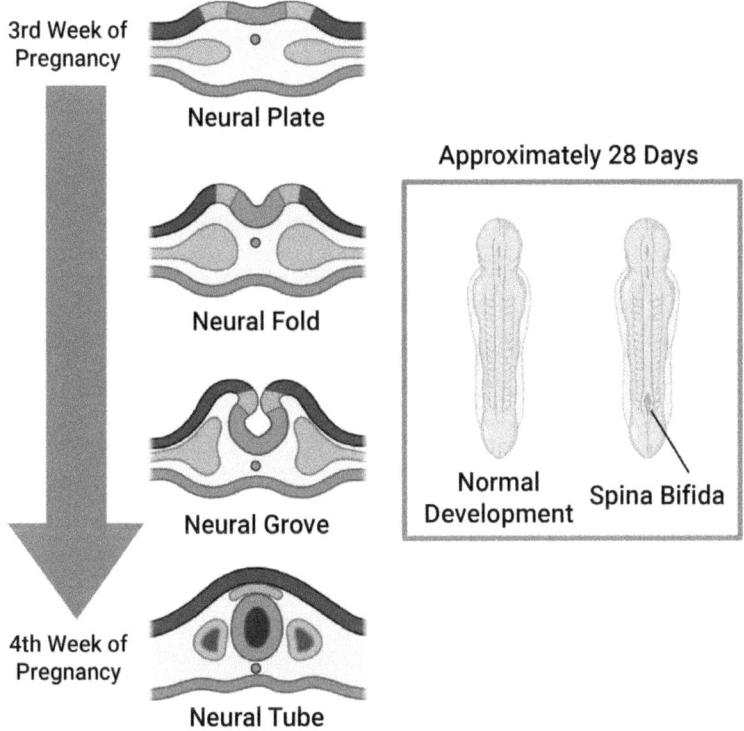

Figure 3.2 The development of the neural tube. Image created with BioRender.

cord, leading to nerve damage and impaired motor function in the lower portion of the body.

Proper nutrients and vitamins are crucial for the intense cellular growth and differentiation required to form healthy cells. Folate plays a central role in brain development by supporting DNA synthesis and methylation, processes essential for the rapid cell replication needed for a developing brain.

During prenatal development, cells multiply at an extraordinary rate, progressing from a single cell to approximately 40 trillion cells by birth—around 100 billion of which become neurons in the brain. During peak brain development, the fetus generates 250,000 neurons per minute. This rapid replication demands precise DNA synthesis, as every cell must receive an exact copy of the genetic material which contains about 6 billion base pairs. Folate provides the building blocks for this process, and a deficiency can result in DNA replication errors, potentially leading to developmental abnormalities and genetic mutations.

Beyond DNA synthesis, folate is vital for gene methylation, a biochemical process that regulates when and how genes are activated or deactivated. During brain development, gene methylation acts like a genetic "switchboard," ensuring that genes are turned on and off in the proper sequence. This coordination is critical for transforming a simple cluster of cells into a fully functioning brain.

For instance, the gene REELIN becomes active around the 12th week of gestation. This gene directs the placement of cells in the developing brain. If improperly deactivated, brain structures can form incorrectly, with layers of the brain being "upside down." This example highlights the importance of proper methylation in ensuring the correct formation, placement, and function of brain cells.

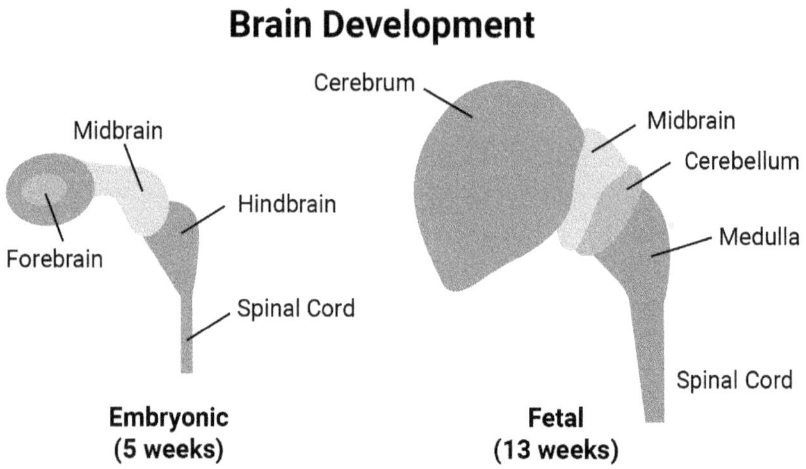

Brain Development

Embryonic (5 weeks): Forebrain, Midbrain, Hindbrain, Spinal Cord

Fetal (13 weeks): Cerebrum, Midbrain, Cerebellum, Medulla, Spinal Cord

Figure 3.3 Fetal brain and nervous system development.

As the neural tube develops, it begins producing neural stem cells, which differentiate into neurons and supportive glial cells. The neural tube also divides into distinct brain regions, each with unique functions. The brainstem, responsible for automatic functions like heart rate and breathing, matures first. In contrast, the cerebrum, where higher-order functions such as language and reasoning occur, matures later. Stressors like infections during pregnancy can disrupt brain development, with the timing of the stressor determining which brain region is affected.

Folate also plays additional roles in brain development, such as supporting neurotransmitter production and promoting myelination, the protective insulation around neurons that enhances signal transmission. These functions are critical both before and after birth for healthy brain development. Insufficient folate levels can result in abnormal nervous system development and impaired neuron function.

Folinic Acid (Leucovorin) – The Chemistry

Folinic acid is a reduced and biologically active form of folate. When used as a medication, it is referred to as leucovorin. Leucovorin is not a specific brand name but rather the generic name for the chemical compound.

As a pharmaceutical, leucovorin is typically manufactured as a salt (ionic mixture) to improve its solubility and absorption into the bloodstream. Physicians often specify the ionic formulation when prescribing leucovorin, with the most common forms being leucovorin calcium and leucovorin sodium.

Many chemical compounds, including leucovorin, can exhibit chirality. Chirality means that the molecules can exist in two mirror-image forms, much like how a person's left and right hands are similar in structure but not interchangeable. Chiral molecules are classified based on their orientation: molecules oriented to the left are known as "levo-" (L-isomer or L-form), while those oriented to the right are referred to as "dextro-" (D-isomer or D-form).

Most formulations of leucovorin are a racemic mixture, meaning they contain both the L-form and the D-form. However, some formulations, known as levo-folinic acid or levo-leucovorin, contain only the L-isomer.

Levo
Left-oriented isomers, also known as the L-isomer or L-form

Dextro
Right-oriented isomers, also known as the D-isomer or D-form

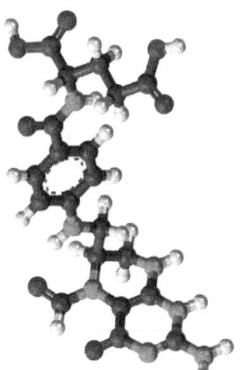
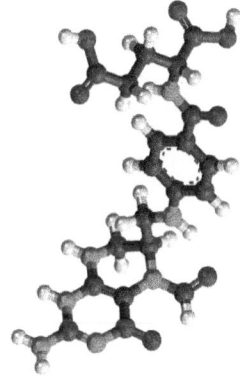

Folic Acid versus Folinic Acid

Folate, also known as vitamin B9, is an essential nutrient crucial for various bodily functions, including DNA synthesis, cell division, and growth. Vitamin B9 can exist in several forms, including folic acid and folinic acid. Both are water-soluble, meaning they cannot be stored in the body and must be consumed regularly. While their similar names can cause confusion, folic acid and folinic acid have distinct differences that are important to understand.

Folic acid is a synthetic form of folate that is not naturally found in foods—it is man-made. In the United States, folic acid is widely used in dietary supplements and food fortification programs because of its stability and ease of incorporation into processed foods. In contrast, folinic acid is a naturally occurring form of folate found in whole foods such as leafy green vegetables, legumes, and citrus fruits.

The primary differences between folic acid and folinic acid lie in how they are absorbed and utilized by the body. Folic acid is the oxidized form of folate, while folinic acid is a reduced form. (For more information, see "Understanding Oxidation and Reduction" in Chapter 2.)

Folic acid must undergo activation before it can be readily used by the body. This process involves converting folic acid into tetrahydrofolate (THF), a reduced form of folate. Once converted, THF can be absorbed, utilized, or further converted into other activated forms of folate, such as folinic acid or 5-methyltetrahydrofolate (5-MTHF).

Another key distinction between folic acid and folinic acid lies in their typical uses. As mentioned earlier, folic acid is a synthetic, stable, and inexpensive form of folate. Due to these qualities, it is commonly included in over-the-counter prenatal vitamins to reduce the risk of birth defects during pregnancy. Additionally, folic acid is widely used in fortification programs, where it is added to grain products like bread, pasta, and cereals in many countries

In contrast, folinic acid is often recommended for specific medical conditions. Like other reduced folates, it can be absorbed directly by the body without requiring activation. The prescription form of folinic acid, known as leucovorin, has been used for decades to counteract the harmful effects of antifolate medications such as methotrexate, which are commonly used in cancer treatments.

Leucovorin is also beneficial for individuals who have difficulty absorbing folate or are at risk of folate deficiency, such as those with celiac disease or Crohn's disease. In these cases, leucovorin is sometimes administered intravenously at high doses to address specific medical needs effectively.

As the folate cycle is discussed in this chapter, the differences between folic acid and folinic acid will become even clearer.

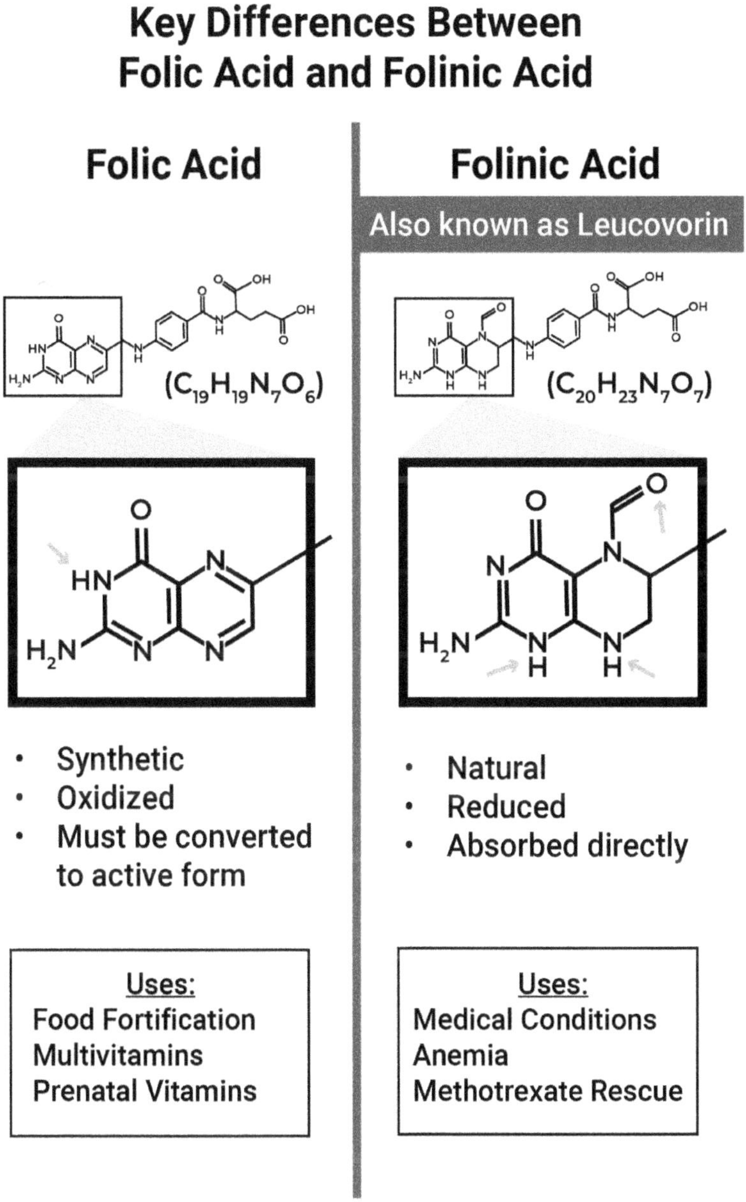

Key Differences Between Folic Acid and Folinic Acid

Folic Acid

$(C_{19}H_{19}N_7O_6)$

Folinic Acid
Also known as Leucovorin

$(C_{20}H_{23}N_7O_7)$

- Synthetic
- Oxidized
- Must be converted to active form

- Natural
- Reduced
- Absorbed directly

Uses:
Food Fortification
Multivitamins
Prenatal Vitamins

Uses:
Medical Conditions
Anemia
Methotrexate Rescue

Figure 3.4 Folic Acid versus Folinic Acid (Leucovorin).

Chapter 3. - Folate: The Workhorse Vitamin - 31

The Folate Cycle

To better understand the differences between folic acid and folinic acid, it is helpful to examine their behavior in biochemical processes, particularly within the folate cycle, a central pathway involved in many critical cellular interactions occurring in the cytosol of cells.

Folate enters the cycle at various points depending on its form. Folic acid, the synthetic form of folate, is an oxidized version that must first be reduced to an active form by the enzyme dihydrofolate reductase (DHFR). This activation process is necessary for folic acid to participate in the folate cycle. However, genetic variations (polymorphisms) in the DHFR enzyme can reduce its efficiency, impairing the conversion of folic acid into its bioavailable form. This can result in the accumulation of unmetabolized folic acid (UMFA) in the body. Some researchers suggest that the liver has a limited capacity to process and reduce folic acid, resulting in the DHFR enzymes becoming overwhelmed by a large amount of folic acid. This may contribute to UMFA buildup, raising questions about the widespread fortification of foods with synthetic folic acid.[21]

Emerging research indicates that UMFA may inhibit folate metabolism, a problem that is not observed with folinic acid. High levels of UMFA, particularly when excess folic acid is consumed, can occur due to the saturation of DHFR, the rate-limiting enzyme in folic acid activation. This issue is especially significant in individuals with DHFR polymorphisms.[22] The resulting accumulation of UMFA may inhibit DHFR further, exacerbating the problem and causing the buildup of UMFA, which slows down the folate cycle and potentially impairs MTHFR (methylenetetrahydrofolate reductase) function by accumulating dihydrofolate (DHF).

Several extensive studies have identified negative impacts associated with UMFA. Research suggests that UMFA can induce genetic errors in mouse models,[23] reduce natural killer cell cytotoxicity in postmenopausal women,[24] and increase the risk of autism spectrum disorder (ASD).[25] Excessive folic acid supplementation during pregnancy has also been linked to conditions such as asthma,[26] insulin resistance,[27] and aberrant methylation of critical genes, including the Insulin-like Growth Factor 2 gene,[28] neurodevelopmental genes,[29] immune response genes, and those regulating cellular proliferation.[30] In animal models, high folic acid intake during pregnancy has been shown to alter cortical development,[31] impair learning,[32] and increase seizure susceptibility,[33] potentially due to disruptions in normal methylation processes.

Unlike folic acid, folinic acid does not face the same limitations, as it readily converts to 5-formyl-THF, which can either enter the folate cycle directly or support the purine synthesis pathway (discussed further in the next section). The distinct metabolic pathways of folic acid and folinic acid have contributed to con-

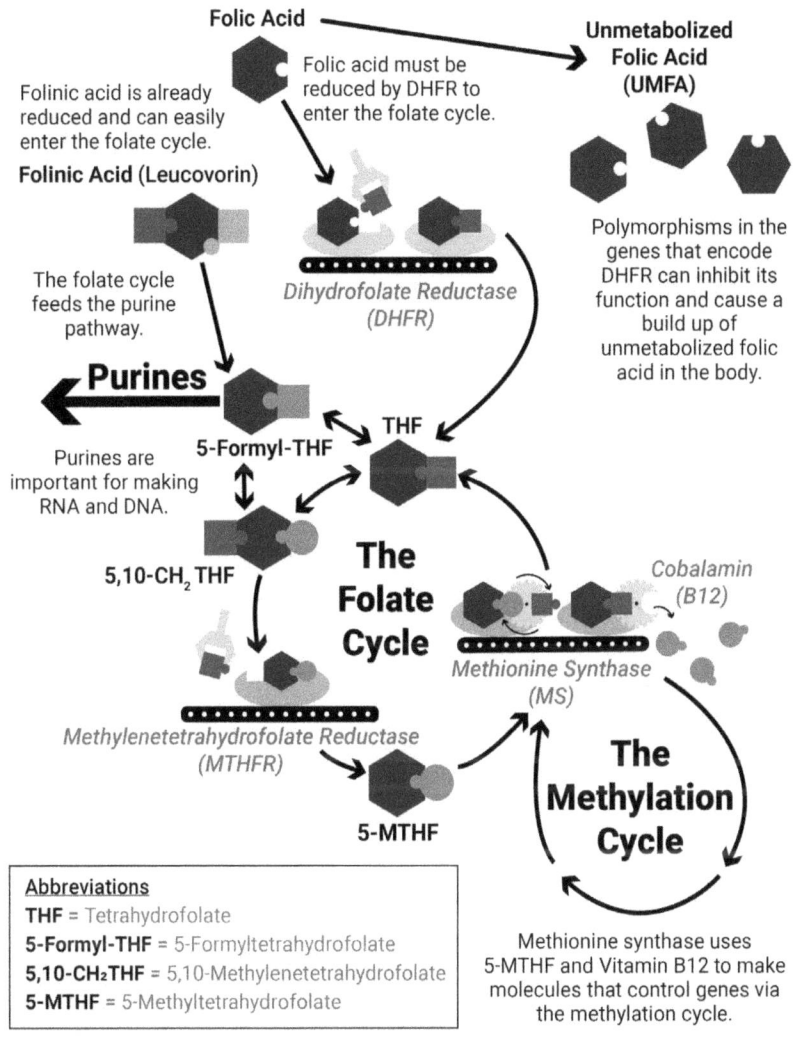

Figure 3.6 The Folate Cycle.

fusion in folate research. While some studies suggest that folate supplementation reduces the risk of conditions such as ASD and certain cancers, others indicate that high levels of folate in the blood may actually increase the risk of these same diseases. These conflicting findings have led some clinicians to question the safety and overall benefits of folate supplementation. However, detailed blood analyses often reveal elevated levels of UMFA in such cases, highlighting the importance of using reduced folates like leucovorin, which the body can process more efficiently.

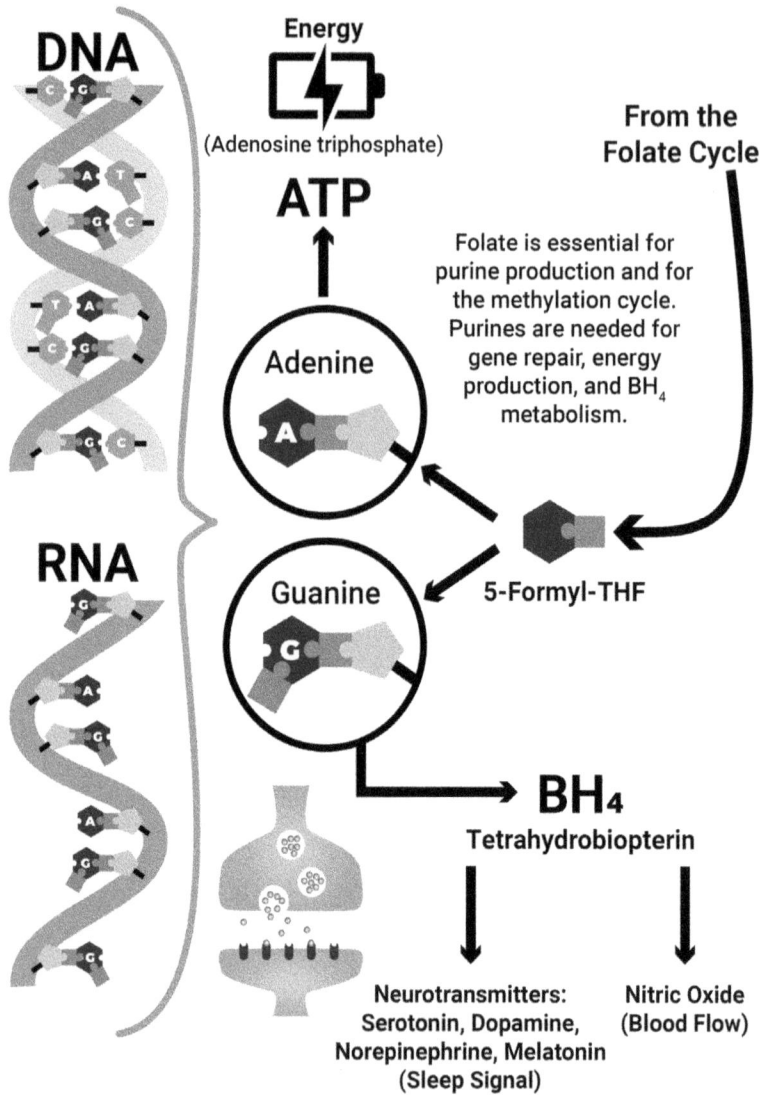

Figure 3.7 The most well-known purines, adenine (A) and guanine (G), are fundamental components of nucleotides, which serve as the building blocks of DNA and RNA. In DNA, adenine pairs with thymine (T), while in RNA, it pairs with uracil (U). Guanine pairs with cytosine (C) in both DNA and RNA. Beyond their genetic roles, adenine is a key component of adenosine triphosphate (ATP), a purine nucleotide that functions as the primary energy carrier in cells. Similarly, guanine forms guanosine triphosphate (GTP), which serves as a precursor for tetrahydrobiopterin (BH_4).

BH_4 is essential for the synthesis of neurotransmitters, such as serotonin and dopamine, and for the regulation of nitric oxide, a molecule crucial for preventing oxidative stress and maintaining vascular health. This underscores the vital importance of folate in the body. Without adequate folate, purine production is impaired, disrupting several key metabolic pathways that are fundamental to genetic stability, energy metabolism, and overall cellular function.

Purine Metabolism

As mentioned earlier, one of the key pathways of the folate cycle is the purine pathway. Purines are essential building blocks of DNA and RNA, which comprise our genetic code. The purines adenine and guanine represent two of the "letters" in this code, A and G, and are critical for maintaining proper genetic function.

Purines play a vital role in DNA replication, a process required for cell division and the formation of new cells. DNA is also present in mitochondria—the powerhouse of the cell—which replicate frequently. Insufficient purine levels can lead to errors in DNA replication, potentially causing mutations. Furthermore, a lack of purines can impair the accuracy of gene repair, compounding the effects of genetic errors when they occur.

Purines are equally important for RNA synthesis, which serves multiple critical functions in the body. RNA transmits the DNA code to the cell's machinery, enabling the production of essential proteins, including enzymes that sustain cellular function. Without RNA, cells would be unable to operate.

Additionally, RNA acts as a regulatory molecule; specialized forms like microRNAs control cellular messages by binding to other RNAs, a function that is particularly important for proper brain development during prenatal stages of development.

Guanine, one of the purines, is also a precursor for tetrahydrobiopterin (BH_4), an important cofactor in the body. BH_4 plays a role in breaking down the amino acid phenylalanine and in synthesizing key monoamine neurotransmitters, such as serotonin, dopamine, norepinephrine, as well as melatonin (the sleep hormone) and nitric oxide (which regulates blood flow). Low levels of BH_4 can impair nitric oxide production, increasing the presence of harmful molecules that damage cells.

Adenine, the other primary purine, is essential for energy metabolism. It forms the base of adenosine triphosphate (ATP), the primary energy carrier of the cell, which delivers energy from the mitochondria to other parts of the cell. Without ATP, cellular functions would come to a halt. Adenine also forms part of other energy-related molecules, such as nicotinamide adenine dinucleotide (NAD) and coenzyme A, both of which are critical for metabolic processes.

In addition to these roles, both adenine and guanine contribute to cellular communication. Molecules like cyclic adenosine monophosphate (cAMP) and cyclic guanosine monophosphate (cGMP) act as "second messengers" inside cells. These molecules relay external signals to the cell's interior, activating specific cellular responses and coordinating essential activities.

Purine Production

As discussed previously, folate is crucial for a wide range of essential metabolic processes, particularly for purine production and the methylation cycle. As shown in Figure 3.6, when leucovorin enters the folate cycle, it can either continue within the cycle or take a detour to contribute to purine synthesis. If leucovorin continues in the folate cycle, it is converted into 5-methyltetrahydrofolate (5-MTHF) by the enzyme methylenetetrahydrofolate reductase (MTHFR). Genetic variations, or polymorphisms, in the MTHFR gene are relatively common. For example, approximately 35% of the population carries the C677T polymorphism, which reduces the enzyme's efficiency. This polymorphism typically does not cause problems unless an individual inherits two copies of the polymorphism (homozygous), which can result in up to a 70% reduction in MTHFR activity. This significant reduction in enzyme function may increase the risk of certain health conditions, such as cardiovascular disease.

The Difference Between Polymorphisms and Mutations

Polymorphism: Little variations in our genetic code that make a body work more or less efficiently. When these are relatively common (they affect more than 1% of people), they are called polymorphism. Sometimes polymorphisms can be involved in disease states, but in very complex ways which may not be completely elucidated by medical science in many cases.

Mutation: Genetic changes that are relatively rare highly likely to cause disease.

It is important to note that having the C677T polymorphism does not guarantee health issues. Instead, it serves as one of several potential risk factors. Individuals with this polymorphism are more likely to experience related health problems if their folate intake is insufficient. For most people, these common variations are not problematic as long as they maintain an adequate folate intake through diet or supplementation.

Methylation Metabolism

In the folate cycle, the enzyme MTHFR converts leucovorin into 5-MTHF, which then links the folate cycle to the methylation cycle. In this next step, methionine synthase (MS) uses 5-MTHF along with cobalamin (Vitamin B12) to create molecules that help regulate gene activity.

The genetic code can be thought of as the cell's instructions, but not all instructions are active at once. The process of controlling which genetic instructions are turned on or off is known as epigenetics. Similar to following a recipe, where each step must be done at the right time, cells regulate the timing and activity of gene instructions through a process called methylation.

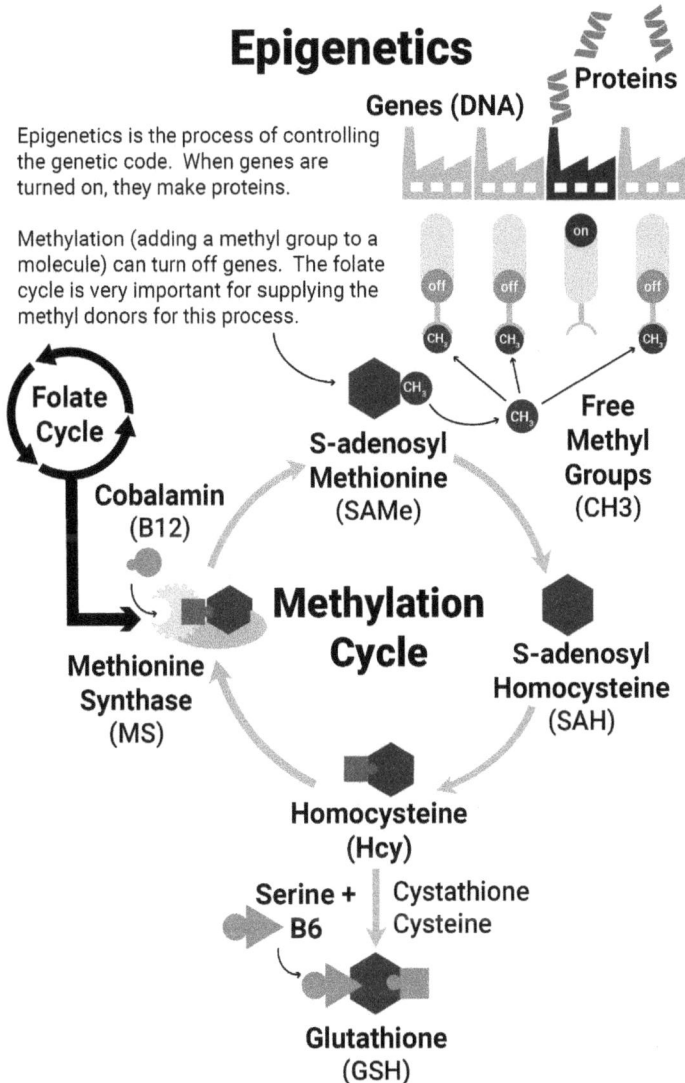

Figure 3.8 Epigenetics and the Folate Cycle.

Methylation involves adding a methyl group (one carbon and three hydrogen atoms) to a molecule, effectively creating "off switches" for genes that aren't needed. The methylation cycle generates these methyl donors, providing the fuel needed for these off switches. If the methylation cycle isn't functioning properly, gene instructions may be activated or silenced at inappropriate times. Folate and the folate cycle are essential for supporting this process, ensuring that gene regulation occurs accurately and in sync with the cell's needs.

Redox Metabolism

One important downstream effect of the methylation cycle is redox metabolism, which is essential for the production of glutathione (GSH)—the body's primary antioxidant. GSH plays a critical role in protecting cells from harmful reactive molecules and in detoxifying the body. In the liver, GSH binds to heavy metals and toxic compounds, converting them into water-soluble forms that can be safely excreted through the kidneys.

The mitochondria, responsible for generating cellular energy, naturally produce reactive oxygen species (ROS) as byproducts of energy metabolism. To prevent oxidative damage, mitochondria rely on GSH to neutralize these ROS. Importantly, the synthesis of GSH itself requires energy and takes place in two ATP-dependent steps, with mitochondria supplying the necessary ATP.

N-acetylcysteine (NAC) serves as a precursor to cysteine, which is also needed for GSH synthesis. NAC contains an acetyl group (composed of two carbon atoms, three hydrogen atoms, and one oxygen atom), which is removed to yield usable cysteine. By increasing cysteine availability, NAC impacts GSH levels.

When GSH levels are low, mitochondrial function can decline, reducing energy production and further impairing GSH synthesis. This creates a vicious cycle of oxidative stress (when the production of ROS exceeds the body's ability to neutralize them), energy deficiency, and cellular damage. Without adequate levels of GSH, cells accumulate toxins and suffer oxidative damage, which can compromise their function.

If methylation metabolism is dysfunctional, redox metabolism is also adversely affected. Similarly, when redox metabolism is overburdened by excessive toxins or reactive molecules, it can disrupt methylation metabolism. Since the folate cycle is a key driver of the methylation cycle, folate is essential for maintaining effective redox metabolism.

These interconnected processes—methylation, redox metabolism, and the folate cycle—are highly interdependent, with each regulating and supporting the others. When patients present with symptoms of metabolic dysfunction, understanding these complex interactions can help clinicians interpret abnormal lab results and connect them to clinical symptoms.

With the foundational role of folate in metabolism established, the following chapters will delve into the consequences of insufficient folate on key biological processes.

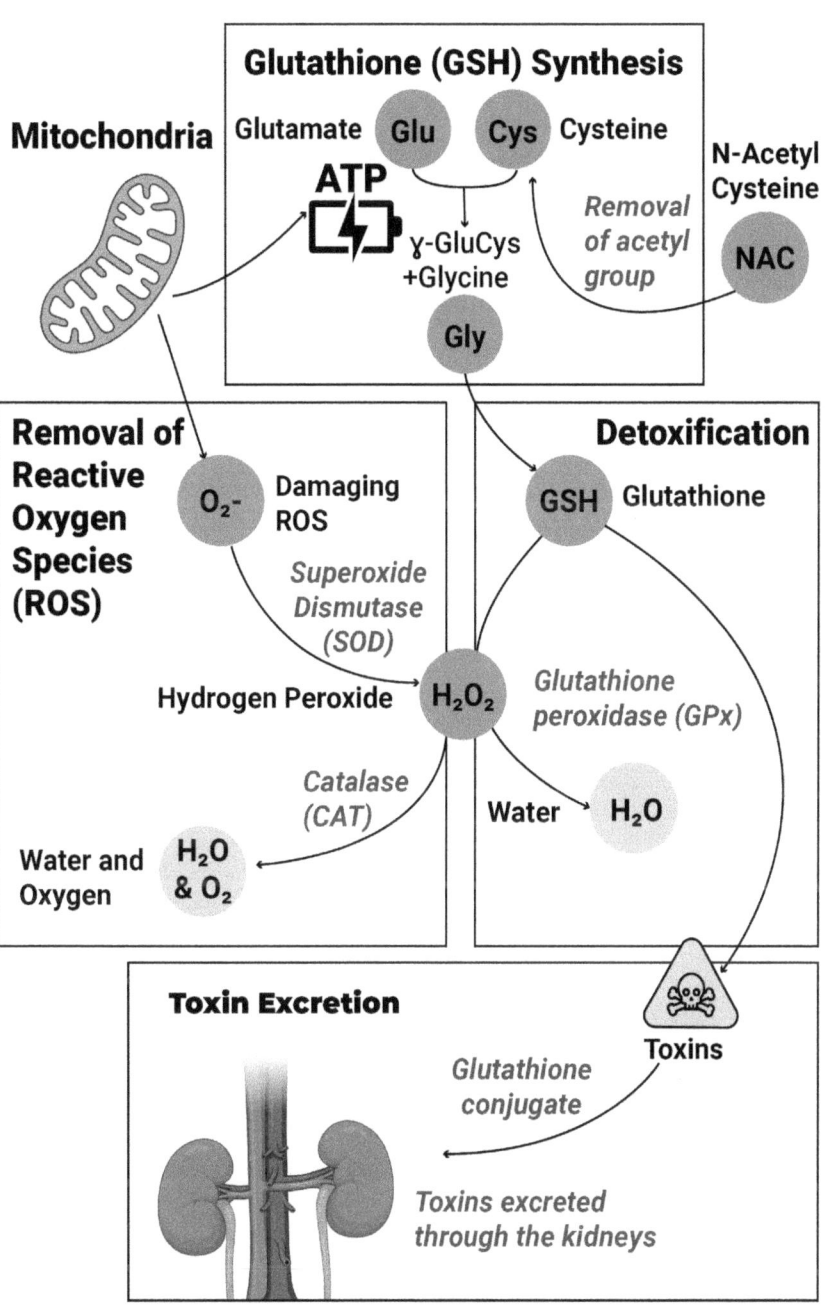

Figure 3.9 Glutathione and Redox Metabolism. Image created with BioRender.

PART II.

IF THE BRAIN LACKS FOLATE

Thus far, this book has explored the importance of vitamins, with a particular emphasis on the essential roles of folate and its key cofactors throughout the body. The profound impact of folate on the central nervous system and brain function cannot be overstated. But what happens if the brain lacks the folate it needs?

Answers to this question have emerged over decades of research and, perhaps most poignantly, through the lived experiences of individuals affected by specific forms of folate deficiency. Much of what we know about folate's role in the body has been shaped by unique cases and medical mysteries presented by individuals with puzzling symptoms. Doctors have greatly benefited from the insights, observations, and detailed accounts of dedicated family members and caregivers who documented and shared unusual symptoms. Their keen observations have been invaluable in advancing our knowledge and guiding researchers, healthcare providers, and others affected by these conditions.

In the chapters that follow, I will share the broader story of folate, blending the history of scientific research with personal narratives to illuminate folate's critical role in neurological health. Most of these stories are grouped by common themes, such as related comorbidities or co-occurring conditions that impact patients. Please note that some identifying details have been modified to ensure patient privacy.

Each chapter will open with a summary of current research on folate-related topics, followed by patient stories and a "Physician's Perspective," where I will apply scientific literature and clinical experience to help interpret and highlight the nuances of each case presented.

CHAPTER 4.
Cerebral Folate Deficiency

Background

Over two decades ago, Dr. Vincent Ramaekers, a European child neurologist working in Germany, documented the first cases of abnormally low folate levels in the central nervous system (CNS) associated with a neurodevelopmental disorder.[34] In his clinical practice, Dr. Ramaekers investigated why several children under his care were experiencing severe neurodevelopmental symptoms (discussed in detail in Chapter 14).

To better understand these cases, Dr. Ramaekers collaborated with Dr. Blau, a scientist renowned for his expertise in analyzing the neurochemistry of cerebrospinal fluid (CSF). CSF, the fluid that surrounds and cushions the brain, is an ideal medium for assessing nutrient and metabolite levels within the brain. Dr. Blau examined the CSF from Dr. Ramaekers' patients and found something interesting. All of the patients had low 5-methyltetrahydrofolate (5-MTHF) concentrations in their CSF. Folate, especially in its active form 5-MTHF, is transported into the CSF before entering brain tissue. Thus, measuring 5-MTHF in the CSF provides a reliable indicator of brain folate levels.

At that time, it was well known that whole-body folate deficiencies can cause neurological symptoms. These deficiencies, typically caused by poor diet or absorption issues, are detectable through blood tests and are often accompanied by other abnormalities, such as anemia. However, the patients under Dr. Ramaekers' care had normal blood folate concentrations, ruling out systemic folate deficiency as the cause of their symptoms. Instead, their folate deficiency appeared to be confined to the central nervous system. As he identified more cases with similar patterns, Dr. Ramaekers coined the term Cerebral Folate Deficiency (CFD) to emphasize the brain-specific nature of the abnormality.[35]

Lumbar Puncture (Spinal Tap)

Most commonly, a lumbar puncture (LP) is performed in the emergency room to look for infections in the central nervous system, as these can be life-threatening.

Other times the procedure is performed under non-emergent conditions, usually to confirm suspected inflammatory conditions, determine if there is a metabolic disorder, or to test the pressure in the brain. In this procedure a long, thin needle is inserted in the lower back between the vertebrae of the spine.

A small hole is made in the outer layers of the meninges, which are the protective membranes that cover the brain and spinal cord. Luckily the body has extra space in this region to allow fluid to be removed safely. The procedure does not have a danger of hitting the spinal cord because the needle is inserted below where the spinal cord ends.

Removing spinal fluid is safe because the amount needed for testing is very small, and the body replenishes CSF regularly. For testing levels of metabolic markers and vitamins, a lumbar puncture must be performed very carefully. If the needle does not go straight into the space between vertebrae, it can pick up some blood and carry it into the CSF.

Although this will not cause harm, it will contaminate the sample so that the measurements of the CSF will not be accurate. Thus, it is advisable to sedate the patient and use a technique called fluoroscopy to visualize the vertebrae with x-rays to make sure there is direct hit with the needle.

Ideally LPs are best performed non-emergently so that everything can be carefully planned and executed to obtain the cleanest sample possible.

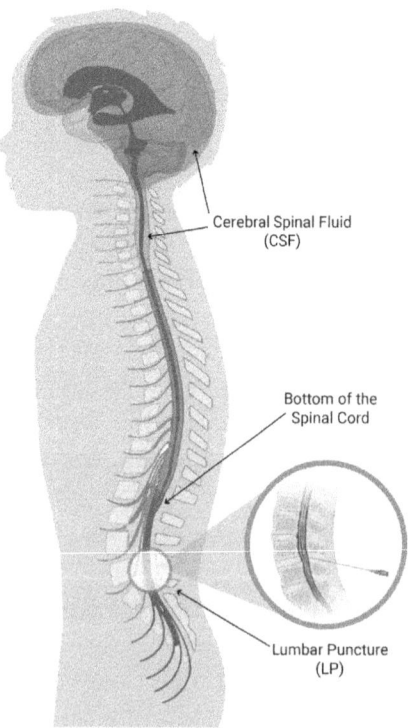

Figure 4.1. A Lumbar Puncture (LP) is used to test the fluid which surrounds the brain known as the cerebrospinal fluid (CSF). Image created with BioRender.

CFD as a Syndrome

Cerebral Folate Deficiency is classified as a syndrome, meaning it represents a cluster of symptoms observed in patients. In syndromes, the specific symptoms can vary widely among individuals—some patients may exhibit all associated symptoms, while others may show only a subset. This variability often perplexes experts, making diagnosis complex and not always straightforward. Consequently, medical specialists play a crucial role in recognizing the broad spectrum of presentations associated with syndromes.

Whenever possible, syndromes are ideally diagnosed using definitive biological markers rather than relying solely on clinical observations. For instance, genetic syndromes like Down syndrome have specific genetic markers that enable accurate diagnoses. By contrast, syndromes such as fetal alcohol syndrome lack such distinct markers and are diagnosed based on a constellation of physical and behavioral characteristics.

Fortunately, classic CFD syndrome can be diagnosed using measurable biomarkers. A definitive diagnosis is made when a patient has below-normal 5-MTHF concentrations in the CSF while maintaining normal folate concentrations in the blood (see Chapter 15 – Diagnosing CFD).

Despite this clear diagnostic criterion, obtaining CSF for testing is invasive and often requires sedation. Determining the folate concentration in the brain involves collecting a sample of CSF through a lumbar puncture, commonly referred to as a spinal tap (see Figure 4.1).

While the diagnostic criteria for CFD is well-defined, generally before CFD is confirmed, it must first be suspected. This starts with the identification of neurological symptoms that are commonly reported in CFD. In young children, these appear as one or more developmental symptoms, whereas in adults, they more commonly manifest as psychiatric symptoms. Figure 4.2 shows a chart of symptoms commonly reported with CFD. Both children and adults manifest neurological symptoms when CFD is severe and, in adults, severe CFD appears to be associated with patients that have multiple neurological symptoms.[36]

In both cases, the presence of these neurological or psychiatric symptoms alone does not necessarily raise suspicion of CFD. In fact, many of these symptoms are often explained by much more common conditions. However, if there is no identified cause of the symptoms or if the symptoms do not respond to the conventional treatments for the more common conditions, then it is reasonable to consider CFD as part of a differential diagnosis.

While a confirmed diagnosis of CFD helps to guide treatment, a lumbar puncture is not always necessary. Luckily patients with CFD often respond to well-tolerated, relatively safe treatments; therefore, in situations where symptoms do not improve from the conventional treatments, a suspected diagnosis of CFD should be entertained. If the patients improve with treatment for CFD, then this provides further evidence for the diagnosis of CFD, even in the absence of a lumbar puncture (see Chapter 15 – Diagnosing CFD).

Children	Adults
• Sleeping Problems	• Memory Loss
• Irritability	• Cognitive Impairments
• Developmental Delays	• Psychosis
• Neurodevelopmental Regression	• Schizophrenia
• Deceleration of Head Growth	• Depression
• Hypotonia	• Suicidal Ideation
• Ataxia	• Sensory Deficits
• Pyramidal Symptoms	• Weakness
• Seizures	• Pyramidal Symptoms
• Dyskinesias	• Movement Disorders
• Loss of Vision	• Cerebellar Syndrome
• Loss of Hearing	• Intellectual Disability
• Autism Spectrum Disorder	• Complex Neurological Disorder

Figure 4.2 Symptoms reported with CFD syndrome.

The Scientific Evidence

The CNS is safeguarded by a system of barriers that regulate the passage of substances from the blood to the brain and its surrounding fluids. Two of the primary barriers are the blood-brain barrier (BBB) and the blood-cerebrospinal fluid barrier (BCSFB). The BBB is formed by the endothelial cells lining the brain capillaries. It is responsible for selecting nutrients and molecules to enter the brain tissue while keeping out harmful toxins and pathogens.

The major site of CSF formation is the choroid plexus, a network of cells in the brain's ventricles. In the choroid plexus, a layer of endothelial cells with tight junctions forms the BCSFB, which regulates the exchange of substances between the blood and the CSF. This is the main entry point of folate into the CNS.

Upon discovery of CFD, Dr. Ramaekers hypothesized that the underlying problem was folate's inability to enter the CNS through the BCSFB barrier. Like other nutrients, folate requires a transporter to enter the CSF. The main carrier of folate into the CNS is the folate receptor alpha (FRα). Based on the lab findings that showed his patients had normal folate concentrations in the blood but abnormally

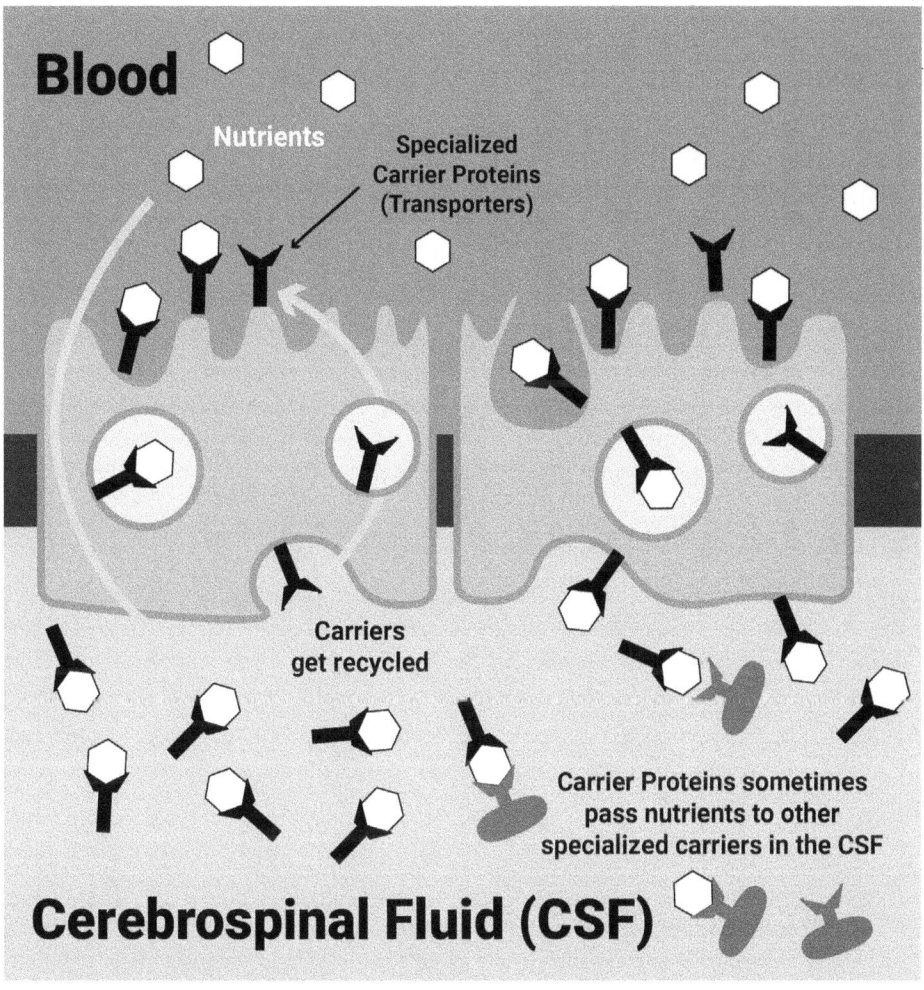

Figure 4.3 Nutrients crossing the Blood-CSF Barrier (BCSFB). Since the central nervous system is very sensitive to its chemical and nutrient environment, it is protected by barriers. The BCSFB prevents most substances from entering or leaving the CSF, and special proteins called carriers transport specific chemicals across it. Before CFD was described, other brain development disorders due to carrier dysfunction were known. The most notable of these involves a problem with transporting glucose, the brain's main fuel. Lack of glucose can lead to seizures in newborns that are difficult to treat with typical drugs. Without treatment, the brain grows more slowly and becomes smaller relative to the child's body, resulting in microcephaly (a small head). Fortunately, there is a treatment if diagnosed quickly, though it involves testing the CSF.

Chapter 4. - Cerebral Folate Deficiency - 47

low folate concentrations in the CSF, Dr. Ramaekers knew the patients were having trouble transporting folate into the brain, which strongly suggested a problem with the FRα.

Dr. Ramaekers had published a paper a couple of years earlier describing female patients with a genetic form of ASD known as Rett Syndrome who had CFD.[37] He felt that perhaps a different genetic explanation was possible for the CFD patients. He suspected that they may have a genetic mutation affecting the form or function of the FRα.

The most likely suspect was the FOLR1 gene. This gene provides the body with instruction for making the FRα. Mutations in FOLR1 can impact folate transport, brain development, and could easily explain CFD found in these patients. However, after examining the FOLR1 gene in multiple patients, Dr. Ramaekers found no errors in the genetic code. He then analyzed the FRαs in the patients' CSF samples and discovered they were not functioning, though the cause was unclear.

He proposed that either the cells had problems producing a functional FRα transporter, or something was blocking folate from binding to the FRα. If the latter, it was possible that the body's immune system was producing antibodies to the FRα transporter, which interfered with its ability to work.

Folate Receptor Autoantibodies (FRAAs)

Dr. Ramaekers then teamed up with Dr. Edward Quadros, a cellular biologist from the State University of New York (SUNY) at Downstate in Brooklyn. During his research into the causes of prenatal birth defects, Dr. Quadros discovered that the body's immune system could produce antibodies that blocked the FRα from working. These antibodies, known as autoantibodies, mistakenly target a person's own tissues or organs, disrupting normal function. This discovery played a crucial role in understanding how the immune system contributes to CFD.

Dr. Quadros discovered two distinct autoantibodies that were preventing the FRα from working properly. He called the first one the "binding autoantibody" and the other the "blocking autoantibody." The blocking autoantibody was found to block folate from attaching to the FRα while the binding autoantibody was found to bind to the FRα, causing it to not work correctly. Together these are known as Folate Receptor Alpha Autoantibodies (FRAAs).

In 2005, Dr. Ramaekers and Dr. Quadros published a landmark medical research paper defining CFD in the *New England Journal of Medicine (NEJM)*,[38] one of the world's leading medical journals. By examining many patients, they could report what type of symptoms and neurological disorders were consistently found with this condition. The patients diagnosed with CFD seemed to have very similar characteristics including the regression (loss) of developmental skills, irritability,

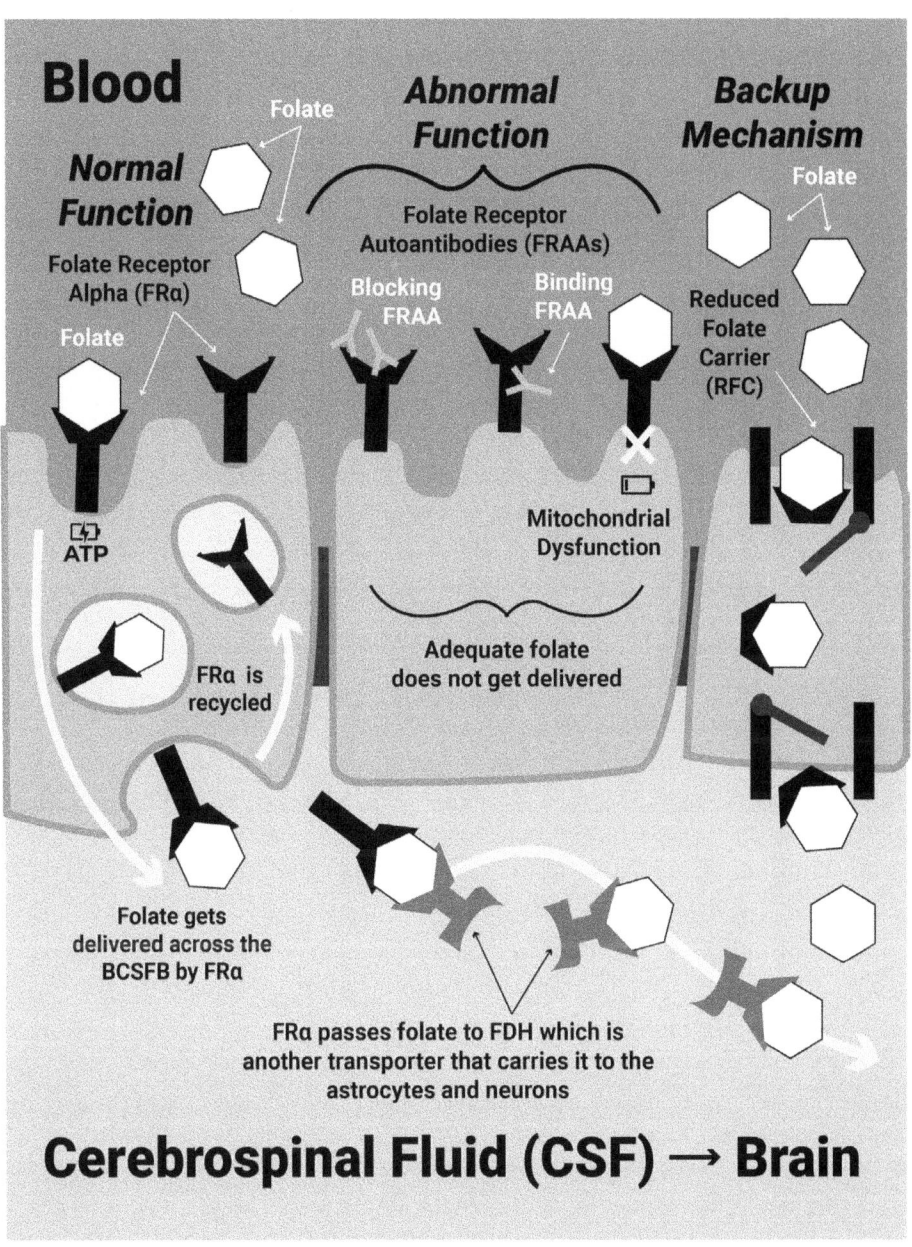

Figure 4.4 Folate needs one of two transporters to cross the blood-cerebrospinal fluid barrier (BCSFB), folate receptor alpha (FRα) or the reduced folate carrier (RFC). These transporters work to pull folate from the blood into the CSF. This figure shows the two transporter types: the FRα, which has a greater affinity for folate, and the RFC, which is used when the FRα is not functioning properly due to folate receptor autoantibodies (FRAAs) or mitochondrial dysfunction. Once inside the CSF, folate-dependent hydroxymethyltransferase (FDH) carries folate to the astrocytes and neurons.

Chapter 4. - Cerebral Folate Deficiency - 49

seizures, and involuntary movements starting at about one year of age (See Chapter 14 for more detailed description of symptoms).

Other Causes of CFD

In addition to the *NEJM* article about FRAAs, Dr. Ramaekers published other articles about genetic causes of CFD. He had also collaborated with researchers at the Baylor College of Medicine in the United States to describe the first case of CFD in a non-genetic form of ASD.[39]

Two years after the seminal *NEJM* paper, Dr. Ramaekers found that children with disorders of the mitochondria also manifested CFD, even in the absence of FRAAs.[40] Because the brain requires concentrations of folate that are 2-3 times higher than that of the blood, maintaining these levels requires active transport, an energy-dependent process. These transporters work to pull folate from the blood into the CSF and are powered by ATP made by the mitochondria. It is believed that without appropriate mitochondrial function, the FRα cannot operate efficiently, thereby causing a secondary CFD.

Cerebral Folate Deficiency Treatment

One encouraging aspect of CFD is that it is treatable. All known causes of CFD stem from the reduced ability of the FRα to transport folate into the brain. Because folate is so critical to the CNS, the body has a secondary mechanism to compensate: the reduced folate carrier (RFC). Research using mouse models has shown that when the FRα is absent, the production of the RFC increases.[41]

However, unlike FRα, which has a high affinity for folate, the RFC has a lower affinity for folate. This means that for the RFC to function effectively, blood folate concentrations must be significantly higher than normal. Additionally, as its name implies, the RFC requires folate in its reduced forms to work properly (see Chapter 2 for more on Reduced Folates).

The FRα's role extends beyond transporting folate into the CSF. It also acts as a binding protein, facilitating the movement of folate through the CSF to the ependymal cells lining the brain tissue. Once in the CSF, FRα works with the enzyme 10-formyltetrahydrofolate dehydrogenase (FDH) to ensure the availability of active folate forms needed to meet the brain's high metabolic demands.

Proper functioning of both FRα and FDH ensures that active folate is delivered to neurons and astrocytes.[42] Consequently, the loss of FRα not only disrupts folate transport into the brain but also impairs its distribution within the brain.

As discussed in previous chapters, a prescription form of folate known as leucovorin has been used for decades, primarily in oncology (the branch of medicine that studies and treats cancers). Although often associated with cancer treatments, leucovorin is not a chemotherapy drug. In fact, it is used at high doses to rescue the body from the harmful effects of chemotherapy (see Chapter 17 for details).

Due to its long-standing use in oncology, the safety and dosing of leucovorin are well established. Equally important, its ability to cross the BBB and enter the CNS has been thoroughly studied. An over-the-counter (OTC) version of leucovorin, known as folinic acid, is available in some multivitamins, although typically at much lower doses than the prescription form.

Dr. Ramaekers treated his CFD patients with leucovorin, achieving variable results. Encouragingly, some patients experienced remarkable recovery. He observed that outcomes were better when treatment began at a younger age. Younger patients often showed profound improvement in neurological symptoms after starting leucovorin. In contrast, patients who were not treated early frequently developed additional symptoms, such as vision and hearing loss, highlighting the importance of early intervention.

Caroline

Caroline was the first known case of CFD in North America.[43] She was diagnosed in 2003 at age five, at a time when the condition was commonly referred to as "low 5-MTHF in the cerebrospinal fluid." It wasn't until a year later that her condition would be officially named "Cerebral Folate Deficiency."

In an unrelenting quest to find help for her daughter, Caroline's mother, Elizabeth, played a pivotal role in advancing the medical and scientific understanding of this disorder. She collaborated closely with scientists conducting laboratory tests, doctors treating the condition, and pharmaceutical companies manufacturing medication for CFD. Thanks to her mother's tireless efforts, Caroline received the treatment she needed and reached milestones that were once unimaginable.

Caroline's remarkable recovery demonstrated to the scientific community the potential of leucovorin treatment for CFD. In 2005, her clinical journey was published in the medical journal <u>Neurology</u>.[44]

Tragically, Caroline passed away at 18 years of age due to a seizure disorder caused by a rare genetic mutation. Although her life was short, Caroline's journey inspired many. Her case was not only documented in medical journals but also shared widely in parent blogs[45] and was featured in major news outlets like "Good Morning America."[46] Her mother, Elizabeth, shares her story here...

Caroline's Story
By Elizabeth DeLuca, Caroline's Mom

Caroline was born healthy, but at two days old she stopped breathing and required mouth-to-mouth resuscitation. She was admitted to the hospital, where it was discovered that she suffered from epilepsy, requiring medical interventions.

Then, suddenly, at three years old, Caroline began screaming uncontrollably and arching her back at night, refusing to be held. She also struggled with crawling and seemed weak. Exhausted with worry, I took her to our pediatrician, who assured me she looked fine.

Over the following weeks, Caroline seemed unable to retain anything she had learned the day before. One morning, she woke up unable to move the entire left side of her body. I returned to the pediatrician and asked, "Could a baby have Alzheimer's Disease?" This time, both the pediatrician and her neurologist were concerned and ordered an MRI. The MRI revealed brain atrophy—essentially, a loss of brain tissue—in the white matter of her cerebellum. It seemed her brain was shrinking.

Caroline's condition continued to deteriorate. By age four, she could no longer swallow food or even her own saliva, requiring a feeding tube. She lost muscle function, bowel control, and the use of her hands. She was as limp as a noodle, barely able to hold up her head. Then, the seizures returned—over 1,000 a day. Her eyes wiggled back and forth in constant motion. Everyone told us that nothing could be done for our bright-eyed little girl. I was beside myself.

I knew I had to find her diagnosis, but I had no medical background. My only grasp of neurology came from the seizure medications we were using. By day, I was a homemaker and mother; by night, I was a medical researcher, looking endlessly for answers.

My husband pleaded with me to stop and come to bed, to accept the situation. The doctors agreed, saying I was in denial. But I wasn't giving up on my daughter, especially when they said she had maybe three months to live. All I had to do was look at her lying on the couch, limp and too quiet, and I knew I had to keep going.

One day, a friend called and told me to turn on The Oprah Winfrey Show. She said there were two kids on the show who looked like Caroline. To my surprise, they were showing a brother and sister who had been as sick as Caroline and had gotten better—"jumping on a trampoline" better. They had a condition called Dopamine Responsive Dystonia, so I researched it thoroughly that night. We tried the treatment, L-Dopa, but it didn't relieve Caroline's symptoms.

While L-Dopa wasn't effective, it gave me a clue and hope to continue. I researched dystonia, dopamine, and pediatric neurotransmitter disorders. I found a test for diagnosing these disorders called a spinal tap, which we hadn't done yet. We scheduled the procedure, and when the results came back, they showed that Caroline had low levels of 5-methyltetrahydrofolate (5-MTHF) in her cerebrospinal fluid (CSF).

At the time, this condition was so new and rare that it didn't even have a formal name beyond "Low 5-MTHF in CSF." The doctor recommended a drug called leucovorin, typically used for cancer treatment. Since little was known about Caroline's condition, no one was sure of the correct dosage or possible side effects. But I knew the risk of not trying was death, so I began crushing leucovorin tablets and putting them through her feeding tube.

Five days after starting treatment, Caroline could move one hand. After a week, she could stand while holding on to the coffee table. Three weeks later, my little girl, who couldn't hold her head up before, was standing on her own two feet. I said, "Caroline, if you lift your foot, you can walk." And she did—one foot in front of the other. She walked across our family room and out the door. She walked two city blocks before her little legs finally buckled. All the neighbors came out to see, and I cried with joy.

I called our geneticist to share the news. He sounded skeptical and asked us to come in. Caroline's condition had been so dire just three weeks before. When we arrived, she ran ahead of me off the elevator, stunning the staff who knew her. "Is that Caroline?" they asked in disbelief. In a room full of doctors, Caroline's recovery was met with astonishment. I later learned that the only available information on her disorder was a five-page paper published in Europe.

I had no idea that she was the first in North America to be diagnosed with this condition. Upon learning this, I did something quite uncharacteristic of me: when the doctors left the room, I searched through her medical file and stole her spinal tap analysis paperwork to find the lab where it was conducted.

Once back in my car with a very happy and energetic Caroline, I called the researcher who signed her report. He immediately knew of our case, and he admitted that he had advised against leucovorin. He felt that Caroline's 5-MTHF levels weren't low enough to warrant treatment. Thankfully, her doctors had gone ahead with it anyway, saving her life.

He explained the rarity of her condition and mentioned the same European paper. The next morning, I reached out to Dr. Vincent Ramaekers, the author of that paper. We agreed he should come to Houston, so I bought his ticket and arranged for his stay. When he arrived, he spoke at Texas Children's Hospital, and we hosted a reception for him.

Dr. Ramaekers, Caroline's medical team, and our family all agreed that we needed to spread the word about this newly identified condition. Although we felt we had solved the mystery for Caroline, we knew there were likely other children who could benefit from learning about CFD. As a result, Caroline and I were featured on Good Morning America and Inside Edition, helping to raise awareness. Shortly afterward, more children were diagnosed and treated for CFD.

Caroline thrived on leucovorin for several years, but over time, its effects began to wane. A pharmacologist friend suggested trying Isovorin, a similar drug available in Europe, to which Caroline responded well. However, we soon learned that Pfizer planned to discontinue Isovorin.

Upon hearing this, I sprang into action, making persistent calls until I reached Pfizer's CEO. Once he understood that children like Caroline relied on Isovorin to treat CFD—a use of the drug they were unaware of due to its "off-label" status—he arranged for its continued production. He connected me with the medical director, who ensured that children would maintain access to the drug. We alternated between leucovorin and Isovorin, a combination that proved effective for Caroline.

Years later, Caroline experienced another regression. She suddenly lost the ability to walk and swallow, requiring hospitalization. Her medical team suspected that she might have an additional, yet unidentified disorder. I had been reading about whole-genome sequencing and asked if it could be performed for Caroline. After a few discussions, my request was granted, and Caroline underwent genome sequencing.

The results revealed a genetic error in the 9q34.11 region, but I was told it was unlikely to be a disease-causing mutation. I was also strongly advised against researching it further. Naturally, I did my own research. As I read more, I became convinced that this mutation could account for many of Caroline's challenges. Studies showed that this genetic mutation was associated with catastrophic epilepsy—which she experienced—muscle weakness, and other symptoms that matched her condition.

Again questioning the "rarity" of Caroline's diagnosis, I asked her geneticist to email his colleagues across the country to see if they had encountered a similar clinical picture with this genetic defect. Replies came in from all over—five children shared the same symptoms and mutation as Caroline! This meant we were likely dealing with a syndrome. I asked the geneticist to share my contact information with these doctors so that other parents could reach out. One mother contacted me, and together we set out to find more families affected by this condition. Our early efforts have helped connect many parents of children diagnosed with what is now known as STXBP1 or STYX (pronounced "Sticks") from around the world.

Recognizing the need for further research, my husband and I decided to fund a lab at Texas Children's Hospital dedicated to STYX, with the hope of finding a treatment. Caroline contributed blood and muscle tissue samples. Under the guidance of the brilliant Dr. Mingshan Xue, the STYX lab has since developed a mouse model for the condition, created a potential treatment, and is now on the path toward a cure. With clinical trials for children with STYX set to begin this spring, we are increasingly hopeful.

Like many other children and teens with STYX, Caroline tragically succumbed to her syndrome, leaving us heartbroken yet more determined than ever to fight this devastating disease. From the extraordinary life of my brilliant and courageous daughter, I've learned to never give up, to keep trying, and to embrace each day as an opportunity to learn something new, even when the challenges seem insurmountable.

A Physician's Perspective

Caroline had a rough start in early life, first having epilepsy and then a sudden loss in motor skills. She became quite sick before a treatable medical diagnosis was found. Her mother was instrumental in exploring the potential medical conditions that might be affecting Caroline and advocating for her at every turn, highlighting the important role that parents play when faced with unusual symptoms that escape current medical knowledge.

The first diagnosis that Caroline's mom suspected, Dopamine-Responsive Dystonia, is a disorder where the body does not make the neurotransmitter dopamine. Her intuition was leading her in the right direction. Interestingly, because folate is needed to make dopamine and other monoamine neurotransmitters, CFD's presentation can overlap with dopamine deficiency disorders.

Because of her mom's persistence, a lumbar puncture was performed and CFD was found, which in itself is miraculous because 5-MTHF concentrations were not routinely tested at that time. Once they realized that Caroline had low folate in her CSF, 34 nmol/L (compared to normal range for her age 40-128),[47] many of her symptoms began to make sense, and more importantly, a treatment finally became possible.

Caroline had refractory epilepsy from early in life, a condition that usually has a poor prognosis. Refractory epilepsy is known to be drug-resistant, meaning that normal anti-epileptic medications are ineffective at controlling the seizures. When CFD is the cause, leucovorin can sometimes prevent further seizures.

CFD is also associated with neurodevelopmental regression (NDR), which means that a child loses previously-acquired skills. Caroline had this unique symptom, when she began losing motor skills. Sometimes loss of white matter in the brain (leukodystrophy) can be seen on an MRI in patients with CFD, which was also the case for Caroline.

It is clear that her mother's search for the diagnosis of CFD and subsequent leucovorin treatment gave Caroline many quality years of life. In addition to the sudden and positive changes witnessed by her family, medical testing also showed incredible progress with leucovorin. After months of treatment, her CSF 5-MTHF increased to 113 nmol/L (well within the normal range), her EEG showed no epileptiform discharges, and her motor skills and hand use improved significantly. She was able to thrive and gain new skills, which defied her earlier prognosis.

It is impossible to know what caused Caroline to stop responding well to leucovorin after so many years of successful treatment. The drug Isovorin®, that her mother referenced, is the specific Pfizer brand of a drug more commonly known as levo-leucovorin. As her mother explains, Isovorin® is not commonly used in the

United States. While both leucovorin and levo-leucovorin are types of folinic acid, they have chemical differences. Leucovorin is a racemic mixture, meaning that it has a combination of L and D isomers (see Chapter 3 for explanation), whereas levo-leucovorin only contains the L isomer. Because both drugs were developed for and tested on chemotherapy patients, research comparing their efficacy and safety has primarily been conducted in cancer settings. A 2009 comprehensive literature summarized randomized, controlled trials in patients with gastrointestinal tract malignancies and found no differences in efficacy or tolerability between the two drugs when used with chemotherapeutic agents.[48]

Leucovorin is easily accessible in the United States and has been very commonly used as a rescue therapy for cancer patients for decades. Because of this, the dosage, safety profile, and metabolic pathways have been well-studied, which informed some of the clinical trials for CFD which are covered extensively in this book. Specific studies comparing leucovorin and levo-leucovorin for CFD patients, and more specifically for children with or without FRAAs, is an important area of research. Studies with levo-leucovorin are ongoing for ASD.

At this time, there are no studies that offer a clear explanation for why Caroline responded differently to levo-leucovorin after several successful years on leucovorin. The driving biological factors causing CFD can fluctuate, making the CFD better or worse at different times. As discussed later in this book, the dose of leucovorin needs to be adjusted from time to time. Without performing repeated lumbar punctures, it is not possible to easily follow the true CSF 5-MTHF concentrations, so many times empirical adjustments must be done.

In summary, Caroline's recovery inspired the medical community to continue researching the causes, diagnostic procedures, and treatments for CFD. As her mother explained, after genome sequencing, Caroline was also discovered to have a mutation in the syntaxin-binding protein 1 gene (STXBP1). This genetic disorder does not have any known treatment, so although the CFD could be treated, the ultimate underlying condition could not.

In 2012, Caroline's case was included in a publication about children with the 9q34.11 deletion.[49] Her family continues to support STXBP1 research and help other children impacted by Caroline's rare genetic disorder. They have also founded The Caroline School, an educational facility for children with special needs and complex medical conditions in Houston, Texas. Her medical case contributed significantly to the interest and understanding of CFD, and we are appreciative that her family generously continues to share her remarkable story.

Marley

The story told by Marley's mom is one that many parents may easily relate to - struggling to find a doctor who is knowledgeable enough about CFD to run the appropriate tests and deliver a treatment, if warranted.

This story also illuminates something that researchers are starting to investigate more - the connection between the mother's pregnancy history and the likelihood of a child having CFD.

For Marley, while treating CFD led to improvements in her health, her story also demonstrates that some children may not respond favorably to leucovorin and will require specialized formulations or other combinations of medications to receive the full benefits of leucovorin treatment.

Marley's Story
By Kelly S., Marley's Mom

My pregnancy was awful. I was terribly ill and threw up ten times per day the entire pregnancy. I needed intravenous fluids more times than I could count. Baby Marley was born at 33 weeks gestation after my water broke. The NICU did several tests. One revealed sleep apnea, so they ordered a head ultrasound. It revealed a grade 4 Intraventricular hemorrhage. Interestingly, Marley developed normally over the next 18 months except that she had poor motor skills due to her brain bleed.

She was followed by a special infant care clinic every two months because of her prematurity. At her 17-month visit, they deemed her on track. At her 19-month visit, (post 18-month MMR, chicken pox, DTaP vaccinations) she was referred for autism testing. She would no longer make eye contact, do things on command, sit still, or use her words (she lost all of them). She also had nonstop explosive poop after the 18-month shots. The GI problems didn't stop. They went from severe diarrhea to severe constipation. It's still a battle to this day.

Initially, we were referred to a neuro-developmental pediatrician. He told me that we needed to start saving our money to institutionalize her because she had severe autism. This was 2005 and was the beginning of our long journey of trying to find answers.

I would fly to autism conferences and sit in the back row and listen and take diligent notes, then go to my hotel room alone after a long day and sob.

In 2012 at a conference, I heard a topic that piqued my interest - Cerebral Folate Deficiency. At that time, CFD was not a well-known condition. Following the conference, I read all of the available studies about CFD. The more that I read, the more alarmed I became - everything was hitting home in a very scary way. There were so many red flags in both my own history and my baby's history.

First of all, I learned that folate problems are known to be linked to pregnancy issues. My pregnancy history included the use of birth control pills, followed by trouble conceiving, a miscarriage, an ectopic pregnancy, terrible morning sickness, and premature labor in multiple pregnancies. Interestingly, while pregnant with my second and third children, I took 5-MTHF, which improved my symptoms and enabled me to carry the babies longer after premature labor had started.

At the time I was learning about CFD, much about Marley's history was also lining up. She had been diagnosed with severe, low-functioning autism. Low-functioning, regressive autism is a sign of CFD. Marley also has genetic markers indicating problems with folate metabolism including FOLR1, FOLR2, DHFR, MTHFR A1298C, and SLC19A1.

There was no doctor that helped me with CFD. I did it all on my own. I trialed 1 mg of 5-MTHF with Marley at age 2.5 years old, and she walked down the stairs independently for the first time. This supplement also ended her staring spells. She stayed at about 2 mg of 5-MTHF until 2014, when I took her to my local neurologist at age 11 years of age.

Luckily, we live in a city with great medical resources and a fabulous, well-known hospital and there just happens to be a pediatric neurologist on staff who knew about and understood CFD and its link to autism. I made an appointment, and after assessing Marley and listening to the information that I presented to him, he agreed that she needed a lumbar puncture right away.

We went into the hospital early in the morning. They used Versed and Fentanyl to sedate her, but she was hard to sedate and even with the maximum dosage of both sedatives, she sang to them during the procedure.

Recovery was hard. She was in extreme pain for two days. She was dizzy and couldn't stand. We had her lie flat on her back and pushed fluids like crazy to get her body to reproduce more spinal fluid. She also had headaches, and the symptoms were more severe than I had anticipated, but after six days, most symptoms had subsided and after nine days, she had fully recovered.

We were on vacation when I got the call from the pediatric neurology resident who had done her lumbar puncture. She said, "We have about half of Marley's results in, and everything is normal."

I was shocked. I said "Define normal. Tell me her numbers."

She told me Marley's 5-MTHF is a 44 with a normal range between

PATIENT STORIES

40 and 120. I exclaimed, "That's not normal! That is very low! It is half of what it should be. We want her to be between 78-82. Especially considering she has been dairy free and supplemented with 5-MTHF almost all her life!"

The pediatric resident just told me to take my argument to the attending doctor whom we had met originally. I did. After hearing my argument, he agreed with me that she needed to be treated for Cerebral Folate Deficiency. I could tell he had little experience treating CFD because I had to tell him the dosage of Leucovorin that should be used, and he easily agreed with me after trying to prescribe a much lower dose.

While this neurologist was somewhat helpful in getting us to the right diagnosis, we left his care and made an appointment to see Dr. Dan Rossignol, a family medicine doctor who specialized in autism and had recently published articles about CFD.

We flew to Florida to see him, and he started her on Leucovorin immediately. Even though Marley's level of folate in her CSF was low, she did poorly on leucovorin. I was shocked. I thought I had found her answer. I added in lithium orotate and riboflavin and she started to tolerate it a little better. But the best improvements came when we added in prescription Levocarnitine. It was like a light bulb went on and she was suddenly finishing my sentences. Over time, instead of only leucovorin, we found that high dose leucovorin paired with high dose 5-MTHF was a winning combination for her.

The biggest improvements we saw with folate treatment were lowered anxiety and increased cognition. We slowly added more mitochondrial supports which have delivered huge improvements as well. Marley graduated from high school with a regular diploma and is an accomplished singer with the local women's choir. She still has autism and cognitive difficulties, but she is a sweet and conversational young lady. She currently has a part-time job doing data entry.

A Physician's Perspective

Marley also had a rough start as an infant by being born prematurely and suffering a bleed in the brain. Despite these challenges, Marley did well as an infant until she experienced neurodevelopmental regression and began to have symptoms of autism. Guided by maternal intuition, Marley's mother started giving her 5-MTHF as a supplement to see if it would help, and it did. Again, this demonstrates how parents are often the driving force in a child's recovery.

Both Caroline's and Marley's cases provide an introduction into the not-so-uncommon course of identifying and treating CFD. Both families struggled to find a diagnosis, and even when there were clues, the disorder was dismissed. This is not uncommon in medicine for new diagnoses as medicine is very conservative and moves slowly for good reasons – doctors do not want to do anything unproven as it might hurt their patients and the Hippocratic oath binds physicians to "first do no harm."

CFD is not yet taught in medical school; therefore, most doctors do not know about it. Additionally, many doctors think of leucovorin as a "cancer drug," not a safe type of folate. A significant challenge in medicine is that some physicians believe children with ASD, cerebral palsy, refractory epilepsy, and genetic disorders cannot be effectively treated. These children endure years without effective treatments. Many experts are skeptical that a simple and safe vitamin could address these complex and persistent disorders.

CFD syndrome was first described in the early 2000s, and since then, our understanding of CFD has evolved. Early treatments showed success, but the best approach is still being refined and varies for each patient. Depending on the cause, treatment may need to be lifelong.

The way in which CFD manifests itself clinically is extremely variable. Epilepsy starting early in life is usually a sequela of complications during birth. When it isn't associated with birth complications, epilepsy can be very refractory and often has a poor prognosis. (In medicine, "refractory" refers to a condition that does not respond to treatments and typical medical interventions).

CFD is a rare cause of early-onset epilepsy. While clinicians recommend genetic testing, including the FOLR1[50] gene, for children with early-onset epilepsy, most CFD cases do not have a genetic cause. CFD is often linked to genetic disorders that do not directly affect the folate pathway, making a lumbar puncture necessary for diagnosis in many cases. For instance, even though genetic testing could have identified Caroline's mutation, which has no known treatment, it might not have revealed her CFD. This could have led to the workup ending without exploring other treatable causes of epilepsy.

Several cases have documented white matter loss in CFD, and one study found that the severity of white matter abnormalities is linked to the severity of CFD.[51] Other studies have shown that these abnormalities can significantly improve with proper treatment.[52]

CFD is linked to neurodevelopmental regression (NDR), typically occurring before a child's first year of life. However, in the cases mentioned, the children lost skills after a year. NDR is connected to both CFD and ASD. Two studies have tracked 5-MTHF concentrations in children with CFD and ASD, suggesting that folate concentrations in the CSF may slowly deplete over time, with symptoms appearing only when levels drop critically low.[53,54]

Doctors may hesitate to perform a lumbar puncture, and families often feel nervous about them. This leads many families to ask why a lumbar puncture is necessary for diagnosis instead of simply trying a folate supplement. While lumbar punctures are safe when done by trained professionals, they can have complications, as seen in Marley's case. The most common issue is a headache, caused by the needle leaving a hole in the dura (the protective layer around the brain and spinal cord) that does not close properly. This headache usually goes away with rest and hydration, but if it persists, a procedure called a blood patch may be needed. In this procedure, a small amount of the patient's blood is injected near the puncture site to stop the leak by clotting. While this process can be inconvenient, it is sometimes necessary.

There are several benefits to doing a lumbar puncture before starting treatment. First, once treatment begins, it can be hard to interpret the CSF results accurately. For example, in Marley's case, the CSF folate concentration was at the lower limit of normal. Since Marley was already taking folate supplements, it's unclear if the measurement truly represents the level of folate in the CSF at baseline (before supplements were started). This creates uncertainty and can lead to differing interpretations and opinions.

Second, if the treatment doesn't work as expected, it can be hard to tell whether the treatment is the issue or if the wrong condition is being treated. In Marley's case, she didn't respond well to leucovorin initially, which could be due to various reasons (see Chapter 17). Without a clear diagnosis, it can be challenging to decide whether to continue the treatment.

Many physicians experienced with treating CFD use the folate receptor autoantibody test (FRAT) to determine whether CFD might be a possible diagnosis. Unlike a lumbar puncture, the FRAT does not measure the concentration of folate in the CSF, but this test will detect the presence of autoantibodies blocking folate from entering the nervous system. A positive result may indicate a lower level of folate in the brain.

Leucovorin is the standard treatment for many reasons, but most of all because the dosing and possible adverse effects are well known. Leucovorin is usually increased slowly to minimize side effects. There are many nuances to treating CFD and using leucovorin, including alternative dosing and adding adjunctive treatments like L-carnitine (See Chapter 17).

In our clinical trials, we've seen improvements in many symptoms, with the most noticeable improvement in language. When starting leucovorin, some children demonstrate hyperactivity, but this is generally transient. We have found that hyperactivity generally improves better than baseline (before treatment) within about six weeks. Many children continue leucovorin treatment for years. For some, initial gains are lost if the leucovorin is weaned.

We have found that problems with brain folate metabolism impact various neurodevelopmental disorders like ASD, Down syndrome, and epilepsy. The upcoming chapters share patient stories that show how these folate issues affect children with a wide range of symptoms. These stories emphasize the need for accurate diagnosis and treatment, encouraging further investigation to improve lives.

CHAPTER 5.

Autism Spectrum Disorder

Background

Autism spectrum disorder (ASD) is a behaviorally defined condition that affects an estimated 2% or more of children in the United States. Despite decades of research, healthcare professionals still do not fully understand the cause of ASD in most cases, and effective treatments remain limited.

Over the past 20 years, the Centers for Disease Control and Prevention (CDC) has established a network to monitor ASD and has made significant efforts to educate both the medical community and the public about recognizing the disorder. However, the average age of diagnosis has not improved and remains around four years old. This delay is critical because treatments like applied behavioral analysis (ABA) are most effective when initiated early, ideally around two years of age.

The prevalence of ASD has steadily increased over time, from 1 in 10,000 children in 1970, to 1 in 1,000 in 1995, to 1 in 150 in 2000, and most recently to 1 in 36 in 2020.[55] While increased awareness and improved diagnostic practices partially explain this rise,[56] other unknown factors likely contribute, though none have been definitively identified.

Optimal care for children with ASD includes 40 hours of behavioral therapy per week, as well as speech and occupational therapy. This level of care requires a dedicated, full-time behavioral therapist for each child. Additionally, one parent often must devote significant time to caregiving, which can make holding a job challenging. As a result, ASD has far-reaching effects not only on the child but also on their family and support network.

The costs associated with ASD are staggering. Between 1990 and 2019, an estimated 2 million cases of ASD in the United States cost approximately $7 trillion USD.[57] If the current prevalence rate continues, these costs are projected to rise to

$11.5 trillion by 2029. However, if the prevalence continues to increase at its historical rate, costs could escalate to nearly $15 trillion by 2029, placing a significant financial burden on families, individuals, and society as a whole.

ASD is defined by behavior rather than biological markers, meaning there are no blood tests or definitive diagnostic tools available. Diagnosis relies on the expertise of highly trained professionals who assess the child's observable behaviors, making the process complex and multifaceted.

Several factors contribute to the complexity of ASD diagnosis. First, many symptoms are developmental, meaning they depend on the child's age and maturity. For example, behaviors like pointing are expected at specific stages, and their absence cannot be assessed until the appropriate age has passed. Since children develop at different rates, doctors may delay evaluation to avoid misdiagnosis, leading to significant delays in identifying ASD. Second, some symptoms only appear after certain skills have developed. For instance, repetitive movements, a common symptom of ASD, may not emerge until motor skills are sufficiently developed. Similarly, echolalia—where a child repeats words instead of responding appropriately—only occurs after speech has been acquired.

Lastly, some behaviors associated with ASD, such as toe walking or hand flapping, can occur in young children but often resolve as they age, making them unreliable indicators of ASD in infancy. Adding to the complexity, the diagnostic criteria for ASD have evolved over time, further complicating diagnosis.

Autism was first described in the 1940s. In 1943, Leo Kanner published a report titled "Autistic Disturbances of Affective Contact," detailing children with symptoms resembling modern ASD. Around the same time, Hans Asperger described children with a high-functioning form of autism, later termed Asperger's disorder.[58] Significant interest in autism did not emerge until the 1960s, when two prominent figures offered contrasting views on the condition. Bernard Rimland, founder of the Autism Research Institute and the Autism Society of America, argued in his book *Infantile Autism: The Syndrome and Its Implications for a Neural Theory of Behavior* that autism was a neurological disorder. In contrast, Bruno Bettelheim, in his book *The Empty Fortress: Infantile Autism and the Birth of the Self*, proposed the controversial "Refrigerator Mother Theory," suggesting that a lack of maternal warmth caused autism.

Despite this growing interest, autism was not officially recognized as a "Pervasive Developmental Disorder" until 1980 in the 3rd edition of the *Diagnostic and Statistical Manual of Mental Disorders (DSM)*, an authoritative guide for classifying psychological and psychiatric disorders. Even after its formal recognition, it wasn't until 1987 that Ivar Lovaas developed the first evidence-based treatment for autism: Applied Behavioral Analysis (ABA).

The Diagnostic and Statistical Manual of Mental Disorders (DSM)

The DSM is a reference guide used by doctors and mental health professionals to diagnose and understand various mental health conditions. It provides descriptions of all recognized mental disorders, with each one having its own set of diagnostic criteria, including specific symptoms and behaviors. If a person's symptoms align with the criteria for a particular disorder, a diagnosis can be made. The DSM is regularly updated to incorporate new research and insights into mental health. Since autism was not included in the DSM until 1980, it was not officially recognized as a psychiatric disorder before then and lacked formal diagnostic criteria.

The defining characteristics of autism transformed from the DSM-III to the DSM-5-TR. Perhaps the best-known definition of autism come from the DSM-4-TR where the diagnosis was defined by three sets of symptoms:

A. Deficits in verbal and non-verbal communication

B. Deficits in social interactions

C. The presence of repetitive and restricted behaviors and interests

In the DSM-4-TR these symptoms were used to classify three different diagnoses:

- Autistic Disorder, the most severe form, defined by having all three categories of symptoms.

- Pervasive Developmental Disorder - Not Otherwise Specified (PDD-NOS), a milder form of autism where symptoms might be missing or one category of symptoms may be mild.

- Asperger's disorder, usually a more high-functioning form of autism where the individual did not have any early language delays.

As more professionals began using these definitions for autism, it became clear that the diagnostic categories were unstable, with individuals often shifting between them over time. Additionally, it was difficult to clearly separate communication and social function symptoms.

Sensory disturbances, such as hypersensitivity or hyposensitivity, were also recognized as common in autism and were not appropriately addressed by the prevailing definitions. As a result, the DSM-5-TR redefined autism using two categories of symptoms:

- Deficits in social communication.
- The presence of repetitive, restricted patterns of behaviors, interests, or activities, and/or sensory abnormalities.

The three diagnostic categories for autism were eliminated when it was recognized that autism exists on a spectrum. As a result, it was officially renamed Autism Spectrum Disorder (ASD). Additionally, a key criterion was added: to be diagnosed with ASD, an individual must experience functional limitations caused by ASD symptoms. In other words, it is not enough to exhibit symptoms of ASD; these symptoms must significantly impair the person's ability to function.

The severity of ASD is classified into three levels:

- Level 1: Requiring support.
- Level 2: Requiring substantial support.
- Level 3: Requiring very substantial support.

The variation in symptoms and characteristics among children with ASD is perhaps best illustrated by the three developmental trajectories they often follow: About one-third of children with ASD show developmental challenges from infancy. Another one-third appear to develop typically during the first year of life but then suddenly stop progressing. The final one-third experience neurodevelopmental regression (NDR), where they develop normally but later lose skills they have previously acquired. This regression may occur suddenly—sometimes linked to an illness or seizure—or more gradually over time, and it most commonly happens in the second year of life.[59]

Despite ASD's high prevalence and significant impact, only two medications, risperidone and aripiprazole, are currently approved by the Food and Drug Administration (FDA) for its treatment. Both drugs are antipsychotics that help manage behavioral symptoms but do not address the underlying biological causes of the disorder.

There is a pressing need for treatments that not only improve core ASD symptoms but also target the underlying biological abnormalities. This chapter explores the connection between Cerebral Folate Deficiency (CFD) and ASD, offering hope that some children with ASD may benefit from treatments aimed at improving their quality of life.

The Scientific Evidence

In 2004, not long after the initial publications about children with CFD, Dr. Ramaekers wrote the first paper describing ASD in CFD. In this paper, he discussed that 7 out of the 20 children with CFD also had the diagnosis of ASD.[60] In 2005, he wrote a seminal paper about CFD in *The New England Journal of Medicine* (NEJM), where he reported a similar finding showing 5 of the 28 CFD patients were also diagnosed with ASD.[61] After this *NEJM* article called attention to the overlap between CFD and ASD, new case reports started appearing in the literature. In 2005, an article was published that described a six-year-old girl with neurodevelopmental regression (NDR), seizures, intellectual disability, and autistic features.[62]

The same research group published a follow-up report in 2008 on a series of seven patients with ASD symptoms, NDR, intellectual disability, epilepsy, and a movement disorder.[63] Separately, but around the same time, Dr. Ramaekers published a case series of 25 patients with early-onset low-functioning ASD.[64] Of these ASD studies, Dr. Ramaekers' was the only one that measured FRAAs. He concluded that these autoantibodies could explain CFD in most of the observed cases. These early reports seemed to suggest that CFD could be found in children with ASD who were low functioning (meaning that they also had intellectual disability) with and without NDR.

Additional studies were conducted looking at children who had more variability in their severity of ASD symptoms. In one study, clinicians performed lumbar punctures on 16 children who had ASD to measure their 5-MTHF concentrations in the cerebral spinal fluid (CSF). None of the children had levels below normal; however, the concentrations were at the lower limits of normal.[65]

Another large study of 61 children with ASD measured CSF 5-MTHF concentrations over time.[66] This larger study found that 16% of children with ASD had a CSF 5-MTHF concentration below normal in at least one sampling period during the study. Interestingly, another finding was that 5-MTHF decreased over time in many children, which suggested that CFD may develop progressively. Lastly, a more recent study demonstrated that 21% of 38 children with ASD had CFD when their CSF was examined.[67] (See Chapter 15 for more information).

A meta-analysis was performed to try to extract more insights from these series of studies. A meta-analysis is a statistical technique used to combine and analyze data from multiple studies to derive a more comprehensive and precise estimate of an effect or relationship. Each study was evaluated for its inclusion and exclusion criteria, sample sizes, variability between the groups of children, and more. When all studies were considered, the results showed that the overall prevalence of CFD in ASD was 38%, and FRAAs were estimated to cause the CFD in 84% of the cases.[68]

As a pediatric neurologist who often treats patients with ASD, I worked with Dr. Daniel Rossignol, another autism-focused clinician, to further explore some of the recent findings. Given that FRAAs may cause CFD in children with ASD, we wanted to see how many of our pediatric patients with ASD had FRAAs.

In our pioneering study, we discovered that 60% of the children with ASD had blocking FRAAs, and 44% had binding FRAAs. In total, 75% of the children with ASD in our study had at least one of these autoantibodies.[69] (Refer to Chapter 4 for more on blocking vs. binding FRAAs and see the Figure 5.1 for details).

Following our original study, several other studies have also looked at the prevalence of FRAAs. The most recent meta-analysis, which summarized all results, found that 71% of children with ASD have FRAAs, specifically 46% have the blocking type and 49% have the binding type.[70] These percentages are compared to typically developing peers who do not have siblings with ASD, where only 15% have FRAAs.

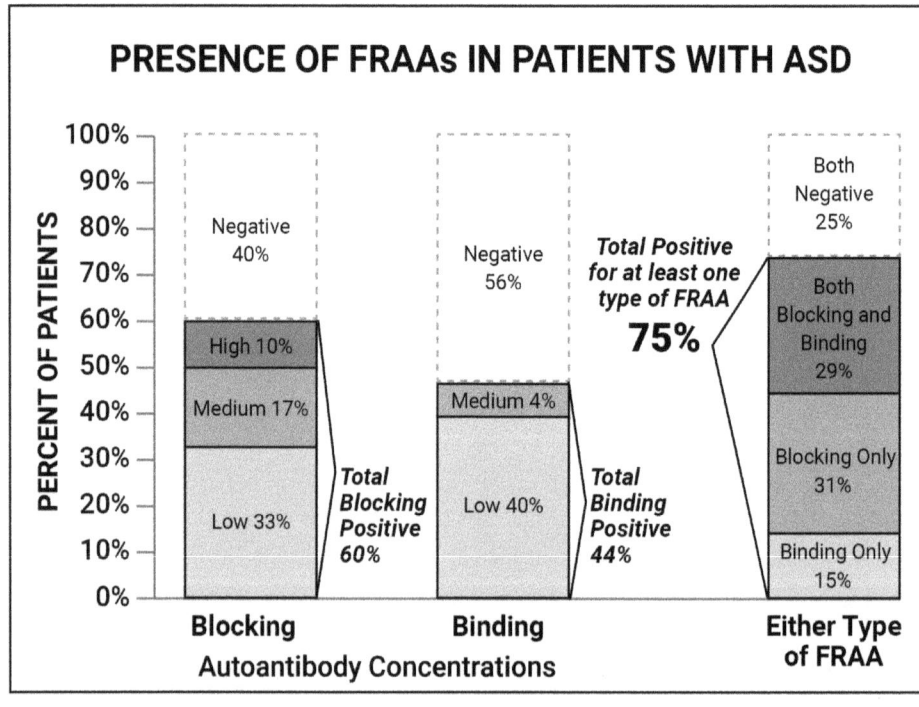

Figure 5.1 Prevalence of the Folate Receptor Autoantibodies (FRAAs) in children with ASD in our initial study

Explanation of Different Types of Studies	
Meta-Analysis	A statistical technique used to combine and analyze results from multiple independent studies on a specific topic to obtain a more reliable and generalizable conclusion. It involves finding relevant studies, extracting the data, weighting the results, assessing consistency, and evaluating possible biases across each study.
Systematic Review	A comprehensive review of every paper published on a certain topic to ensure unbiased reporting of the conclusion of previous research. Standardized techniques are used to ensure the quality of the systematic review as well as document the thoroughness of the review. Many times, such a review will rate the quality of the individual research papers and the overall quality of the evidence supporting or refuting a research conclusion.
Uncontrolled Study	An uncontrolled study examines the effects of an intervention or treatment on a single group without comparing it to a control group. This means there is no separate group for comparison, making it harder to determine if the effects are due to the intervention or other factors. Uncontrolled studies are often used for preliminary insights.
Controlled Study	In a controlled study, researchers compare an intervention or treatment group with a separate control group that does not receive the intervention. The control group helps determine whether any observed effects are due to the intervention itself or other factors. This design helps provide more reliable evidence on the effectiveness of the intervention.
Blind Clinical Trial	In a blind clinical trial, participants do not know whether they are receiving the actual treatment or a placebo (a fake treatment). This helps prevent their expectations or beliefs from influencing the results. The study can be single-blind, meaning only the participants are unaware, or double-blind meaning that the staff conducting the study and the participants are unaware of which participants receive the active treatment.
Randomized Trial	In a randomized trial, a random number is used to assign participants to one of several groups so there is no bias in group assignment.
Double Blind Clinical Trial	In a double-blind clinical trial, neither the participants nor the researchers know who is receiving the actual treatment and who is receiving a placebo. This design minimizes bias from both the participants and the researchers, providing more accurate and reliable results regarding the effectiveness of the treatment.

Figure 5.2 Different types of scientific studies with explanations for each

Over the years, the use of leucovorin to treat ASD has been investigated in different groups:

1) Individuals with ASD and confirmed CFD

2) Individuals with ASD who test positive for FRAAs

3) Individuals with ASD regardless of FRAA status or CFD presence

In the first group, nine uncontrolled studies evaluated leucovorin treatment at doses ranging from 0.5 mg/kg/day to 3 mg/kg/day. Leucovorin appears to have alleviated CFD symptoms for many patients[71] (see meta-analysis summary in Figure 5.3). Neurological symptoms such as ataxia, epilepsy, and pyramidal signs improved in most patients, while ASD symptoms improved in about two-thirds (see Chapter 14 for symptom details).

Irritability and movement disorders showed improvement in about half of the patients. While these studies provide valuable insights, they cannot account for other factors that might affect the results, such as dosage variations, concurrent medications, and comorbidities. These confounding variables limit our ability to draw definitive conclusions from uncontrolled studies. Nonetheless, the data suggesting that leucovorin could benefit many children with ASD and CFD is quite compelling.

The percentage of children with ASD and CFD who improved with leucovorin treatment			
Symptoms	Improvement	Symptoms	Improvement
Autism	67%	Ataxia	88%
Irritability	58%	Pyramidal Signs	76%
Epilepsy	75%	Movement Disorders	47%

Figure 5.3 Meta-analysis results showing the percentage of children with ASD and CFD whose symptoms improved with leucovorin treatment

Recognizing that the FRAA could be used as a biomarker for CFD, one of our studies treated children with ASD who were FRAA-positive in a controlled fashion and measured the change in nine symptoms from the start of treatment.[72]

These children were compared to similar FRAA-positive children with ASD who did not receive leucovorin or make any changes to their existing treatment regimen (Discussed further in "A Physician Perspective"). This study found significant improvements in receptive and expressive language, verbal communication and attention.

Three placebo-controlled studies have examined leucovorin's effects in the general ASD population—one conducted by my team,[73] another in France,[74] and a recent study from India.[75] Our study was the first to use a randomized double-blind placebo-controlled design, with one group receiving leucovorin and another receiving an identical-looking but inert substance.

We specifically measured verbal communication and treated the patients with 2 mg/kg/day (up to a maximum of 50 mg) in two divided doses over 12 weeks. The results showed significant improvements in verbal communication for children treated with leucovorin compared to those receiving the placebo. Additionally, behavioral improvements were noted as measured by the Aberrant Behavior Checklist (ABC). Importantly, there were no differences in adverse effects between the two groups.

Because we enrolled children from the general ASD population, some had FRAAs and some did not. Having these two different groups allowed us to answer an important question: Does having FRAAs predict a response to leucovorin treatment in a child with ASD? The answer was definitely "Yes." Results summarized in Figure 5.5 show the higher rates of response in the FRAA-positive group. A positive response to treatment was defined as gaining language equivalent to the standard results from intense behavioral interventions.

Antibody Status	Leucovorin Response	Placebo Response	Compared to Placebo	Odds	Number Needed to Treat (NNT)
Negative	50%	29%	21%	2.5	4.7
Positive	77%	22%	55%	11.7	1.8

Figure 5.5 Clinical trial response based on status of having (Positive) or not having (Negative) FRAAs. The number needed to treat (NNT) shows how many people with that status would need to be treated to have one patient experience a positive response.

Exactly half of the children without FRAAs responded to leucovorin, while a significantly higher percentage (77%) of those with FRAAs showed a positive response. Both groups were then compared to the control groups who were receiving a placebo. The FRAA-positive group had a 55% higher response rate to leucovorin compared to placebo, whereas the FRAA-negative group had only a 21% higher response rate compared to placebo. The odds ratio of 11.7 for the FRAA-positive group versus 2.5 for the FRAA-negative group indicates that those with FRAAs are much more likely to benefit from leucovorin.

Additionally, we calculated the number needed to treat (NNT), which is the number of patients that must be treated for one patient to experience a positive response. While some might assume the NNT should be 1.0 (indicating every patient responds), in reality the NNT for many drugs ranges from four to six. This means that four to six patients need to be treated to achieve one positive response.

Our study's data suggests that for children who are FRAA-negative, five need to be treated to get one to respond to leucovorin. For children who are FRAA-positive, fewer than two need to be treated to achieve at least one positive response. These insights help clinicians to practice more personalized medicine, determining which patients are most likely to respond to treatment.

The French leucovorin study, which was also randomized placebo controlled, examined whether leucovorin treatment helped ASD symptoms. This study examined 19 children using a lower dose of leucovorin (5 mg twice a day) than our study. ASD symptoms were measured using the Autism Diagnostic Observation Scale (ADOS), which is a gold-standard diagnostic instrument for ASD. ADOS total scores and subscales were found to significantly improve, demonstrating that general ASD symptoms diminished with leucovorin treatment.

The study conducted in India used a randomized double-blind, placebo-controlled design to study 80 children with ASD. This is the largest study to date. They treated the children with the same dose of leucovorin as our original study but treated the children for 24 weeks. The Childhood Autism Rating Scale, a standard instrument to rate ASD severity, decreased more in the children treated with leucovorin as compared to the children treated with placebo. Improvement was more pronounced for those children with higher FRAA titers. In addition, behavior, as measured by the Child Behavior Checklist, a standard parent-completed questionnaire, improved significantly in the children treated with leucovorin as compared to the children treated with the placebo.

Building on these findings, we have conducted additional studies to evaluate other aspects of folate metabolism in patients with ASD. Another potential biomarker that we recently evaluated is something called the soluble folate binding protein (sFBP) that is sometimes found in the blood of children with ASD. We looked at 110 patients from our ASD clinic and found that 14 of them (13%) were positive for sFBP. Half of these children also had the binding FRAA. Our analysis showed that sFBP-positive patients often had severe ASD, gastrointestinal issues, and exhibited self-injurious or aggressive behavior.[76]

Twelve of the 14 patients with the sFBP started treatment with 25 mg of leucovorin, twice a day (which is considered a standard dose), but half of the children required the dose to be doubled to 50 mg, twice a day for a clinical response. Significant improvements were found in ASD symptoms as measured by two standardized tests - the Social Responsiveness Scale (SRS), which measures ASD symptoms, and the ABC, which measures behavior. Based on our findings, we believe that the sFBP could be a useful biomarker for identifying severe cases of ASD. In our study, most patients with positive sFBP results started with high scores in the "severe" range on the SRS, indicating severe ASD, and had high scores on the ABC, indicating many concerning behaviors.

With treatment, these patients showed slow but positive progress on the SRS, indicating improvement in ASD symptoms, and often experienced rapid improvements on the ABC, indicating significant improvement in disruptive behaviors. This was especially encouraging for families, as many of these severe patients had not made progress before starting the treatment. Over months and years, the improvements were significant, leading to dramatic benefits for both the individuals and their families.

In our previous clinical trial, we discovered that patients with FRAAs were more likely to benefit from leucovorin treatment. To investigate this further, we conducted another study and found that binding autoantibodies predicted improvements in ASD symptoms.[77] The following graph shows the average change in social behavior for patients based on their binding FRAA titers. For individuals with very high binding titers (3.0 OD), the social awareness subscale on the SRS improved by an average of 16 points, while the social cognition, communication, and motivation subscales on the SRS improved by about 8 points. In some cases, these improvements were sufficient to change the classification of the patient's condition from severe to moderate, moderate to mild, or mild to typically developing, depending upon their initial level.

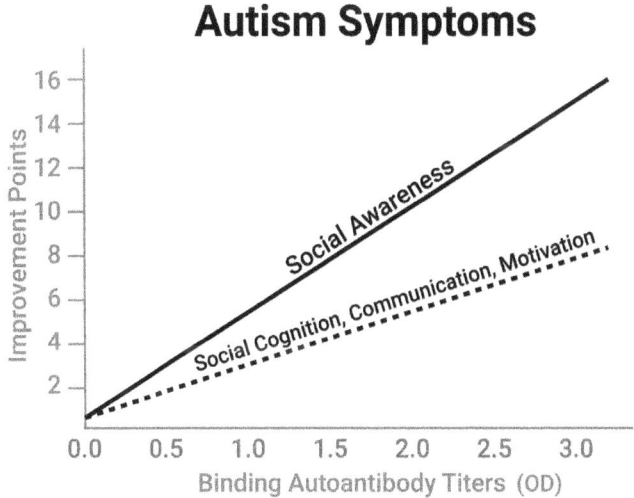

Figure 5.6 Improvement of ASD symptoms based on binding FRAA titers

Chapter 5. - Autism Spectrum Disorder - 77

These promising findings naturally lead to further questions, such as the predictability of other folate biomarkers like blocking FRAA and sFBP. Unfortunately, current studies have not included large enough sample sizes to draw statistically significant conclusions. This underscores the need for larger studies to improve the diagnosis and treatment of CFD.

The research conducted so far provides preliminary but promising evidence that leucovorin can address a range of ASD symptoms. Additionally, the presence of FRAAs and sFBP appears to be predictive of treatment response. The studies indicate that children have primarily shown improvements in verbal communication and social functioning. Given the lack of medical treatments for core ASD symptoms, leucovorin offers hope to families seeking ways to enhance their children's lives.

Evan

Evan's story is one of mysterious symptoms, and no known unifying diagnosis, despite several doctors performing multiple tests to search for answers. The persistence of Evan's parents eventually led them to a CFD diagnosis, and Evan responded well to treatment.

Parents who have watched their children suffer through seizures and other difficult challenges will be able to relate to the urgency and desperation felt by Evan's family. This story provides encouragement for other parents to see what is possible when folate issues are adequately addressed.

PATIENT STORIES

Evan's Story
By Tina C., Evan's Mom

I was 36 years old when I found out I was pregnant with Evan. We were overjoyed at the prospect of having a second child. Our first child, Kyle, had been such an easy baby, and at two years old, he was excited to become a big brother. Because of my age, my obstetrician suggested we pursue high-risk pregnancy care. I welcomed the additional oversight, as it seemed prudent.

My pregnancy with Evan began much easier than with Kyle—no morning sickness, slower weight gain, and far fewer cravings. I thought I had pregnancy figured out until we had the screening test for Down syndrome. The doctor informed us that Evan had a chance of having Down syndrome and recommended that we have an amniocentesis for confirmation. I was frightened and had many unanswered questions but waited patiently through the process. On the day of the amniocentesis, our obstetrician told me that if I were his daughter, he would advise me to abort the baby. Just like that. "There are too many Down syndrome babies in the world. They drain their parents and live too long," he said.

I was shocked, confused, and hurt. We went home from the test exhausted after a full day at the hospital. We lay in bed and cried. Then we prayed together, asking God to guide us in caring for this baby regardless of the challenges he might face. This was my first real disappointment with a doctor responsible for caring for Evan, and it is one I will never forget. We immediately changed doctors and never regretted our decision to do so, nor did we ever regret our decision to have Evan and face any challenge that came our way.

One day, while folding laundry and watching a CNN report on the increasing number of children affected by ASD, I was about six months pregnant with Evan. I remember thinking, "Thank God that's not a problem for us." I already knew Evan had certain challenges because he didn't move as much as my older son. And after all, he might have Down syndrome. We were seeing specialists at a large national children's hospital. They ran tests on his heart, lungs, and kidneys to ensure he was growing and functioning properly. I thought their approach was a bit excessive, but I was relieved when they repeatedly told me that his test results were normal. When I asked why he wasn't moving much, none of our physicians could provide a clear answer. "Some babies don't move much," they would say. I knew in my heart there was a problem. I welcomed the little movement I did feel but worried day and night that something was wrong.

The rest of my pregnancy was stressful. I had to wear a belt around my stomach connected to a device that would detect the baby's movements. My family had many questions that I couldn't answer: Would he be alright? What was wrong? Did he have Down syndrome?

When I finally got a date for induction at 40 weeks of pregnancy, I was relieved that I would finally get to meet my baby. During labor, his heart rate kept decreasing to unsafe levels. The nurses instructed me to change positions, lie on my side, or move from side to side, believing the heart rate changes were positional. Little did I know there would be many other instances of bradycardia for Evan. After seven hours of labor, Evan was born and cried beautifully! As the nurses cleaned him and checked his vitals, they seemed concerned, but when I asked questions, they told me not to worry. I noticed that his breathing was a bit labored, but again, I was told not to worry. The doctor thought it might be due to excess fluid.

I was relieved to see that there were no visible signs of Down syndrome. My baby was healthy, and we were happy. However, overnight, Evan's hearing was tested, and he failed the newborn hearing screening. They repeated the test the next day, and he failed again. I couldn't believe Evan couldn't hear and thought the test must be wrong.

The first few weeks with Evan were challenging. I had breastfed my first son and wanted to do the same for Evan. He struggled to latch on and didn't seem to be getting enough milk. We brought in a lactation nurse, but nothing she suggested made much difference. She recommended supplementing with formula, but Evan still couldn't seem to get milk from the bottle. We repeatedly asked the pediatrician for advice, and he suggested making bigger holes in the bottle nipple so that Evan didn't have to work so hard. This helped get the milk into his mouth, but if it came out too quickly, he would choke and spit up most of what he had taken in.

Evan cried almost constantly in those early days, and I couldn't seem to soothe him. No matter what I did, he seemed uncomfortable.

PATIENT STORIES

I made more calls to the pediatrician but received the same response each time: "Some babies take a little longer to catch on. It's nothing to worry about," he'd say. As the weeks went on, it seemed that Evan's eyes did not track evenly. He was very weak and slept more than I thought was normal. I was consumed by worry for him. I wasn't sleeping and could only focus on whether he was alright.

One day, while grocery shopping with my older son and Evan, a woman in the store remarked on how wonderful it was to have a newborn. When she looked at Evan's face, she gasped and somewhat rudely asked, "What's wrong with him?" I was devastated. Evan's facial features were unusual compared to his older brother's. There were many such interactions that led me to stay home more to protect Evan from the world. In a way, it was also a way to protect myself. My heart broke every time a stranger made comments about Evan's appearance. My heart broke a lot.

At our four-month check-up, the pediatrician told me he didn't think there was anything seriously wrong, but if it would make me feel better, he would refer us to a neurologist. I was relieved that he seemed to be taking my concerns seriously. He acknowledged that no one knows their baby like a mother does and assured me he would help me get some answers.

I immediately scheduled the appointment but was told we would have to wait nine months to be seen! I knew Evan couldn't wait that long, so I pushed with repeated calls and managed to get an appointment with a neurologist in two months. Evan was six months old at our first visit.

The day was packed with appointments. We saw a social worker, a dietitian, a general practitioner, and finally the neurologist. While moving from place to place, we saw many sick children—those with cancer, missing limbs, or cerebral palsy. It was heartbreaking, and I thought I could never return to a place so filled with sadness. But I learned that day that everyone we met was dedicated to caring for children with all kinds of special needs. They were some of the happiest clinicians and staff I had ever encountered. I realized that, as difficult as it was to see other children affected by lifelong illnesses, this was exactly where we needed to be.

Our first visit ended with orders for testing and a commitment to thoroughly evaluate Evan. This was the beginning of what seemed like endless testing for a variety of conditions. My in-laws frequently stayed at our house to watch our older son while we went for our long medical visits. When we returned home, they asked: What did they find? What will they test for next? When will he get better? We had as many questions, too, and very few answers.

In the meantime, Evan was missing every milestone and struggling with swallowing. He wasn't rolling over and seemed to lack strength. He couldn't grasp anything, and I had to feed him slowly to prevent choking. He was still difficult to comfort, but when I held him, I knew he was happy.

We began physical therapy at home to help Evan gain some strength. We saw our therapist three days a week for hour-long sessions. Our therapist told us that Evan had a unique challenge—motivation. He was highly motivated to be propped up against the couch and would stand as long as he could while she supported his hips. Then he would plop down and immediately raise his hands to try again. My older son would model what Evan should do, and during these sessions, their inseparable bond was solidified.

Evan's neurologist suggested occupational therapy since he was unable to grasp objects. Despite his motivation, he was still not progressing as hoped. And there were more tests. It seemed that every test came back negative. It became a dinner-table topic: "What are we testing for next?" my father-in-law would ask. My husband would respond, "It doesn't matter, Dad. It will be negative." We all tried to laugh it off, knowing that eventually, we'd get an answer.

Each hospital visit for testing was exhausting, and it seemed there was no benefit. Evan was uncomfortable in the car and screamed every time they drew blood. His veins were so difficult to access that it almost never happened on the first try, making it harder for him—and for us.

At nine months, we took Evan to a new hearing specialist for another hearing test. This time, the physician suggested surgically implanting tubes in his ears to see if he might be able to hear. We scheduled the surgery, not realizing it would be the first of many for Evan. I remember feeling so nervous and helpless about what he had to go through. After the surgery, I spoke to him as usual, and he responded with laughter! It was the most amazing sound I had ever heard. Evan had never responded to my voice before; I had always wondered if he could hear at all since he had failed every hearing screening. Now I knew he could hear, and I couldn't wait to get home and show Kyle and his brother that he could respond to sound.

Chapter 5. - Autism Spectrum Disorder - 83

The next several months were filled with joy as we conclusively knew that Evan could hear. The missed milestones became less concerning because we believed he would eventually catch up or that we'd find an intervention to help him reach new levels of functionality.

Our next visit was with Evan's neurologist. At 14 months old, we were following up on the latest round of testing. The neurologist admitted he was at a loss. He had tested Evan for everything he could think of, and since all results were negative, he didn't know what else to do. We were still facing many seemingly unconnected medical issues. Evan couldn't swallow easily, which made eating very difficult. He was very weak with low muscle tone, his eyes didn't track evenly, and we were unable to comfort him. He had no speech and couldn't stand without assistance. The neurologist suggested that we take Evan to a large national medical center across the country for further evaluation. He assured us that the medical center was much more extensive than our local one and that we would likely get answers there.

Once again, we went home feeling confused, exhausted, and perhaps this time, a bit hopeful. We discussed whether we could relocate across the country to be near the new medical center and start a new life with our boys, giving Evan a chance to thrive. My husband was at a point where he could take early retirement, and I worked for a company headquartered in the new city. I had traveled there frequently for work and decided I would visit the medical center on my next trip. That night, we decided to move.

In March 2007, during my business trip to the new city, I also looked at houses. We knew it would be impossible to bring the boys with us, as we had never flown with Evan before. I was the scout, tasked with finding our new home. On this trip, I stayed with a coworker and her husband and had scheduled viewings of several houses over three days with a realtor. The prospect of getting answers was incredibly inspiring for us as a family.

While I was at dinner with my coworker, my husband called to tell me that Evan was being rushed to the hospital. He had had a grand mal seizure. I was terrified and went into an immediate panic. Was he okay? How would I get home? I didn't realize that this would be the first of hundreds of seizures that would complicate Evan's life even more.

The next several months were filled with doctor's visits that yielded no answers. Initially, Evan's seizures were diagnosed as being caused by a high fever, yet he had no fever on the day of the seizure or on the days preceding it. As we made our plans to move, we prayed that Evan would be well and free of seizures.

We moved without any problems and immediately started our journey with one of the nation's largest children's hospitals. Initially, we saw several specialists who wanted to re-run every test we had previously done. We were not in favor of this, as we had already put Evan through so much testing and knew the results. After several months, we met with a neurologist who was very impatient with us as a family. Evan struggled to wait patiently during doctor visits, and the process was stressful for all of us. I was relieved when we found a pediatric neurologist and hoped we could reason with her about how stressful it was to have to repeat all the tests we already had.

Unfortunately, during our first visit, she said that Evan had no issues other than me. I was stunned. She went on to say that my stress was causing Evan to appear as if he had medical issues when, in fact, he did not. I didn't know how to respond but went home feeling emptier than ever before. And still without answers.

My husband and I both found employment. My husband worked as a security director coordinating security with the city's police department, and I was an information technology director. One day, I saw a patient story about a little boy who had a similar facial structure to Evan. It was about a patient with CFD and spoke about how much he improved after seeing Dr. Richard Frye, a pediatric neurologist at one of the large hospitals. I knew in my heart that we needed to see Dr. Frye, and many years later, I knew I was right.

When we had our first appointment with Dr. Frye, he reassured me that he could help us and noted that Evan exhibited certain characteristics suggesting he might have CFD. Dr. Frye recommended a lumbar puncture, a test not previously considered by other doctors, to measure the level of folate in Evan's CSF. This test confirmed Dr. Frye's suspicion—Evan had CFD. We began Evan on a course of leucovorin, and within weeks, we noticed a difference!

Before seeing Dr. Frye, Evan was unable to walk and had significant speech delays. He remained difficult to calm and seemed irritated by noises and bright lights. Dr. Frye also diagnosed Evan with ASD and explained that it was common for children with ASD to have both CFD and seizures.

The effects of leucovorin were almost immediate. We observed improvements in Evan's strength and his ability to speak more words.

Chapter 5. - Autism Spectrum Disorder - 85

PATIENT STORIES

Within six months of starting the medication, Evan began to walk independently. Although he still had significant muscle weakness, which caused him to fall after only a few steps, he showed consistent progress.

Of course, Evan has continued to face challenges over the years. Despite therapies that helped manage his folate issues and seizures, he still experienced seizures that were difficult to control. We tried various treatments, including intravenous immunoglobulin, with some success. However, it was not until he had a vagus nerve stimulator (VNS) implanted that we saw significant improvement. The VNS, which stimulates the vagus nerve with regular, mild pulses of electrical energy, ultimately helped reduce his seizures. Fewer seizures allowed us to focus more on learning and skill acquisition without as much disruption. Eventually, the seizures stopped completely, and we were able to reduce some of his seizure medications.

Evan also underwent scoliosis surgery to correct a 72-degree curve in his spine, which eliminated the need for a wheelchair. Although he would frequently tire while walking and sometimes fall, the wheelchair had kept him safe and allowed us to engage in activities outside the house for longer periods.

The growth in Evan's skills and his increased happiness have brought immense comfort to our family. Evan has always approached each day as a new adventure and seeing him seizure-free and relieved from scoliosis pain has made us believe there are no limits to what he can achieve.

Recently, we transitioned him to a new adult program. Evan has embraced this change and is ready for more grown-up activities. As a mother of a non-verbal autistic child, I have had many fears about his inability to be completely independent. However, I've adapted to his new level of independence, which he so desperately wanted and needed. The transition has been challenging for both of us, but I know the time is right, and I am confident he will continue to flourish.

Our breakthrough came with diagnosing CFD and starting leucovorin treatment. This experience confirmed that our efforts to find answers and improve Evan's life were worthwhile.

PATIENT STORIES

Kai

Many people do not know that it is possible for a child to lose their ASD diagnosis. Kai's story is a remarkable example of a child who met the criteria for severe ASD, only to be "undiagnosed" years later after seeking appropriate treatment for CFD.

Like many children with CFD, development can stall or move backwards, leading to NDR. Kai's mother shares an encouraging story about Kai's recovery.

Kai's Story
By Kai's Mom

When I was 39 weeks pregnant, my OB/GYN noted that my amniotic fluid was low but not yet alarming. Out of concern, we attempted to induce labor, but it was unsuccessful. At 40 weeks and 4 days, we tried inducing again, and Kai was born! I had a vaginal delivery, but my OB/GYN had to use forceps to assist with Kai's delivery. This intervention resulted in an injury to Kai's neck, which developed into torticollis (tightness of the neck muscles) and caused plagiocephaly (flattening of the head on one side). Kai was also jaundiced but did not require treatment.

Kai was born with significant lip and tongue ties, which made breastfeeding difficult. We had to supplement with formula from birth, and I pumped for six months to provide him with breast milk. At three months old, Kai began experiencing severe diarrhea.

By seven months, he was congested, had a cough, and developed a bilateral ear infection, for which he was prescribed amoxicillin. Despite this, his bowel movements remained problematic, and at nine months, his doctor suggested it was likely viral and advised waiting for it to resolve on its own.

At nearly ten months old, Kai developed a fever, tested positive for influenza B, and also contracted hand, foot, and mouth disease. He was prescribed Tamiflu. Unfortunately, Kai's diarrhea persisted well past his first birthday, and he began experiencing mucus in his stools, frequent bloating after eating, and increased gas. He also developed pimples on his buttocks and eczema on his cheeks and thighs.

Despite these health issues, Kai was a good eater and sleeper from the age of three months and remained a generally happy and easygoing baby. He enjoyed interacting with people and his dog and met all his developmental milestones up until 18 months. At that age, he was saying about eight words, such as "mama," "dada," and "uh oh," but his speech development then seemed to plateau.

We also observed that he stopped using some of the words he had previously said and became increasingly distant, with reduced eye contact. His sleep patterns changed; he took much longer to fall asleep and occasionally woke during the night, which was unusual for him. Additionally, his balance deteriorated, leading to frequent stumbling, and he became constipated, sometimes going days without a bowel movement.

At 21 months, Kai experienced two alarming episodes of unresponsiveness, followed by severe exhaustion within just two days. We were referred to a neurologist, who recommended a series of tests, including a brain MRI, prolonged EEG, genetic testing, and bloodwork. Despite all the results coming back normal, I couldn't shake the feeling that something was seriously wrong. It was heartbreaking to watch Kai, once a perfectly happy and healthy child, decline so rapidly.

I expressed my concerns to Kai's pediatrician about his speech regression and reduced eye contact. The pediatrician suggested we seek an evaluation through our local early intervention agency. After assessing Kai, the agency identified developmental delays and raised concerns about his limited speech, minimal interactions, and reduced eye contact. However, they felt it was too early to provide a definitive diagnosis.

Kai began occupational, speech, and play therapy soon after. Determined to explore every possible avenue, I arranged consultations with various specialists, including an ENT, a developmental pediatrician, a craniofacial specialist, an ophthalmologist, and a gastroenterologist. The developmental pediatrician, addressing our concerns about ASD, diagnosed Kai with ASD Level 3 and recommended therapy as the primary course of treatment.

The diagnosis didn't sit well with me—I felt like something was missing. Not long after, Kai began to twitch throughout the day, tilting his head toward his shoulder repeatedly. Desperate to help him, I turned to his diet, as it was one thing I could control. After researching, I decided to remove dairy entirely from his meals. Remarkably, the twitching stopped the very next day.

Determined to dig deeper, I found a functional medicine doctor in my area, someone trained to look at the whole body and its functions. During our initial appointment, she suspected CFD based on Kai's history and behavior. She prescribed 30 mg of leucovorin daily when Kai was 2 years and 1 month old. We also tested for FRAAs, which revealed that Kai's titers were extremely high—his blocking FRAA measured 8.02 pmol blocked per ml, and his binding FRAA was 0.684 OD units.

Chapter 5. - Autism Spectrum Disorder - 89

PATIENT STORIES

Within just one month of starting leucovorin, we saw significant improvements. Kai began using sign language, saying more words, pointing, and engaging more meaningfully with others. When he was 2 years and 9 months old, we increased the leucovorin dosage to 90 mg daily, and his progress continued across all areas. Eventually, the same developmental pediatrician who initially diagnosed Kai with ASD re-evaluated him. After a thorough assessment, the team of professionals concluded that Kai no longer met the criteria for an ASD diagnosis.

Kai is now five years old, fully conversational, and ready to start 1st grade!

Had we not discovered Kai's CFD when we did, he wouldn't be where he is today. We were overwhelmed with confusion and fear when he started to decline, unsure of what was happening. Now, you would never guess what our reality once was. Kai continues to follow a gluten- and dairy-free diet, and he will always be under the care of a functional medicine doctor.

Recently, we repeated the FRAA test after two years, and Kai tested negative! Throughout this journey, we consulted many professionals in search of answers, yet none suggested additional testing to explore what might be missing. I truly believe that our commitment to periodic lab work, the right supplementation, and a tailored diet led us to the optimal treatment. Today, Kai is thriving!

Mason

Mason's story is not unusual. He initially showed signs of severe language delay, but it wasn't until unmistakable symptoms emerged that his parents felt compelled to pursue an ASD diagnosis on their own.

Determined to explore every possible treatment, Mason's parents enrolled him in our leucovorin trial. Mason responded remarkably well to the treatment, making significant progress, and has since continued leucovorin therapy.

PATIENT STORIES

Mason's Story
By Caroline C., Mason's Mom

We had a challenging journey to conceive, eventually seeking help from a fertility specialist. The doctor prescribed levothyroxine to support my thyroid function and Clomiphene for my husband due to his low sperm count. We were fortunate that intrauterine insemination (IUI) was successful on our first attempt—something that's not very common.

The pregnancy went smoothly, and I continued working right up until delivery. At 33 weeks, however, I was in a car accident and was taken to the hospital to check on the baby. I felt fine, but, unbeknownst to me, I was having contractions. To stop them, the doctors gave me Terbutaline, though I was unaware at the time of its black box warning and its association with autism spectrum disorder (ASD).

The delivery itself was wonderful: just six hours of labor and twenty minutes of pushing, and our perfect baby boy was born. We named him Mason. There were no complications, and he was a great eater and sleeper. I loved breastfeeding and continued until his first birthday, exclusively giving him breastmilk for the first four months of his life.

Mason reached all his milestones in his first year and was a happy, easygoing baby. It wasn't until after his first birthday that we began to notice he wasn't speaking yet, unlike some other babies his age who were beginning to talk. At 18 months, he still hadn't spoken, so we filled out the autism screener at our pediatrician's office.

Despite his lack of speech, our pediatrician wasn't concerned. Yet, we started to notice other signs: hand-flapping and spinning when he was excited, and he would dash away without looking back when we called his name. Still, we waited, hoping his speech would develop. Finally, at two and a half, we decided to have him evaluated. Mason was diagnosed with ASD Level 2.

A few days after the diagnosis, a friend notified us about a clinical trial looking at the effects of leucovorin in children with ASD. We had read an online story about the remarkable progress that a young girl had made taking this medication, so we were eager to participate.

After some testing and questionnaires, we were sent home with our bottle of hope. The trial was a double-blind placebo study, so we didn't know if we'd receive leucovorin in the first phase, but within days we felt sure we had the real thing. One night at dinner, while feeding snacks to his little brother, Mason looked directly into my eyes and said, "more." I was stunned. Motivated by the snack sharing, he had spoken a word!

Mason's language and awareness continued to improve, and a blood test revealed that he was FRAT positive—meaning he had a folate receptor autoantibody that prevented his body from properly transporting folate to his brain and into cerebrospinal fluid. This led to the suspicion of Cerebral Folate Deficiency (CFD), along with mitochondrial dysfunction, which he also showed signs of in his lab work.

We had the rest of the family FRAT tested, I learned that I carried one type of autoantibody, while everyone else tested negative. I often wish I could go back in time and have been tested during pregnancy. If I had taken leucovorin then, Mason might have developed neurotypically.

As time went on, Mason continued to make strides. As the clinical trial was ending, we were anxious to continue his leucovorin treatment. I remember trying to squeeze every last drop from the bottle. Determined to keep Mason on this path, after the clinical trial, we became patients of Dr. Frye at Rossignol Medical Center so Mason could continue receiving treatment.

Reflecting on this journey, I realize how fortunate we were to have started leucovorin at such a young age, knowing it's something he'll likely need for the rest of his life. Dr. Frye once told me, "It's food, mortgage, and leucovorin."

Today, we are hopeful that by the time he reaches kindergarten, he will be ready for a mainstream educational environment, as we've heard is possible for other children on leucovorin. Everyday life is much easier now that our son can verbally communicate his needs. While his speech still has a way to go, we have come so far from that very first word.

The Overlap between Cerebral Folate Deficiency and Autism Spectrum Disorder

These three stories highlight the wide variation in symptoms and characteristics among children with ASD and CFD. While Evan exhibited developmental issues very early, Kai experienced a marked neurodevelopmental regression, and Mason's symptoms emerged in toddlerhood. These cases underscore both the challenges parents face in uncovering the root causes of their children's symptoms and their determination to pursue every possible avenue to find effective support.

The stories also illustrate the diverse recovery trajectories among children with ASD. Evan made significant progress but continued to face substantial cognitive challenges, requiring ongoing applied behavior analysis and other therapies. Mason showed steady, progressive improvement, with promising expectations for continued gains. Kai appears to have achieved an optimal recovery. The reason behind Kai's normalization of FRAA levels remains unclear, though an early shift to a milk-free diet may have contributed, as milk is known to elevate FRAA titers, while a milk-free diet can substantially reduce them.[78] (See Chapter 16 for more about the relationship between milk and CFD).

Despite the differences in their journeys, all three children experienced meaningful improvements, demonstrating how leucovorin can be a transformative treatment for some patients and their families.

A Physician's Perspective

After completing my Child Neurology residency, I pursued two fellowships—one in Behavioral Neurology and Learning Disabilities and another in Psychology. At that time, ASD was just starting to gain wider recognition in the medical community. Because of my specialized training, many doctors and staff assumed I had expertise in ASD. When a family came to the neurology department seeking care for their child with ASD, schedulers would often assign the patient to me. Parents would arrive at my clinic saying, "My child was just diagnosed with autism, but we were told no one knows what causes it or how to treat it." They often added, "Since it likely involves the brain, we thought you might be able to help." I saw this as a meaningful challenge and began immersing myself in the complexities of ASD.

One of my first roles after fellowship was as an assistant professor at the University of Texas Health Science Center at Houston (UTHealth Houston). As my child neurology colleagues learned of my growing expertise in ASD, they began referring all their ASD patients to my clinic. Before long, children with ASD made up the majority of my caseload, leading me to formally name my clinic "The Medically-Based Autism Clinic."

Many of my ASD patients were referred because they hadn't responded to standard treatments. The child neurologists at my center were proactive, committed to comprehensive care and thorough evaluations. As a result, many children underwent an extensive work-up, including a lumbar puncture (spinal tap). In doing so, I began noticing neurochemical abnormalities in these patients, particularly low levels of tetrahydrobiopterin, a crucial cofactor for neurotransmitter production.

Soon, I also identified that many children with ASD had borderline low or below-normal concentrations of 5-MTHF in their cerebrospinal fluid (CSF). I found that high-dose folinic acid (leucovorin) had shown promise as a treatment in the literature, especially given folate's role in producing tetrahydrobiopterin. This connection piqued my interest, especially as I had published a case report on folinic acid-responsive seizures during residency.[79] Shortly thereafter, a colleague presented a case at Grand Rounds about a patient with CFD caused by FRAAs, and it became clear that I needed to begin testing my patients for these antibodies.

I reached out to Dr. Edward Quadros at SUNY Downstate, who developed the FRAA test, to explore collaboration. I also connected with Dr. Daniel Rossignol from the Rossignol Medical Center, with whom I had been working to deepen our understanding of ASD. Both of our clinics had established research protocols to evaluate which treatments were most effective for our patients. Discovering the link between ASD, CFD, and FRAAs led us to collaborate closely on aligning our treatment strategies.

Our findings were remarkable—many children with FRAAs showed significant improvement with leucovorin treatment. After some time, we decided to review these observations systematically to quantify the results. To achieve this, we developed the Parent-Rated Autism Symptomatic Change Scale (see Chapter 18), a 12-item questionnaire that asked parents to rate changes in their child's symptoms since the last appointment using a 7-point Likert scale, ranging from "much better" to "much worse." This tool was administered at each visit, allowing us to track progress in a measurable way.

7-Point Likert Scale

A Likert scale is a psychometric tool used to measure attitudes, opinions, or perceptions. It typically presents a statement followed by a range of responses that span from one end of the spectrum to the other. In our studies, we measure changes in symptoms, with one end of the scale representing improvement in symptoms and the other representing worsening. The scale typically has an odd number of response options (often seven), allowing for a neutral midpoint and ensuring an equal number of responses on each side of neutral to prevent bias in the degree of judgment for either extreme. Parents select the response that best reflects their observations, providing valuable insight into symptom progression.

1	2	3	4	5	6	7
Much Worse	Worse	Mildly Worse	No Change	Mildly Better	Better	Much Better

Focusing on the first nine symptoms in the scale, we analyzed changes following the initiation of leucovorin treatment. To create a control group, we looked at FRAA-positive patients who had not started leucovorin or made any other changes since their last visit. These were typically patients returning to receive FRAA test results, unaware of whether they tested positive or negative. (See 2-page spread on next page summarizing the results).

The findings confirmed what we had observed in the clinic. Many children with ASD who tested positive for FRAAs and were treated with leucovorin showed notable improvements.[69] Specifically, two-thirds of the patients experienced gains in expressive and receptive language, as well as verbal communication (see Figures 5.7 and 5.8). While improvements were observed across other areas, hyperactivity worsened in some cases, though this was usually transient. Adverse effects were minimal and infrequent.

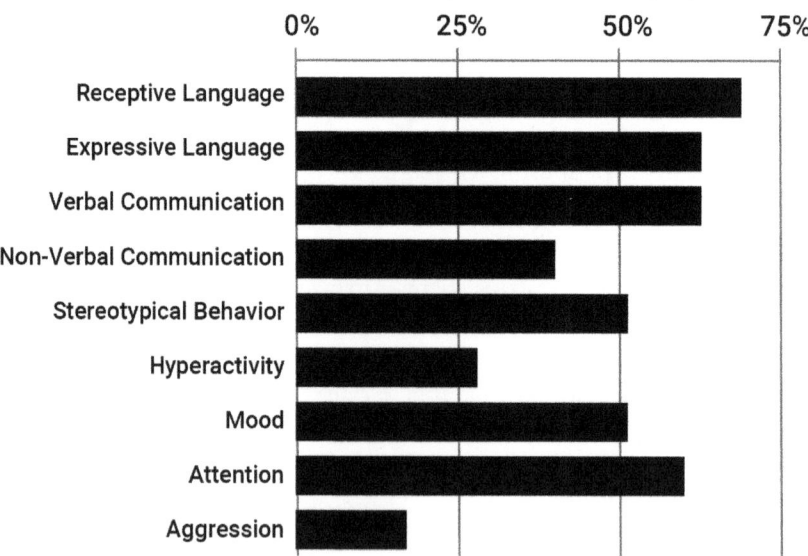

Figure 5.7 Percent of patients with improvement in symptoms with leucovorin

In 2011, I accepted a position at Arkansas Children's Hospital to lead their ASD program. One of my first initiatives in this role was to launch the first double-blind placebo-controlled trial of leucovorin in children with ASD. Based on the previous open-label trial, where most children showed improvements in language, we hypothesized that language would be the primary symptom to improve in the controlled trial.

Language was an ideal focus because there are established tools that can qualitatively measure it using trained examiners. However, we encountered a challenge with the existing tools for measuring language in a clinical trial setting. Many of the children had language skills far below what would be expected for their age. Since most language assessment instruments are age-based, we needed to develop a method for selecting the right tool to accurately measure language based on the child's current abilities rather than their age. Fortunately, I was able to assemble a top-tier team, solve these issues, and successfully move the study forward.

The double-blind placebo-controlled study demonstrated that leucovorin improved verbal communication to a much greater extent than the placebo (See Figure 5.8). We also found that it improved irritability, social withdrawal, stereotypy, hyperactivity and inappropriate speech.[80]

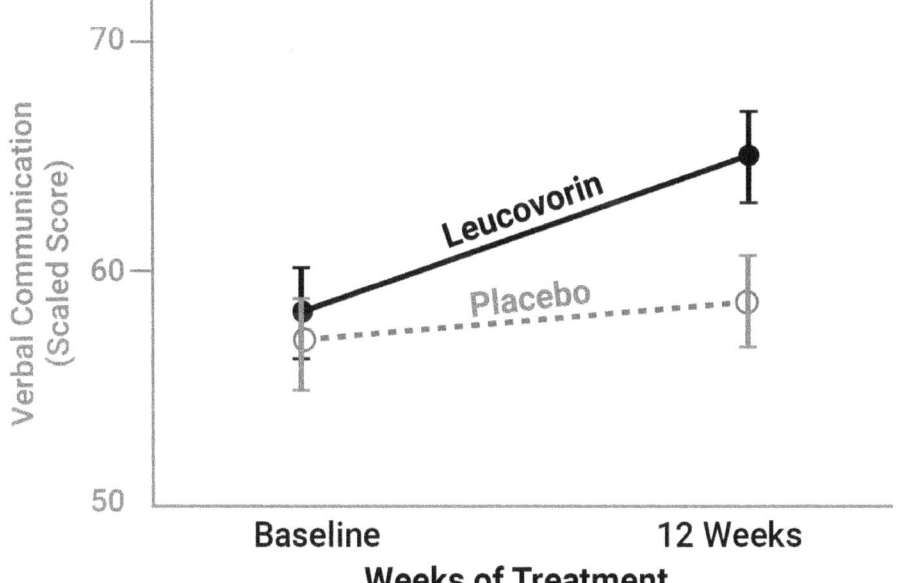

Figure 5.8 Outcome of language assessment for children on leucovorin versus placebo during our double-blind controlled study

Although hyperactivity generally improved, we wanted to investigate whether a subset of individuals experienced increased hyperactivity when given leucovorin. Throughout the study, we tracked specific potential adverse effects every three weeks. While we didn't ask specifically about hyperactivity, we did inquire about agitation and excitement (See Figure 5.9).

Chapter 5. - Autism Spectrum Disorder - 97

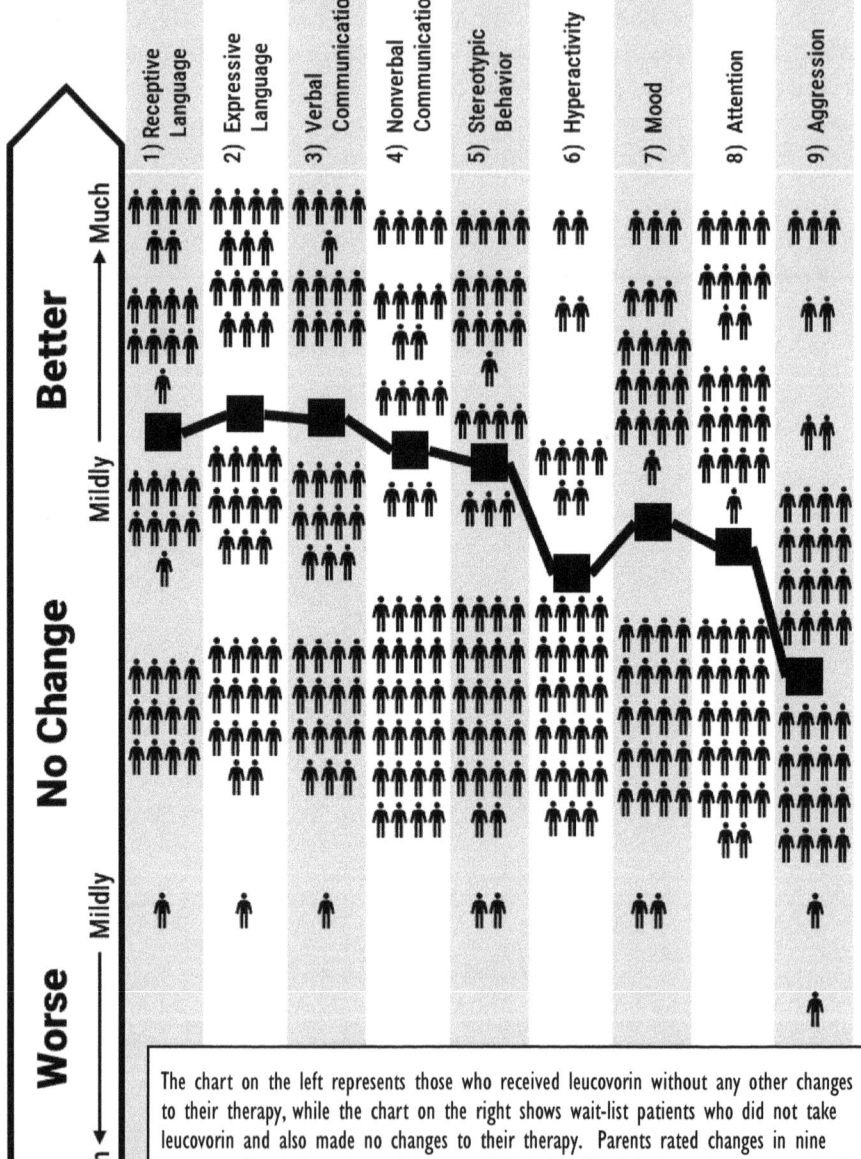

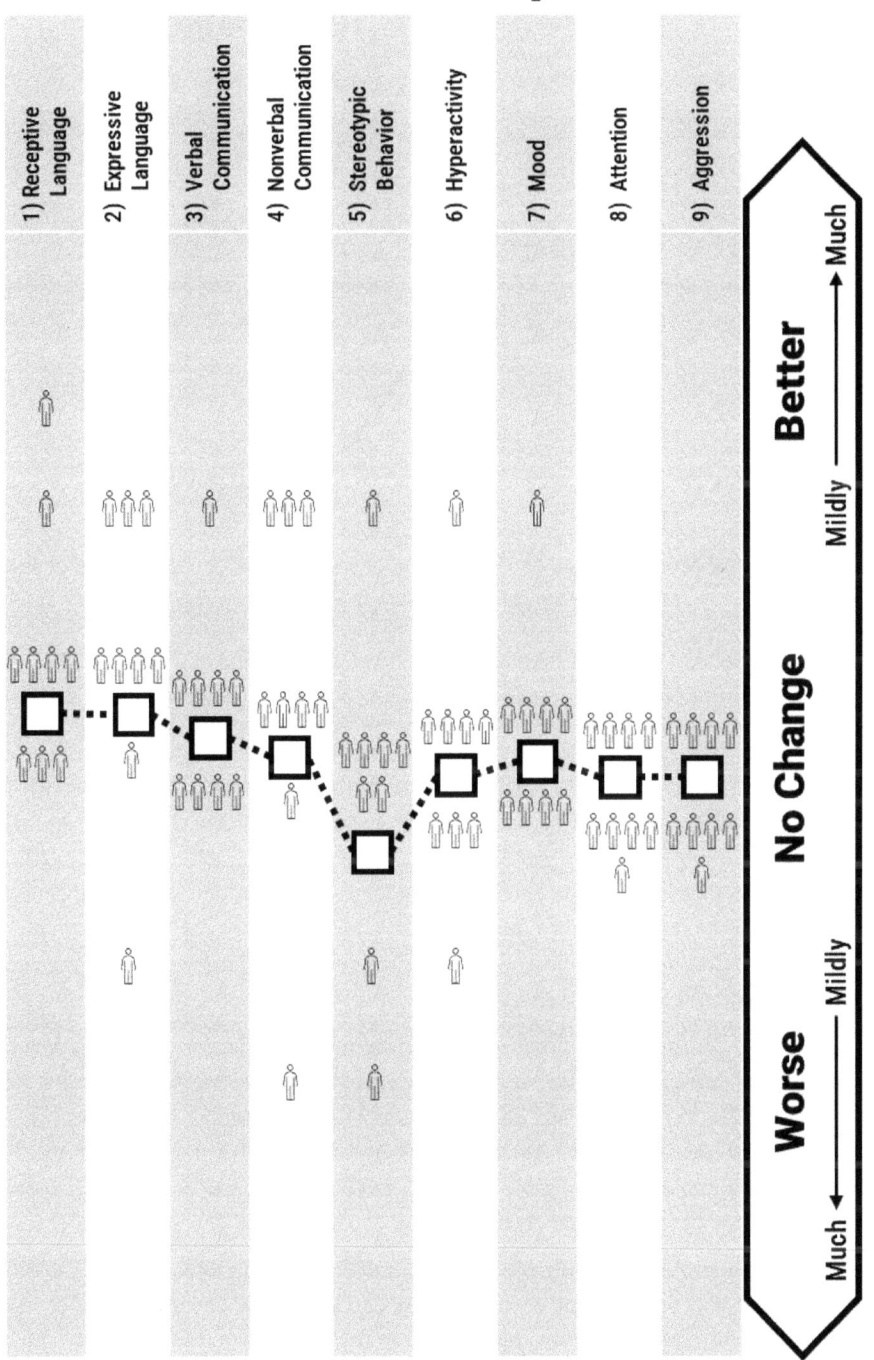

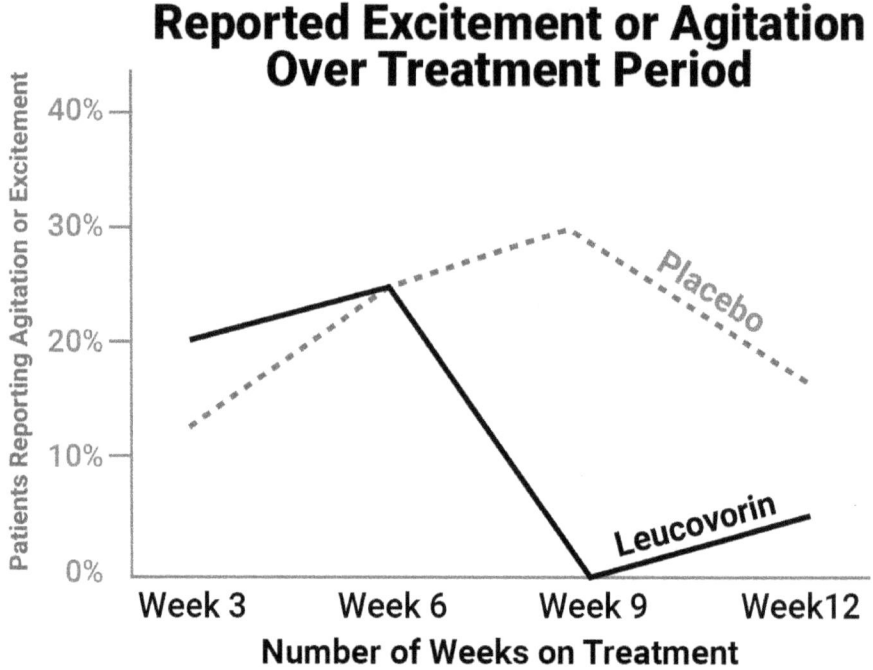

Figure 5.9 Excitement or agitation over treatment period compared to placebo

When we analyzed how many patients reported these symptoms over the 12-week period, the numbers were similar between the leucovorin and placebo groups until around week nine. At that point, the number of families reporting agitation or excitement dropped to zero for those taking leucovorin, whereas about 20% of children on the placebo continued to exhibit these symptoms.[81] This suggests that leucovorin may have a calming effect, though the benefit appears to be delayed up to two months after starting treatment. In practice, when this hyperactivity occurs, it seems to resolve within 3-4 weeks.

The results of our first controlled trial on leucovorin were promising, but further validation was needed. To build on these findings, we have launched several multicenter trials to confirm our earlier results and explore the efficacy of leucovorin in younger children with ASD, specifically those under five years of age. As Mason's mother explained, he was one of the children included in these studies who showed positive effects from the treatment.

We recently published findings on the soluble folate binding protein (sFBP), a biomarker that was known but whose role in CFD or ASD was unclear. Our study suggests that children with this biomarker may respond to leucovorin, though some may require higher doses, and the response may take months or even years.[82]

While this is an important discovery, none of the patients in the study had a lumbar puncture, so it's uncertain if they truly have CFD. Additionally, the current test only detects the presence of sFBP, so further development is needed to better understand this biomarker and its link to folate metabolism.

Another ongoing area of research is the investigation of a special form of leucovorin called levo-leucovorin (l-leucovorin). As explained in Chapter 3, many drugs exist in two mirror-image forms (levo- and dextro-). It is believed that the dextro form may be inactive and cause adverse effects, while the L-form produces the desired therapeutic effect. Regular leucovorin contains both forms, whereas levo-leucovorin contains only the active form of the drug, potentially allowing for lower doses and fewer side effects. More research is needed to fully investigate the use of l-leucovorin for patients with ASD.

In my clinic, I screen all children with ASD and other neurodevelopmental disorders for the FRAAs as well as the sFBP. A positive test suggests that a trial of leucovorin, slowly increased to the standard dose of 2mg/kg/day (max 50mg) in two divided doses, is an option for initial treatment. Also, it is standard to start on a milk-free diet since milk is known to increase the autoantibody titer[83] (See Chapters 16 and 17).

Some patients wish to try leucovorin before performing the FRAA test. I do not recommend this because sometimes children, especially adolescents, may not respond to the initial dose and it might need to be increased. If the FRAA status is not known then it is difficult to increase the dose without confidently knowing that the child is a candidate for the therapy.

Sometimes there is a lackluster response to leucovorin at the standard dose and a higher dose may be necessary. This is often commonly needed in adolescents, most likely because of their size. In such cases, I slowly increase the dose to determine if there is a response. I may do this several times to find the optimal dose. This also might very well be that the leucovorin is not being absorbed well if there are significant gastrointestinal problems, which are common in children with ASD.

Often other supplements are needed to complement leucovorin. Our recent study suggested that L-carnitine, omega 3 fatty acids and subcutaneously delivered methyl-B12 might provide benefits when given with leucovorin[84] (See Chapter 17). Many times mitochondrial targeted treatments, which include L-carnitine, can provide some mitochondrial support. Cobalamin (B12) connects the folate cycle to the methylation cycle, so addition of a B12 supplement can be beneficial. Animal studies have also demonstrated that Vitamin D[85] and PQQ[86,87] up regulate the RFC, which is the secondary pathway for folate to get into the brain when the FRα is blocked.

Although uncommon, some children may experience side effects after starting leucovorin. The most frequently reported are insomnia, hyperactivity, and irritability. It's important to recognize that not all leucovorin formulations are the same—many contain lactose and other additives. Since many children with ASD (and people in general) are lactose intolerant, these formulations can cause irritability. Additionally, commercial leucovorin brands often include other additives, which can also contribute to irritability. In such cases, a compounded version without additives is often needed to minimize side effects.

Transient hyperactivity is another potential side effect. If this becomes an issue, the leucovorin dose can be increased more gradually to help manage it. Insomnia, though not specific to leucovorin, is sometimes linked to B vitamins, which can increase energy levels in some individuals. To address this, I typically advise parents to administer the second dose earlier in the day, usually in the afternoon, which often resolves the insomnia.

Overall, both my experience and that of other physicians suggest that abnormalities in folate metabolism and the presence of FRAAs are commonly found in children with ASD. Many of these children respond positively to leucovorin, offering a promising treatment option for those with limited alternatives. When combined with standard therapies, leucovorin can play a significant role in helping children achieve optimal outcomes.

CHAPTER 6.
Down Syndrome

Background

Most people have 46 chromosomes in their cells, arranged in 22 matching pairs, plus two sex chromosomes that determine biological sex at birth. Interestingly, many of us carry small extra segments (duplications) or missing segments (deletions) of chromosomes. These changes, known as copy number variations (CNVs), often go unnoticed because they typically occur in parts of the genome with no known function. While most CNVs are harmless, the presence of an entire extra chromosome or the loss of a full chromosome can lead to significant developmental or functional issues in the body. Unfortunately, many such cases are not compatible with life, resulting in miscarriages. However, some babies with chromosomal abnormalities are born with unique genetic changes, often referred to as genetic syndromes.

One example of a genetic syndrome caused by an extra chromosome is Down syndrome, also known as Trisomy 21, where there is an extra copy of chromosome 21. This is the smallest human chromosome, which may be why Down syndrome is one of the most common chromosomal abnormalities, occurring in about 1 in 700 live births. It is named after John Langdon Down, the British physician who first described it in 1866.

The exact cause of Down syndrome is unknown, but there are certain risk factors, such as advanced maternal age. While most children with Down syndrome are born to women under the age of 35 (since younger women have more babies), the risk increases for women of advanced material age (35 and older). Prenatal screening for Down syndrome is now standard practice, but not all cases are detected before birth. Even when diagnosed prenatally, many parents choose to continue the pregnancy.

Features of Down Syndrome

Facial Features	•Slightly rounded face •Upward slanting eyes •Small nose and ears •Flat facial profile •Protruding tongue
Body	•Short stature •Low muscle tone
Hands and Feet	•A single crease across the palm •Short fingers •Wide space between the big toe and second toe
Development	Developmental delays in motor and language skills typically start at birth, but with appropriate support and education, new skills can be acquired.
Regression	It has recently been recognized that some children may lose skills in late childhood or adolescence - a phenomenon termed Down Syndrome Regression Disorder (DSRD). In late adolescence or early adulthood, some become non-responsive and develop catatonia. In addition, individuals with Down Syndrome can develop dementia early in adulthood.
Cognitive	Individuals with Down syndrome often have intellectual disabilities, which can range from mild to moderate.
Language	Speech and language development is often delayed and many have difficulty with articulation. Some can communicate effectively using sign language.
Social Development	Individuals with Down syndrome are typically very social and love to connect with others. They are often warm and friendly.
Overall Health	Individuals with Down syndrome can have certain medical conditions, such as: •Congenital heart defects •Cancers like leukemia •Hypothyroidism •Sleep apnea •Hearing and vision problems •Gastrointestinal disorders

One lesser-understood aspect of Down syndrome is the wide variation in intellectual and developmental abilities among individuals. Some have only mild intellectual disabilities and achieve a range of skills and accomplishments, while others face significant cognitive challenges. Down syndrome is marked by a combination of physical, intellectual, and developmental differences, as well as distinct physical characteristics.

Currently there is not any specific medical treatment for Down syndrome itself. However, individuals with Down syndrome often benefit from supportive care, including standard medical treatments for any health issues, and therapies to assist with developmental challenges. That being said, treatments targeting some of the biological abnormalities associated with Down syndrome can significantly improve the quality of life for both the individual and their family.

The Scientific Evidence

People with Down syndrome and children with CFD have some overlapping symptoms. This may cause one to wonder if individuals with Down syndrome have issues with their folate metabolism. A limited number of studies have explored this possibility.

In 2001, Dr Jill James and her colleagues studied folate-related one-carbon metabolism and the glutathione redox pathways in cell cultures from children with Down syndrome. They compared the metabolic activity of 42 children with Down syndrome to that of their 36 typically developing siblings.[88] Dr. James identified multiple abnormalities in the methylation pathway, which regulates gene expression, and in the glutathione redox pathway, critical for detoxifying cells and managing physiological stress.

She hypothesized that these disruptions were linked to the superoxide dismutase gene, located on chromosome 21, which plays a key role in controlling cellular stress. Interestingly, the chromosomes in the Down syndrome cell cultures were hypermethylated, a state that silences genes.

This suggested that these metabolic abnormalities might be preventing many genes from being activated. Most notably, Dr. James found that adding 100 μM of leucovorin, along with other nutrients important to the methylation pathway, improved these metabolic abnormalities in the cell cultures.

The first clinical trial using leucovorin in children with Down syndrome was conducted at University College London.[89] Researchers studied 156 infants under 7 months of age with Down syndrome, treating them with either antioxidants, leucovorin (100 mcg), or a combination of both, and compared these groups to infants receiving a placebo.

Eighteen months after starting the treatment, infants in the treatment groups showed a slight improvement in development compared to the placebo group. However, this 2-point gain in developmental scores was not considered clinically meaningful, as a 6-point improvement was required to be deemed the effect of the treatment clinically meaningful.

Additionally, measures of physiological stress and glutathione production showed no significant differences, suggesting that the treatment did not improve metabolism as expected. This outcome indicates that the dosage or treatment regimen may not have been high enough to produce a measurable metabolic effect.

In the second clinical trial using leucovorin in children with Down syndrome, conducted at the Institut Jerome Lejeune in Paris, researchers treated 113 patients aged 3 to 30 months with 1 mg/kg of leucovorin for 12 months.[90] When analyzing data from the 87 patients who were assessed by the same examiner at both the beginning and end of the trial, they found a significant improvement in development among those receiving leucovorin compared to the placebo group. Notably, patients who were also taking medication for hypothyroidism showed an even stronger effect.

When comparing this trial to the first, some key differences stand out. First, the leucovorin dosage in this study was significantly higher—approximately 150 times greater than in the previous trial. Second, the results suggested a possible interaction between leucovorin and hypothyroidism treatment, which may have contributed to the enhanced effects observed in those patients.

Thus, to confirm their compelling data, the researchers at the Institut Jerome Lejeune designed a trial to replicate and expand their treatment protocol.[91] This was called the Assessment of Systematic Treatment With Folinic Acid and Thyroid Hormone on Psychomotor Development of Down Syndrome Young Children.

In this trial, 175 patients were initially enrolled and received either leucovorin (1 mg/kg), thyroid hormone, both, or a placebo. However, participants with pre-existing hypothyroidism or hyperthyroidism were removed from the study after starting treatment. Overall, the treatment groups showed only marginal and statistically non-significant improvements compared to the placebo group.

Those receiving leucovorin scored approximately half a point higher, and those on thyroid medication scored about one point higher than the placebo group. These results suggest that any potential gains from the treatments in this study were likely not clinically significant.

Brooklyn

Brooklyn's story is a remarkable example of serendipitous discovery. While many medical journeys begin with a diagnosis leading to treatment, hers began with a cancer treatment that worked so unexpectedly well, it sparked curiosity about an underlying condition.

Her mother's keen observations and questions about the "mysterious red liquid" in her IV led to further investigation by the medical and scientific team. This inquiry ultimately launched groundbreaking research. The knowledge gained from Brooklyn's case and the research conducted in Little Rock, Arkansas, has since benefited countless families.

PATIENT STORIES

PATIENT STORIES

Brooklyn's Story
By Dana F., Brooklyn's Mom

When I became pregnant with my daughter Brooklyn at 22 years old, I was working for a pediatrician in Bryant, Arkansas. It was my first pregnancy, and all signs pointed to us having a healthy, typical baby. My tests were normal, the pregnancy was uneventful, and being young, I was considered low risk for complications.

While my husband Brian and I had not yet learned the sex of our baby, I had a vivid dream during the pregnancy that predicted that I was having a girl. In the dream I was at my Mimi's house and there were two ornamental angels hanging from the ceiling, one had the face of what we presume Jesus resemble and had a glowing pink light coming from His hands as He spoke to me and said, "Dana, you're going to have a little girl and she is going to be very special."

Working in pediatrics, I was familiar with children with special needs and knew what happens when a child is born with complications – my boss would leave early and go to the hospital to examine the newborn who had the unexpected issues. This knowledge offered me little comfort when, on the day that I delivered Brooklyn, I learned my boss was already at the hospital when usually he was still seeing patients at clinic. I immediately knew something was wrong – he was there to assess my baby. My husband and I were told our daughter most likely had Down syndrome.

The dream I had during my pregnancy became a source of comfort during this uncertain time. Though the news was overwhelming, my trust in God prepared me for the journey ahead. We took things one day at a time, and fortunately, Brooklyn was born healthy, weighing 5 pounds, 15 ounces, with a beautiful head of dark hair like her father.

Brooklyn was a happy baby and developed well, with few medical concerns other than severe constipation. The doctors recommended Miralax, but it wasn't until many years later that I learned about its possible neurotoxicity and stopped giving it to her. From then on I used natural remedies such as Magnesium, and Cascara Sagrada.

Like many children with Down syndrome, Brooklyn attended

physical, occupational, and speech therapy to help her reach developmental milestones. Her constipation issues turned into explosive diarrhea following her 15-month shots. I vividly recall a trip to Pittsburgh where on the ride back home to Arkansas she soiled 16 diapers. It was so severe it warranted us to stop at a Nashville ER for help because she was so dehydrated. During this time, she also lost her language skills. The diarrhea continued for a full year.

Though she was not speaking, after her GI problems settled down, she was doing very well. Brooklyn became a big sister at age 4 years when we had our second daughter, Blakeley. A couple of years later, I was pregnant again with our third daughter, Brennan.

Brooklyn was about to turn six years of age when her health took a sudden turn for the worse. She began showing signs of illness, including a large unexplained bruise on her back. Assuming she had fallen at school, I spoke with her teacher, but there was no explanation. I took Brooklyn to the pediatrician, who ordered blood tests. The results were devastating—Brooklyn's bloodwork indicated she had cancer. While the type wasn't yet clear, the doctor was certain it was leukemia.

That time was a whirlwind. Brooklyn was admitted to the hospital, where we learned her kidneys were already failing. By 10 PM that night she had a port placed for chemotherapy and underwent a bone marrow aspiration and genetic workup to determine the type of leukemia and the best treatment. Just days before she had been looking forward to her birthday celebration, and then suddenly, she was fighting for her life.

The genetic tests confirmed Brooklyn had Acute Lymphoblastic Leukemia (ALL), the most treatable form of leukemia, especially in girls. She started treatment immediately but battled neutropenia (low immune cells) throughout three years of treatment, which prolonged her recovery.

The chemotherapy drug methotrexate proved toxic for Brooklyn, even at a reduced dosage compared to the standard protocol for children without Down syndrome. She lost her hair three times and suffered from methotrexate toxicity, which caused the drug to leak through her skin, resulting in painful, pox-like pustules both internally and externally.

We referred to her three-day hospital treatments as "psycho chemo" because they included high-dose steroids that made her ravenously hungry. However, a side effect of Vincristine paralyzed various nerve functions, including those needed for her colon to function properly, creating additional complications.

Over the next three years, Brooklyn spent a total of 97 days in the hospital. It was an incredibly challenging period for our family. I was six months pregnant when we initially received her cancer diagnosis. I gave birth to our third baby girl and left the maternity ward within hours to be back by Brooklyn's side.

While we had a supportive family that helped us as much as possible in caring for our children on clinic days or during hospital stays, I was determined to have our family together even if it meant all of us spending the night at the hospital. The stress of being separated or having to choose whether to stay with Brooklyn at the hospital or stay home with our two-year-old and newborn was too much and was avoided as often as possible.

It was during one of Brooklyn's difficult chemotherapy periods that I noticed something remarkable. After receiving a red substance through her IV, Brooklyn, who had been very ill from a treatment, sat up in bed within 30 minutes then signed and said, "eat!" Not only could she verbally express her hunger, but she also felt well enough to eat, avoiding the need for IV nutrition.

Each time Brooklyn had this "red substance," she perked up. The effect was so striking that I started asking the nurses about it and learned it was a mixture of B vitamins, including methyl-B12 and leucovorin. This combination not only helped her recover from the chemotherapy but also improved her speech and cognitive skills and I began inquiring if leucovorin was something she could take long term after she was finished with her chemotherapy.

I wasn't the only one to notice. At Arkansas Children's Hospital, metabolic researchers Dr. Jill James and John Slattery, along with pediatric neurologist Dr. Richard Frye, were studying metabolic and folate abnormalities in children with ASD. They began working together with me and another mom, Laurette Janak, whose daughter also had Down syndrome, leukemia, and a formal diagnosis of autism.

Soon, a small team of interested doctors were in Brooklyn's hospital room, observing firsthand the positive effects of leucovorin on her condition.

By age nine, Brooklyn had beaten cancer. Once off the cancer drugs and steroids, I made further changes to her diet, eliminating gluten and dairy. Though the dietary adjustments were challenging, they helped normalize her gut and improve her behavior.

Today, as an adult, Brooklyn continues to rely on folate supplementation. She takes leucovorin to support her speech, cognition, and behavior, and without it, she regresses.

Brooklyn's journey has been remarkable. Looking back, her cancer battle was terrifying and painful, but it led to groundbreaking research that continues today. Just as my dream had foretold, Brooklyn truly is a special girl. Not only is she a cancer survivor, but she also played a key role in bringing together the right people at the right time.

Part of my hope in sharing her story is to highlight the critical importance of physicians truly listening to their patients and their parents. Too often, we encounter doctors who dismiss our concerns or fail to recognize the value of our insights and experiences—a frustration that no family should have to endure. I am eternally grateful to Dr. Bob Saylors, Dr. Jill James, and Dr. Richard Frye, who took the time to listen and consider my observations, making a profound difference in Brooklyn's care.

PATIENT STORIES

Reeve

Reeve's story highlights some of the difficulties families face when they have a child with a primary diagnosis of Down syndrome. Extra effort must be taken to differentiate symptoms that indicate something beyond Down syndrome is impacting the child.

Providers who are unfamiliar with Down syndrome may assume that what is being observed is an inherent part of Down syndrome, and is therefore, not treatable.

Parents must be diligent about documenting the concerning changes and advocating for their children. Reeve's story also shows how the U.S. medical system is not designed to diagnose or treat complex metabolic disorders.

Reeve's Story
By Shana A., Reeve's Mom

A parent never wishes for their child to have cancer, but in the Winter of 2019, we found ourselves desperate for an answer – any answer – and the diagnosis of cancer had one appealing aspect to it: it came with a treatment plan.

The nurse escorted my husband and I back to a room where we waited while our son was in the operating room undergoing a bone marrow aspiration. The oncologist had already explained that if the biopsy showed abnormalities indicating leukemia, we would be checked into the hospital right away to begin chemotherapy. While that sounded dreadful, the idea of going home without any answers or potential solutions sounded worse.

In the seven months leading up to that moment, we had seen our son deteriorate. Once a healthy and energetic little boy with Down Syndrome, now he was a sickly child. He was unable to go to school, unable to feed himself, unable to speak, unable to walk more than twenty feet, and unable to stay awake throughout the day. His beautiful smile rotted before our eyes. In just a couple of months, he had developed 13 cavities requiring crowns on almost all of his teeth. In the months after that, the rest of the uncrowned teeth rotted, too, despite our steadfast devotion to his oral hygiene.

He had recently been diagnosed with Juvenile Idiopathic Arthritis (JIA), and his knees were frequently swollen and knobby. He now had movement disorders – dystonia and dyskinesias - that made him look like an adult in the advanced stages of Parkinson's Disease. He stared into space, he hallucinated, he covered his ears and turned off the lights. He was always sick with something – fevers, rashes, vomiting, nosebleeds, blotchy skin, and fatigue. So much fatigue. And while doctors generally chalked these up to 'contagious viruses of unknown origin' - nobody else in our house ever caught these "viruses'" that uniquely plagued our sweet boy.

While only a handful of these symptoms fit the diagnosis of leukemia, it was an important disease to rule out. The oncologist explained that children with Down syndrome are at an increased risk of leukemia, and sometimes they present with walking issues in the earliest stages as the cancer replicates in their bone marrow. It made sense. Our son's blood tests showed only mild abnormalities, but the doctor said that if cancer was there, the good news is that we were catching it early.

We sat anxiously in the waiting room, knowing that an answer was within reach. In our minds, we were torn between leukemia and something just as bad as leukemia, but lacking the diagnostic protocols, the shiny hospital wing with pastel paint and beautiful decorations, the empathetic doctors and nurses. Without a name for his illness, we had no community support. We had no ability to learn about research or treatments. If not leukemia, we were left with a basket of debilitating symptoms that seemed to worsen each month as we carried our son and his symptoms from specialist to specialist hoping for an explanation and a cure.

That day, we left for home with the wonderful, and painful, news: our son did not have leukemia. We were released from oncology and scheduled for a six-month follow up with hematology. Other than that appointment, there was no plan, no new insights, no statistical likelihood of recovery, no next steps. We were again on our own.

Over the next two years, we would often find ourselves in this same awkward position of hoping for an undesirable diagnosis, just because it felt like the only way to move forward. It was hard to believe that so many doctors were needed to investigate our son's small 40-pound body. We learned that our primary care physician and our insurance company first had to divide up and retrofit his ailments into the world of specialties, subspecialties, and waiting lists. We would wait a couple months for one person to look in his ears, another to address his gastrointestinal issues, another to monitor his heart, another to investigate his rash (which inevitably had disappeared by the time our appointment rolled around), another to read his genetic test results, and so on…

We learned how the medical system works. More importantly, we learned how it does NOT work when you have a complex medical condition. We learned how it requires frequent recalibration when your child has a pre-existing condition like Down syndrome. Down syndrome seemed to be a preferred catch-all explanation for doctors who were too uncomfortable to admit they had no time for, answers to, or interest in our case.

"Many children with Down syndrome have trouble walking," we were told by one neurologist. "But do children with Down syndrome often LOSE the ability to walk?" I questioned. "Yes, sometimes," he replied expressionless. I knew that was not true.

I had started this path very polite, passive, and compliant. The agony and urgency of caring for my son quickly taught me to be direct, efficient, and skeptical in each appointment. Doctors suggested tests and "work ups" – and we followed any advice that seemed reasonable. Our son underwent numerous blood labs, urine tests, cultures, saliva samples, ultrasounds, X-rays, MRIs, EEGs, EKGs, gait analyses, therapies, and more.

We had a mixed bag of results – mostly normal, but occasionally an "interesting" result would show up: an EEG that showed "cerebral dysfunction and slowing." Blood tests with elevated lactic acid and evidence of ketonuria. A positive ANA test indicating autoimmunity and a slightly elevated C-reactive protein showing inflammation. Low Vitamin D and glutathione levels, and "possible variants of interest" from genetic testing.

The first real result came nearly six months after the bone marrow aspiration. Our son had a lumbar puncture showing a drastically low concentration of 5-MTHF in his CSF. We had no idea what it meant, but it was the first conclusive report we had ever received.

Below his result was an interpretation explaining that this finding was consistent with something called "Cerebral Folate Deficiency." The report pointed to a handful of symptoms like metabolic abnormalities, seizures, and ataxia that were linked to this condition in literature and case studies. We later learned that "ataxia" simply meant difficulty coordinating muscles for movements like walking, eating, and speaking: exactly what we had been seeing.

Armed with this lab result and a name for our son's condition, we felt that treatment was imminent. All we would have to do is show this report to our doctors, and they would smile and say "ah ha! I can't believe we forgot to check for this!", grab their prescription pads, and we'd be on our merry way to recovery. We had no idea that after reading this one-page report and the studies linked in the footnotes, we already possessed a level of expertise about CFD that surpassed that of most neurologists who we would meet.

Over the next few months, we would go to three different neurologists in three different hospitals. They would see our son's symptoms, review the abnormal lab, then suggest totally different tests and work-ups, without ever providing an explanation or a solution to our son's existing lab results.

"The 5-MTHF lab is abnormal, but not enlightening," said one neurologist.

The frustration and ire that we felt after each appointment only strengthened our resolve to find a doctor, THE DOCTOR, who could help. Our son now required a wheelchair, was back in diapers, was spoon-fed like a baby, completely non-verbal, and plagued with fatigue. We were desperate, and at this point, the tests that doctors were suggesting were mere repeats of ones we had already performed. We needed to approach the situation differently.

We printed off all of the scientific studies about Cerebral Folate Deficiency from the last decade and researched who the authors were. Most journal articles were written by PhDs and academics, not clinicians. Some of the doctors treating patients were far away in Europe. But finally, we found a series of journal articles written by Dr. Richard E. Frye, MD, PhD. He was a practicing pediatric neurologist in Arizona who was not only diagnosing, but also treating CFD. To our astonishment, his email address was listed in the publication.

We flew out to Arizona to see Dr. Frye as soon as we could. Our appointment with him was perhaps the most life-changing two hours we experienced since our journey began. We had an in-depth conversation about the potential causes of CFD.

Further workup revealed that our son had high FRAA titers and mitochondrial dysfunction. Knowing the causes of his CFD helped to shape the treatment plan that Dr. Frye recommended. Over the next several months we introduced medications, supplements, and diet changes to address both conditions. The treatment plan was multifaceted, but simple and safe.

At first, changes were slow, but we saw encouraging signs on a regular basis. Fatigue disappeared, exercise stamina increased, movement disorders decreased, cognition improved, and speech returned. Soon our son was less dependent on his wheelchair and could make small trips to the mailbox and back. The mailbox became the end of the street. The end of the street became around the block. One word became two words, two words became phrases, phrases became sentences. His daily naps dropped from three hours to one hour, then thirty minutes, then became non-existent.

About a year after treatment began, we felt that our son had his childhood back. He began achieving therapy goals that he had never achieved before and began using the toilet on his own. He rarely got sick anymore. His recovery was incredible for all who witnessed his journey.

The treatment seemed too good to be true, was it a coincidence? Were we mistakenly crediting this regimen for a recovery that would have come naturally over time?

The answer to this question came several months later when we accidentally filled an old prescription for his primary medication, leucovorin. Our son regressed that month, and we did not know why. It was not until the next month that the pharmacy pointed out that we had refilled the old prescription, which was half the dose, the month prior. At that moment, we understood the power of leucovorin.

The results were again confirmed over the Christmas holiday. We forgot to refill our son's mail-ordered methylcobalamin/folinic acid injections before the holiday, and he went six days without treatment. By the fifth day, he was unable to walk or talk, and he was again plagued by fatigue. That glimpse of our old life was enough to scare us into setting multiple reminders each month for his prescription refills. As soon as the shipment of injections arrived, we resumed treatment, and our son recovered immediately.

At the time of this writing, most people have never heard of CFD. This includes most physicians whom we interact with on a regular basis. The idea of a central nervous system vitamin deficiency causing symptoms on par with leukemia sounds absurd. And yet, that is exactly what happened to our son.

We are terrified to think of what may have happened if we had failed to identify the cause and the treatment for his condition when we did. It was progressive. We wonder how many other children are out there suffering not only from a list of insurmountable symptoms, but also from a lack of knowledge about this highly treatable condition.

We hope that our son's story will help to illuminate the darkness for families and physicians alike. We cannot be more enthusiastic about future research to better understand both CFD and related metabolic conditions. We embrace opportunities to spread awareness and education for what is already known. This knowledge is absolutely life-changing – we say that confidently from our experience.

PATIENT STORIES

Bella

Bella's story illustrates a phenomenon sometimes seen in teens and adults with Down syndrome—the loss of skills and the emergence of new neurological symptoms. While there is ongoing research into a newly recognized condition called Down Syndrome Regression Disorder (DSRD), much remains unknown about why a small subset of individuals with Down syndrome experience this regression.

In Bella's case, it was fortunate that her doctor ordered a more comprehensive lumbar puncture, including a central folate work-up. Without this, her metabolic abnormalities might have gone undetected, and she may not have received the crucial treatment she needed.

Bella's mother's dedication to researching, understanding, and acting on this information played a pivotal role in Bella's remarkable recovery. Her story underscores the vital importance of family advocacy when navigating complex medical conditions.

Bella's Story
By Michelle S., Bella's Mom

I was 37 years old when I found out I was pregnant with my fourth child. Although we knew there was a higher risk of this baby having Down syndrome because of my age, we opted out of prenatal testing. There was nothing unusual about this pregnancy, so I had no reason to believe this baby would be any different from my other three typically developing children. To our surprise, we received an early Christmas present when our beautiful Isabella Grace was born on December 24th, almost two weeks early!

The delivery was extremely fast, and she arrived soon after we got to the hospital. She was 6 pounds, 3 ounces, and had a full head of beautiful hair! A few hours later, our pediatrician told us he suspected she had Down syndrome, which was confirmed by a blood test a few weeks later. Thankfully, she didn't have any heart issues that are sometimes associated with Down syndrome.

Bella's first years of life were relatively uneventful, aside from a few ear infections, croup, and some delayed milestones typical of Down syndrome. Eventually, she had her tonsils and adenoids removed and ear tubes placed to help with drainage. When she was about 3 to 4 years old, she started exhibiting ASD-like behaviors, including repetitive movements such as twirling ribbons and cords, rocking back and forth, walking in circles around the kitchen table, and lining up her toys in long, straight lines. Around this same time, I noticed her right hip was clicking or popping when I would get her dressed or put her on my lap. She didn't seem to be in any pain, but I took her for x-rays just to be safe. Everything looked normal.

Several months later, while playing in her room, her hip dislocated. She screamed in pain as we rushed her to the ER, and she had to be sedated to set it back in place. It happened again a few days later, and again, she had to be sedated. This continued multiple times until she finally had corrective surgery just a few weeks after her fifth birthday. She was in a spica cast (a cast that covers the hips, waist, and abdomen) for six weeks post-surgery. The procedure was successful with no issues until she was twelve years old. She had just started her sixth-grade school year at a new school when her hip dislocated while she was changing for PE class. That led to several more surgeries, and with each one, she was bedridden for several weeks, once again in a spica cast.

Bella was mostly non-verbal, but she had a vocabulary of about 20-25 words that we could understand. As she grew older, she seemed to gradually lose some of those words and other skills she had previously acquired, but we mostly attributed these setbacks to her traumatic hip surgeries and the many weeks she was unable to move.

Bella's teenage years were happy, and she enjoyed going to school and spending time with her friends. Her favorite pastimes were dancing, bowling, and watching movies and videos on her phone. But all of that changed, almost suddenly, when she was 17 years old.

One morning, I sat her on the toilet several times, but she didn't urinate until 2 p.m. that day. The urine retention continued to worsen, and it became a big struggle to get her to urinate even twice a day! She usually needed water stimulation to help her go.

Bella also lost interest in her phone and tablet, which was shocking to us because, for years, she had wanted to be on them 24/7! She had been able to navigate photos, videos, and her favorite apps independently, but she began sitting on the couch doing nothing. She would stare, often looking over her shoulder, and sometimes laugh for no reason. We believe she was hallucinating.

She also stopped feeding herself and drinking independently, only taking a drink when I offered it to her. Eventually, she lost complete use of her hands. She would just lay her hands in her lap, almost as if she were unable to move them. The teachers and staff at her school had to feed her, and we had to feed her at home as well. She lost 20 pounds over the course of about six months.

She started having dizzy spells upon waking and would sometimes sit on the floor after walking only a few feet. One morning, she fainted, and we called 911. By the time the paramedics arrived, all her vitals were normal. We took her to the pediatrician multiple times for bloodwork, but all results came back normal. We took her to a cardiologist to rule out heart issues, and again, all tests were normal. They told us to increase her salt intake and electrolytes and to have her sit up for a few minutes before getting out of bed.

Bella then developed catatonia. She would "freeze" walking down the stairs or while getting into the car. She would just stand there, almost as if she didn't know what to do next. Everything was in slow motion. Standing up from a chair was slow. Getting dressed was slow. She needed multiple prompts, or she wouldn't know what to do next. If I told her to come to the table for dinner, she would look at me like she had no idea what I was saying. I had to go to her, grab her hand, and lead her to the table. She became totally mute—nothing. Not a word or a sound for several months.

One day, I was scrolling on the Facebook page of our local Down syndrome society, and I saw a story about a young girl who was diagnosed with and treated for Down Syndrome Regressive Disorder (DSRD). What? How had I never heard of this before? This girl's symptoms were almost identical to Bella's, and the story told of a doctor who was an expert in treating DSRD. I took the story to my husband and said, "Bella has this disorder, and I want to take her to see this doctor!" We contacted the doctor's office but were told we needed to run a series of tests before we could even schedule an appointment.

Bella was deteriorating quickly, so I was on a mission to get these tests done as soon as possible. Our pediatrician referred us to a local pediatric neurologist, who then recommended four days of in-patient testing to complete everything quickly. She ordered the necessary blood work, a 12-hour EEG, MRI, and a lumbar puncture.

The first abnormal result revealed a severe deficiency of folate in her blood, along with deficiencies in B12 and Vitamin D. This folate deficiency prompted me to investigate why someone would be so deficient in folate. In my research, I learned about variations in the MTHFR gene. Additional testing showed that Bella had two copies of the MTHFR C677T polymorphism. While this genetic variation did not explain her systemic folate deficiency, it did alert me to the fact that Bella may not be able to process folate efficiently.

A few weeks later, we received the lumbar puncture results, and we finally had a diagnosis! Her neurologist called us in and told us this could be the answer to our prayers. Bella's Cerebral Folate Deficiency (CFD) diagnosis was possibly the root of all her issues, maybe even going back to when she was younger. Her cerebrospinal fluid contained only 17 nmol/L of 5-MTHF, far below the standard range of 40-120 nmol/L, confirming the diagnosis of CFD. The doctor had limited experience with CFD before Bella, so she was unfamiliar with the treatment. She walked into the room with a printed sheet showing the treatment as Leucovorin, but she wanted to start on the lower end for her weight, which was 50 mg per day. We had a follow-up appointment a month later. We told her we saw some minor improvements, but nothing significant. She suggested that the dosage likely needed to be increased, and we agreed. We started giving 100 mg per day, and that's when we began seeing many positive changes!

Bella's urine retention and catatonia were the first symptoms to resolve, and she started regaining some of her independent skills. Despite my initial concerns about side effects, even at this high dose, she tolerated it very well. She started picking up her phone again and looked less "zoned out." She began smiling and laughing again, using her hands, and feeding herself! Her words and sounds started to return! The teachers and staff at her school couldn't believe the changes.

I continued researching CFD, which eventually led me to several journal articles written by Dr. Richard E. Frye, MD, PhD. I think I read most of his papers and watched every video he recorded on the subject. There were a lot! That's where I learned about FRAAs and mitochondrial dysfunction, and how to test for these two possible causes of CFD.

We ordered the FRAT (Folate Receptor Autoantibody Test) and the MitoSwab, then waited several weeks for the results. Since our local neurologist wasn't experienced with treating CFD, she agreed that we should consult Dr. Frye for further guidance.

Armed with the lumbar puncture, FRAT, and MitoSwab results, we finally met with Dr. Frye a few months later. The results showed that Bella had a very high titer for binding autoantibodies (2.796 OD) and evidence of mitochondrial dysfunction.

The initial two-hour meeting with Dr. Frye was incredibly informative, and I was amazed that we used every minute of those two hours! He was so knowledgeable about CFD, and we appreciated how he explained everything in a way we could understand. He increased Bella's oral leucovorin dose even more, added a methylcobalamin/folinic acid injection, and a daily "Mito Cocktail" (a multivitamin regimen to support mitochondrial function, plus Ubiquinol CoQ10 and L-carnitine). Within a few months, Bella was nearly back to baseline.

It has been a little over two years since starting treatment, and Bella is now back to where she was before regression, and in some ways, she's even better than before. She is doing things she hadn't done in years!

She started getting out of bed in the morning and walking downstairs on her own—a milestone she hadn't achieved since her first hip surgery at five years old.

Part of me wonders if the multiple hip and ear surgeries, with many hours of anesthesia, contributed to Bella's regression. Last year, after Bella had recovered, she needed to have hardware removed from her hip. We hesitated, of course, but unfortunately, it was something that had to be done. The day after this short procedure with anesthesia, many of her regression symptoms returned. I felt so depleted. Dr. Frye assured me she would bounce back. It took about a month, but she eventually returned to baseline.

Also, as a side note, a special thanks to our local neurologist who ordered the test to check Bella's 5-MTHF levels in her lumbar puncture. To our surprise, that specific test wasn't required in the standard DSRD workup, yet it turned out to be the most crucial test, providing us with the answers we needed!

Had we not discovered CFD, we might have pursued treatment for DSRD, which typically involves intravenous immunoglobulin (IVIG), electroconvulsive therapy (ECT), and/or high-dose psychotropic medications.

I can honestly say Bella's regression was one of the hardest times our family has ever endured. I refused to accept that this was how Bella was going to live for the rest of her life. I knew she was still in there, and THAT is what motivated me to find answers. I hope our story of regression and recovery will help other families find answers and treatment. Now that we understand CFD and how to treat it, we have renewed hope for Bella's future!

The Overlap between CFD and Down Syndrome

These three cases highlight the remarkable impact that treatment for CFD can have on the lives of children with Down syndrome and their families. While these examples are truly inspiring, they raise an important question: Are these isolated instances, or could there be other children with Down syndrome who also suffer from undiagnosed and untreated CFD?

All the children in these cases experienced regression and were diagnosed with CFD through different paths. Brooklyn was among the first to be identified, thanks to her mother's keen observations and relentless pursuit of answers at a time when CFD was just starting to be recognized. Her mother's insistence that the leucovorin infusions provided her daughter with immediate improvements in health and new skills highlighted the need for further investigation. Unlike Brooklyn, whose story began with a treatment that led to a diagnosis, Bella and Reeve's diagnoses of CFD came after extensive testing in response to significant neurodevelopmental regressions, including loss of speech and onset of new movement disorders.

Though each journey is unique, these stories reflect the common challenges families face when navigating the complexities of CFD. When children with Down syndrome exhibit signs of neurodevelopmental regression, many practitioners attribute these changes to "just Down syndrome" rather than investigating further. This can happen even when the symptoms are uncommon for Down syndrome.

Down syndrome is not the only condition affected by these inherent biases. Many children with genetic disorders or other pre-existing conditions have their symptoms overlooked, misdiagnosed, or mistakenly attributed to their existing diagnosis. For children who cannot communicate, the challenge is even greater, as they are unable to describe their symptoms or how they feel. In all three cases, a lack of awareness about CFD led to delayed diagnoses. Fortunately, the mothers in these stories were relentless advocates, ensuring that no stone was left unturned in the search for answers.

As alluded in Bella's story, there is a phenomenon called Down Syndrome Regression Disorder[92] (DSRD) (formerly known as Down Syndrome Disintegrative Disorder or DSDD) that usually occurs in adolescence or young adulthood with regression in cognition, the development of ASD characteristics, insomnia, catatonia, and psychosis.[93] The cause of this disorder is not known but some children have responded to immunomodulatory therapy with IVIG.[94] For Bella, the DSRD appears to have been caused by her CFD. The possible relationship between DSRD and CFD merits a deeper discussion.

When comparing DSRD and CFD, both share many overlapping symptoms. Both conditions are characterized by notable developmental regression and the onset of autism-like behaviors. Bella exhibited both, along with catatonia.

So, what is catatonia? Catatonia is a neuropsychiatric condition marked by both motor and behavioral disturbances. Motor symptoms include rigid muscles, repetitive movements, and posturing. Individuals with DSRD often become mute, lose the ability to speak, or exhibit echolalia, the involuntary repetition of words spoken by others. These symptoms can closely resemble those seen in CFD.

In addition to ASD-related symptoms such as speech disruption, echolalia, and repetitive movements, CFD is often associated with movement disorders and dystonia, which can cause muscle stiffness. This makes it easy to see how Bella's catatonia overlapped with the symptoms of CFD.

Recognizing CFD in patients with movement disorders is crucial as standard treatments for catatonia, such as benzodiazepines, can have significant side effects including sedation and dependence. Leucovorin, a treatment for CFD, offers a safer alternative with fewer side effects compared to these conventional DSRD therapies.

Bella was also reported to have experienced psychosis with hallucinations. Interestingly, Drs. Ramaekers, Quadros and their colleagues described a case series involving 18 patients with schizophrenia who were unresponsive to conventional treatment.[95] One of major symptoms of schizophrenia is psychosis and hallucinations. Of these, 15 (83%) were found to have FRAAs. Additionally, 7 out of 13 (54%) patients who had their cerebrospinal fluid (CSF) tested were found to have CFD along with abnormalities in dopamine and serotonin—two neurotransmitters whose production is dependent on folate. Treatment with leucovorin led to clinical improvements over a six-month period. This suggests that psychiatric symptoms, such as those seen in psychosis, may indeed be indicative of CFD and should be considered in patients who do not respond to standard treatments.

What about treatment with IVIG? Can it help resolve CFD and reverse its symptoms? The answer is yes. For many patients, CFD is caused by FRAAs. IVIG works in several ways, including modulating the immune system and neutralizing harmful autoantibodies, such as FRAAs. This can help eliminate the antibodies responsible for CFD. So, why isn't IVIG the standard treatment for CFD? IVIG requires lengthy infusions, often over several days, and common side effects include rash, nausea, vomiting, and headache. Additionally, IVIG treatments typically need to be repeated monthly, which can be burdensome and costly, especially if not covered by insurance—averaging around $10,000 per month.

Leucovorin, on the other hand, has been found to be effective for treating CFD without the need for IVIG. It is also significantly more affordable, costing approximately $150-300 per month if not covered by insurance. For these reasons, leucovorin is often preferred as a first-line treatment for CFD.

Considering that CFD can occur in individuals with Down syndrome, could it be responsible for some of the developmental or psychiatric symptoms observed in patients with Down syndrome? Is it possible that the wide variation in developmental outcomes seen in children with Down syndrome may be partially attributable to undiagnosed CFD? Additionally, since approximately 40% of children with Down syndrome exhibit ASD-related symptoms[96]—could this be linked to underlying CFD?

Interestingly, low blood folate levels have been linked to an increased risk of Alzheimer's disease.[97] Additionally, studies have shown that individuals with Alzheimer's often have a folate deficiency in the CSF and an impaired function of the folate receptor alpha (FRα) transport system.[98] Early-onset Alzheimer-type dementia is frequently observed in individuals with Down syndrome in adulthood. Could cerebral folate deficiency contribute to this condition?

All of these are important questions that warrant further investigation. With the diverse presentation of Down syndrome, and with disruptions in folate metabolism as the cause of so many symptoms frequently observed in patients with Down syndrome at various ages, it is worthwhile to investigate the potential role of CFD in this population.

Earlier in this chapter, we reviewed scientific studies on leucovorin treatment in children with Down syndrome, which yielded mixed results. Why were the outcomes so variable? One significant issue with clinical trials is that they often apply a uniform treatment approach to all patients, without considering individual differences. Research has shown that the presence of FRAAs in the blood can predict a patient's response to leucovorin.[99] Both Bella and Reeve tested positive for at least one FRAA, which indicates that they were more likely to respond to CFD treatment.

Additionally, both Reeve and Bella exhibited signs of mitochondrial dysfunction. Because folate transport into the brain is an energy-dependent process, patients with mitochondrial dysfunction may require unusually high doses of leucovorin to see improvements, which was the case for these children.

Some of the prior studies showed little to no effect from leucovorin; however, it should be noted that those studies used very low doses of leucovorin. (For perspective, Bella and Reeve were receiving weight-based doses approximately 250 times higher than some of those studies). The unremarkable results in some of the earliest Down syndrome investigations of leucovorin may therefore have been due to inadequate dosing.

Furthermore, clinical trials conducted in France suggested a potential interaction between leucovorin treatment and thyroid medication. In the most recent trial, only children with normal thyroid function were treated with thyroid medication, which contradicts conventional wisdom and may have influenced the results.

As alluded to in the patient stories, not all leucovorin is the same. Some brands contain lactose which can cause irritability in patients with lactose intolerance. Other brands have additives that can interact with leucovorin or cause discomfort. Interestingly, one study estimated that about half of the adverse effects associated with medication can be linked to the additives in the medications.[100]

The key point is that children with neurodevelopmental disabilities, regardless of their specific diagnosis, should be treated with an individualized approach, guided by the principles of personalized precision medicine. More research is needed to understand the biological variations and medical comorbidities in children with Down syndrome so that effective treatments like leucovorin can be used more widely. In the meantime, it is essential to have physicians who are both attentive and well-informed to provide the best possible care for these children.

A Physician's Perspective

My interest in Down syndrome began before I even entered medical school or had the opportunity to work with or care for children with Down syndrome. My interest was sparked in the 1990s when I co-authored the first paper on olfactory function in adolescents with Down syndrome.[101] Several years later, I began working with Dr. Jill James at Arkansas Children's Hospital and became aware of the metabolic disorders often associated with Down syndrome.

Dr. James has an intriguing background in research related to Down syndrome. For much of her career, she focused on cancer research, specifically studying abnormalities in one-carbon metabolism, which includes processes involving folate, methylation, and glutathione production. One day, a parent asked if she could investigate whether children with Down syndrome also had disorders in these metabolic pathways. Her subsequent study confirmed that children with Down syndrome indeed showed such abnormalities.[102]

During this research, she made another significant discovery that would alter the course of her career. While studying both children with Down syndrome and their siblings, she noticed that one sibling exhibited severe abnormalities in these metabolic pathways. Curious, Dr. James asked the mother if there was anything unusual about this child. The mother responded, "This child has autism." This revelation led Dr. James to pivot her research towards autism spectrum disorder (ASD), where she became the first to identify metabolic abnormalities in one-carbon metabolism in children with ASD.

At Arkansas, our center's expertise in the metabolic abnormalities associated with Down syndrome attracted many parents seeking specialized treatments for their children. My first patient with Down syndrome there, Brooklyn, left a lasting impression on me.

Over the years, I cared for about seven patients with Down syndrome. I tested four of them for folate receptor alpha autoantibodies (FRAAs); two tested positive and two were negative. The two patients with positive FRAAs responded well to leucovorin, achieving optimal results at a higher-than-usual dose of 50 mg twice daily. Conversely, one of the patients who tested negative for FRAAs did not respond to leucovorin.

I had not examined the CSF of children with Down syndrome, as the lumbar puncture procedure requires sedation and carries potential risks. We decided that a trial of leucovorin was a better initial approach for patients with suspected CFD, given leucovorin's safety profile. This approach was discussed in our first publication on treating children with ASD using leucovorin.[103] As a result, I couldn't be certain whether the children with Down syndrome I treated had CFD.

Reeve was one of the first patients who convinced me that we were truly on to something. His mother came to my clinic determined and motivated, having finally found a potential explanation for her child's symptoms. I was deeply impressed by both Reeve's mother and the referring physician, who had gone above and beyond to identify the underlying cause of his condition, rather than just addressing the symptoms. Reeve showed remarkable improvement on leucovorin, recovering significantly and continuing to make further gains.

Now, I follow many children with Down syndrome, most of whom are referred to me because they test positive for FRAAs or have CSF findings consistent with CFD. I have consistently observed improvements in these children with leucovorin treatment. However, given my now biased referral base, I cannot say with certainty that every child with Down syndrome will respond in the same way.

To help define the number of children with Down syndrome that might respond to leucovorin, I asked Religen (Plymouth Meeting PA), the company that performs the FRAA test, to review their records to see how many samples from children with Down syndrome were positive for FRAAs. Their initial review showed a small sample size of six patients who were positively coded for having Trisomy 21 (this information is not always provided). Of the children known to have Down syndrome, 100% were positive for at least one FRAA. This does not mean that every child with Down syndrome is positive for FRAAs, as the samples sent are likely children suspected of CFD, not relatively healthy children with Down syndrome. However, it does demonstrate the potential for investigating and treating CFD in this very special population.

CHAPTER 7.
Epilepsy

Background

Seizures are defined as sudden changes in behavior, movements, sensations, or awareness caused by disturbances in the brain's neuronal firing patterns. As illustrated in the diagram on the next page, seizures can present with a wide range of symptoms. While most people associate seizures with dramatic episodes involving a person falling to the ground and experiencing rhythmic movements of the arms and legs, seizures can also manifest in more subtle ways.

These subtler symptoms may include staring spells, pauses in speech, internal sensations like a rising feeling in the chest, or external sensations such as a tingling or numbness in the arm. Seizures can also manifest as flashing lights or unusual sounds or smells.

The two most common types of seizures are generalized seizures and focal seizures. Generalized seizures affect the entire brain, while focal seizures originate in a specific area. Among generalized seizures, the most common type is the generalized tonic-clonic seizure, also known as a grand mal seizure.

This type involves abnormal electrical activity throughout the entire brain, resulting in symmetric, rhythmic movements of the arms and legs. Because the whole brain is involved, the person will be unconscious during the seizure. Afterward, the brain is essentially "stunned," which often leaves the person feeling confused. As they start to regain consciousness, they may be disoriented for some time. It is common for individuals to experience drowsiness, which can last from a few minutes to several hours after the seizure.

Another type of generalized seizure is the absence seizure, which is classified as a non-motor seizure, meaning there are no noticeable changes in movement. During an absence seizure, the person appears to be staring and is unresponsive.

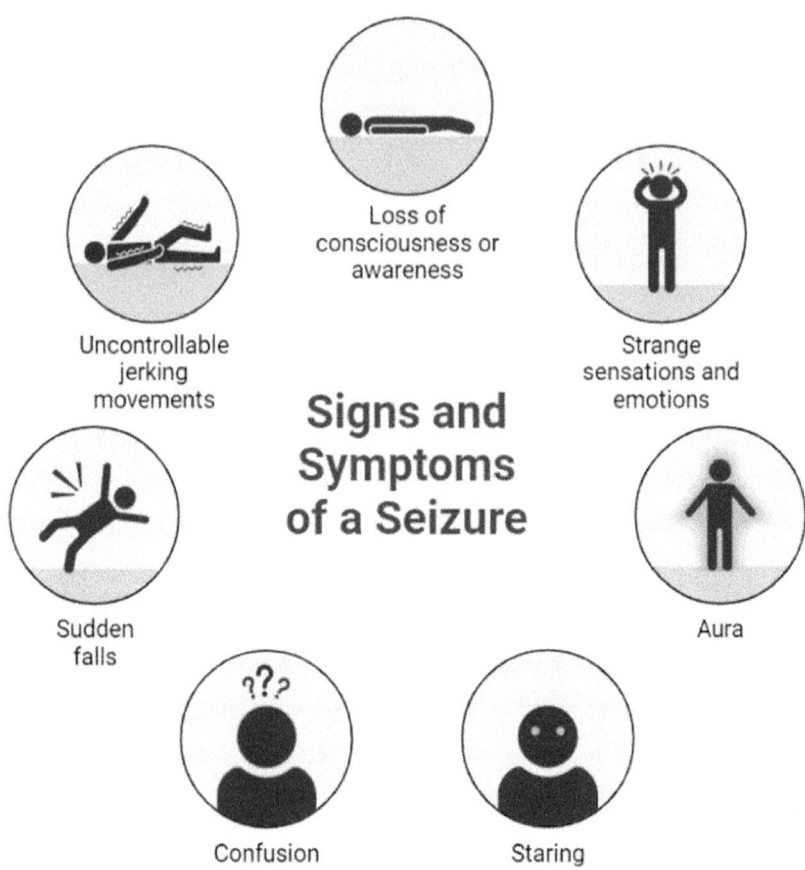

Figure 7.1 Seizures can present with many symptoms aside from shaking. Image created with BioRender.

While many people may have brief staring episodes, they typically respond if their name is called or if they are touched. In contrast, someone experiencing an absence seizure will not respond, even if shaken. These seizures are often brief, lasting only a few seconds, and can easily go unnoticed. Some individuals may experience over 100 absence seizures a day, sometimes leading to misdiagnosis, such as attention deficit disorder, because they appear inattentive.

Focal seizures affect only one part of the brain. Because they do not involve the entire brain, they often do not impair consciousness, allowing the person to be aware of and even feel the seizure as it occurs. However, in some cases, the abnormal electrical activity can spread to other areas of the brain, leading to impaired consciousness resulting in a partial complex seizure. If the seizure activity spreads to the entire brain, it can result in a generalized seizure, known as a secondary generalized seizure.

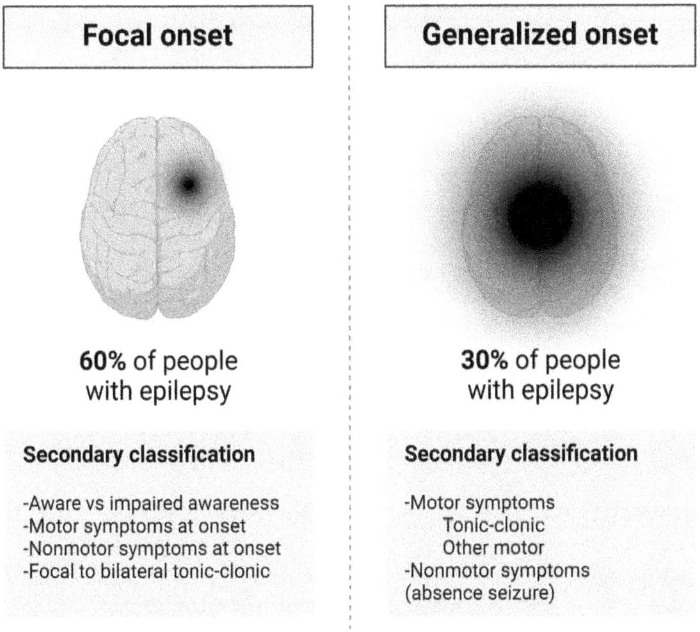

Focal onset	Generalized onset
60% of people with epilepsy	30% of people with epilepsy
Secondary classification	**Secondary classification**

-Aware vs impaired awareness
-Motor symptoms at onset
-Nonmotor symptoms at onset
-Focal to bilateral tonic-clonic
	-Motor symptoms
	   Tonic-clonic
	   Other motor
	-Nonmotor symptoms
	   (absence seizure)

Figure 7.2 Key differences between focal and generalized seizures. Image created with BioRender.

The symptoms of a focal seizure depend on the area of the brain where it originates. Seizures occur in the cortex, the outermost layer of the brain, responsible for complex neuronal processes. The cortex is divided into lobes, each associated with different functions, so a seizure in a particular lobe will disrupt the specific functions controlled by that lobe.

The most recognizable type of seizure is a motor seizure, which involves shaking or jerking movements of the face or one or more limbs. This type of seizure typically originates in the frontal lobe of the brain, which controls not only movement but also behavior and speech. As a result, seizures in the frontal lobe can lead to abnormal behaviors and sometimes an inability to speak.

The parietal lobe processes sensory information from the skin, so a seizure in this part of the brain can cause unusual sensations such as tingling, numbness, or a feeling of heat or cold. The occipital lobe is responsible for processing visual information from the eyes, so seizures in this area may cause visual disturbances like flashing lights or visual hallucinations.

The temporal lobe has many complex functions. It processes sound from the ears and converts it into language, so seizures here can result in the perception of strange noises or ringing sounds. This lobe is also involved in processing smells, so seizures may cause the perception of unpleasant odors.

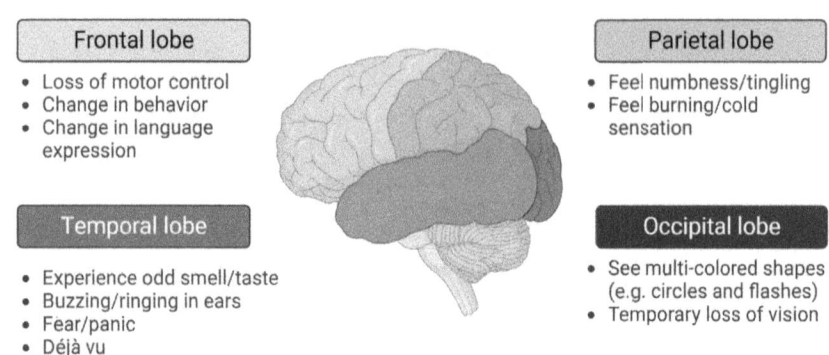

Figure 7.3 Lobes of the brain and associated seizure symptoms. Created with Biorender.

The temporal lobe interacts with other parts of the brain that regulate emotions and communicate with the gastrointestinal tract and other organs. Consequently, temporal lobe seizures can lead to feelings of panic, which may manifest as panic attacks, or cause strange sensations in the stomach, often described as a rising feeling from the abdomen to the chest. A sudden sensation of déjà vu is also unique to temporal lobe seizures.

To diagnose and understand seizures, doctors use an electroencephalogram (EEG) to measure the brain's electrical activity. During an EEG test, small electrodes are placed on the scalp and connected to wires that record the brain's electrical signals. The electrodes do not emit any power, making the test completely safe and non-invasive.

Figure 7.4 shows EEG tracings of normal brain waves as well as brain waves which occur during a generalized seizure and a focal seizure. An EEG measures electrical activity in the two sides of the brain, each of which is called a hemisphere. We can see that the left hemisphere brain waves are on the top of the EEG tracing and the right hemisphere brain waves are on the bottom of the tracing. Each recording electrode is represented by a letter and a number.

The odd number electrodes are recording the left hemisphere while the even numbered electrodes are recording the right hemisphere. The letters indicate that part of the brain is being recorded. F represents the frontal lobe near the forehead, C represents the top of the brain near the border between the frontal and parietal lobe, T represents the temporal lobe and O represents the occipital lobe.

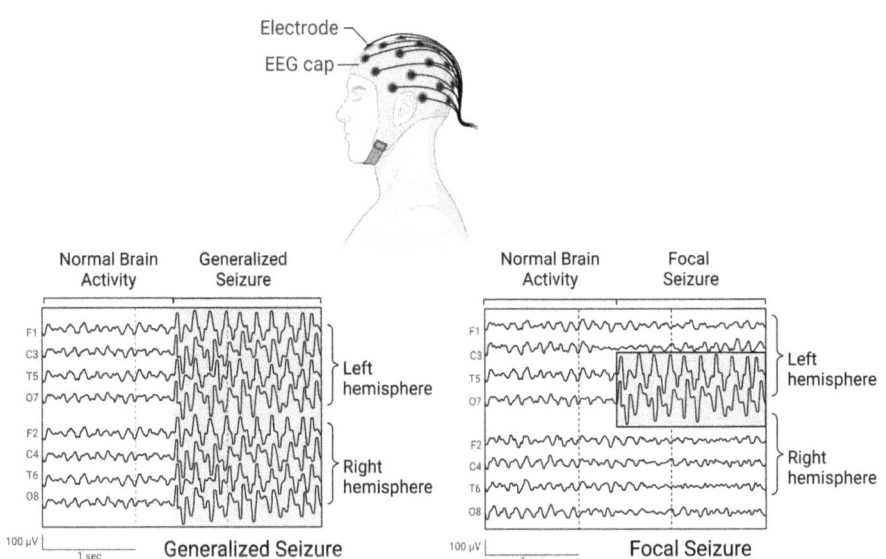

Figure 7.4 Generalized versus focal seizures on EEG. Created with Biorender.

Normal brain waves, which appear as irregular, bumpy patterns on an EEG tracing, are shown on the left side of each example. Under normal conditions, different parts of the brain are engaged in independent activities to process various types of information. This results in the random up-and-down motion of the brain waves, superimposed on a background rhythm, which can be thought of as the brain's "heartbeat." When a seizure occurs, the neurons in the affected area of the brain begin to fire synchronously, which is abnormal, creating large, uniform, sharp waves on the EEG. On the right side of the EEG tracings, you can observe a generalized seizure, where the entire brain exhibits synchronized activity, and on the left side you can observe a focal seizure, where only a specific region, such as the left temporal-occipital area, shows abnormal synchronization.

Seizures can be triggered by various factors such as fever, infection, or metabolic disturbances. When seizures occur without any identifiable cause, the condition may be diagnosed as epilepsy. Epilepsy is defined as having two or more unprovoked seizures. It is often said that people "get one seizure free," meaning that a single seizure during your life is relatively common and does not necessarily indicate epilepsy. In most cases, an individual will have only one seizure and may never experience another.

Epilepsy can affect individuals of all ages, from infants to the elderly, with severity ranging widely. According to the CDC, approximately 1.2% of the U.S. population has epilepsy. In children without underlying neurological conditions, epilepsy often resolves after a few years of treatment with anti-epileptic medications.

If a person remains seizure-free for several years while on medication, a follow-up EEG may be conducted. If the EEG shows normal brain activity, a gradual discontinuation of medication may be possible. While this approach is not always successful, it works in the majority of cases.

Treating epilepsy is critical for several reasons. One major concern is the risk of status epilepticus—a seizure that does not stop—which can be life-threatening. While the body can often withstand a grand mal seizure for several minutes, prolonged seizures can cause severe stress and damage to the heart, lungs, and brain. Sustained rhythmic movements can also lead to muscle breakdown, releasing myoglobin, a protein that can damage the kidneys. For this reason, individuals with epilepsy should have access to rescue medications to stop seizures lasting longer than 3–5 minutes.

Another critical reason for treatment is the danger of having a seizure in high-risk situations, such as driving, swimming, biking, or bathing, where loss of control could result in serious injury or death. Due to these risks, most states impose driving restrictions on individuals with epilepsy, and they must take extra precautions in daily activities. These limitations can significantly impact their independence and overall quality of life.

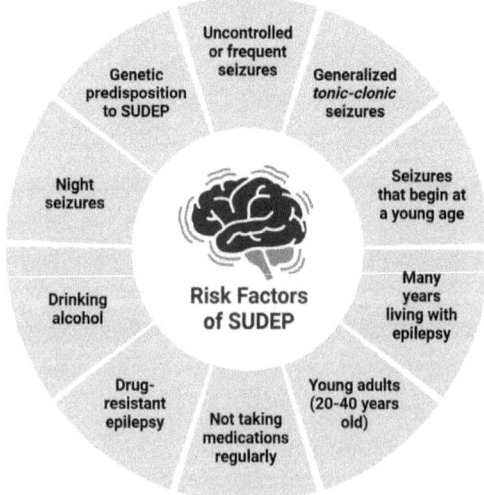

Figure 7.5 Risk factors of SUPDEP. Image created with BioRender.

Finally, there is the risk of Sudden Unexpected Death in Epilepsy (SUDEP). Although rare, SUDEP can occur without warning. Certain controllable factors can help reduce this risk. Maintaining good seizure control and adhering to prescribed medications are critical steps in minimizing the chances of SUDEP. Sometimes epilepsy does not resolve quickly but can be managed with anti-epileptic medications or other treatments. However, approximately 25% of epilepsy cases are classified as refractory, or drug-resistant epilepsy. In children, drug-resistant epilepsy is more common in the presence of neurodevelopmental disorders such as autism spectrum disorder (ASD), genetic syndromes, or brain injuries.

For these refractory cases, additional treatment options may be considered, such as the ketogenic diet, a vagus nerve stimulator (VNS), brain surgery, or other advanced interventions. These cases are often severe, characterized by frequent and difficult-to-control seizures. Unfortunately, in many of these instances, seizures do not fully resolve, and lifelong management is necessary.

Some cases of epilepsy are linked to disruptions in metabolic pathways, such as mitochondrial dysfunction or other metabolic abnormalities. Seizures can also be triggered by deficiencies in essential vitamins crucial for brain function, such as folate or pyridoxine (Vitamin B6). In this book, we will focus specifically on folate-dependent seizures.

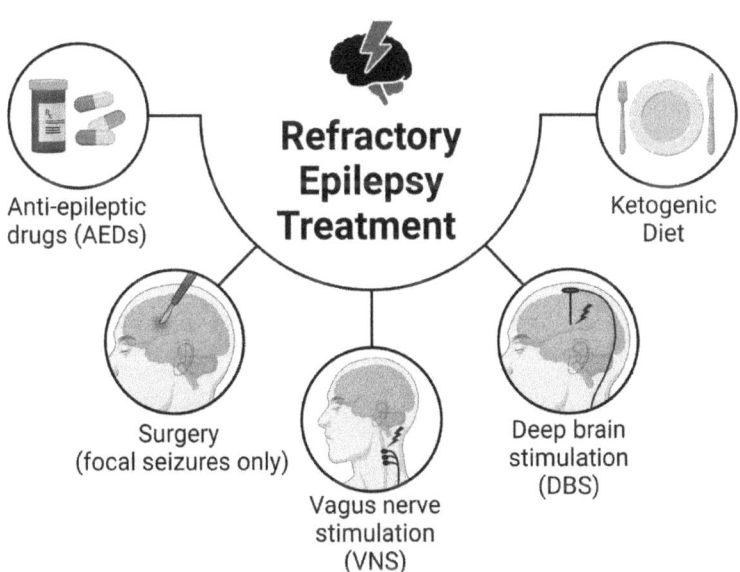

Figure 7.6 Refractory Epilepsy Treatments. Image created with BioRender.

The Scientific Evidence

One of the earliest reports of folinic acid-responsive seizures was published in 1989.[104] The case involved a child with dihydropteridine reductase (DHPR) deficiency, a disorder that impairs the production of tetrahydrobiopterin (BH_4), an essential cofactor for neurotransmitter synthesis. Seizures are a common complication of this condition. The patient also exhibited elevated levels of phenylalanine in the blood, along with reduced levels of dopamine and serotonin, two critical neurotransmitters in the brain.

The following diagram illustrates the role of BH_4 in supporting the function of three critical enzymes known as hydroxylases. These enzymes are essential for synthesizing L-DOPA and 5-Hydroxytryptophan (5-HTP), which are precursors to the vital neurotransmitters dopamine and serotonin. Additionally, one of these hydroxylases is crucial for breaking down phenylalanine, an essential amino acid. Although phenylalanine is necessary for the body, elevated levels can lead to neurotoxicity and a condition known as phenylketonuria (PKU).

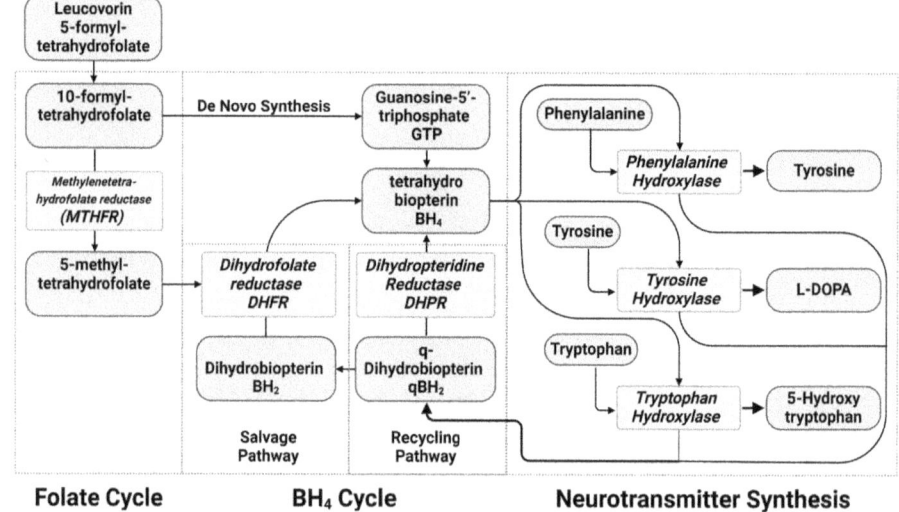

Folate Cycle **BH_4 Cycle** **Neurotransmitter Synthesis**

Figure 7.7 Folate, BH_4 and Neurotransmitter Cycles. Leucovorin enters the folate cycle as 5-formyl-tetrahydrofolate. Central to the tetrahydrobiopterin (BH_4) cycle is dihydropteridine reductase (DHPR). Individuals who have a DHPR deficiency can still generate BH_4 from the de novo and salavage pathways; however this requires additional folate.

Fortunately, most individuals with PKU are diagnosed at birth and placed on a special low-phenylalanine diet to prevent complications. However, in rare forms of PKU, like the one discussed here, the standard dietary treatment may not be effective because of insufficient or absent BH_4. This deficiency hinders the proper function of the hydroxylase enzymes, making it difficult to control phenylalanine levels through diet alone.

As shown in the diagram, the enzyme DHPR is not involved in the production of BH_4 but is crucial for recycling it. This means that individuals with DHPR deficiency can still produce BH_4, but they quickly deplete their supply because it cannot be efficiently recycled. So, how does the body compensate?

There are two pathways to increase BH_4 levels, both of which require folate:

1. **De Novo Synthesis:** Folate serves as a precursor to BH_4. Specifically, 10-formyl-tetrahydrofolate, derived from the folate cycle, is used to produce GTP, which is then converted into BH_4. If sufficient folate is available, this pathway can help maintain normal BH_4 levels.

2. **Salvage Pathway:** BH_4 can also be recycled through an alternative pathway using the enzyme dihydrofolate reductase (DHFR), which requires folate in the form of 5-methyl-tetrahydrofolate.

In individuals with DHPR deficiency, the demand for folate increases significantly to support both the de novo synthesis and the salvage pathway for BH_4 production. Without extra folate, BH_4 levels cannot be adequately maintained, leading to what can be described as a functional folate insufficiency. This is not a typical folate deficiency but rather a higher-than-normal requirement for folate due to the inability to recycle BH_4 effectively.

So, how does this relate to the patient with seizures? In this case report, the physician discovered that treatment with leucovorin resulted in the resolution of both the seizures and the neurotransmitter abnormalities. Additionally, the child's MRI scan revealed abnormalities similar to those seen in disorders associated with central folate deficiency. Upon reviewing the medical literature, the researcher identified five other cases of DHPR deficiency that exhibited the same MRI abnormalities consistent with low folate levels in the central nervous system.

This single case report provided crucial insights, leading to improved treatment strategies for refractory seizures not only in DHPR deficiency cases[105] but also in other genetic conditions involving BH_4 deficiencies.[106] This is particularly significant, as 57% of patients with DHPR deficiency have elevated phenylalanine levels, which is likely a major contributor to their seizures.[107]

Folinic Acid Responsive Seizures

In 1995, Dr. Keith Hyland, a renowned expert in neurotransmitter disorders and brain metabolism, described a new condition called folinic acid-responsive seizures while working at the Baylor Research Institute's Metabolic Disease Center.[108] He observed that infants who developed seizures in the neonatal period and did not respond to standard seizure medications, showed significant improvement with leucovorin treatment.

During his research, Dr. Hyland identified a novel peak in the chromatogram of the HPLC/electrochemical analysis system while analyzing compounds in the CSF of affected children. This unexpected finding suggested the presence of an unidentified compound in the CSF. Remarkably, the mysterious peak disappeared with leucovorin treatment, offering a crucial insight into the underlying mechanism of these seizures and paving the way for more effective therapeutic approaches.

Four years later, Dr. Hyland and his coauthors published another case series describing three infants with the same unidentified compound in their CSF and refractory epilepsy. Despite having normal folate concentrations in their CSF, the infants responded to leucovorin treatment.[109] However, while their seizures improved, they continued to experience significant developmental delays, brain atrophy, and abnormalities in white matter, highlighting the complexity of the underlying condition.

In 2003, I encountered my own patient with folinic acid-responsive seizures.[110] At two months old, the infant, whose neonatal seizures had previously been controlled, experienced a sudden worsening of seizures that did not respond to anti-epileptic medications. The CSF analysis revealed the characteristic compound associated with folinic acid-responsive seizures. Treatment with leucovorin resolved the seizures within 24 hours. Unfortunately, several months later, the seizures recurred and could not be controlled, even with increased doses of leucovorin or additional anti-epileptic medications.

In 2006, a case was reported of an infant boy whose seizures initially responded to pyridoxine (vitamin B6) supplementation as a neonate.[111] Testing of the CSF revealed the same mystery compound. Although the child experienced good seizure control for several months, his seizures became resistant to treatment at four months of age. Leucovorin was then introduced. With leucovorin treatment, a reduction in this unidentified compound was observed, indicating a positive response to the new therapy.

In 2009, a group of doctors reported two cases of neonates with treatment-resistant seizures that responded to leucovorin and exhibited the mystery compound in the CSF.[112] One of the infants was initially treated with pyridoxine, but this had no effect on the seizures. However, the addition of leucovorin successfully controlled the seizures. The child was subsequently weaned off both pyridoxine and leucovorin. Five days later, the seizures recurred and did not respond to leucovorin alone until pyridoxine was reintroduced.

Upon further examination of the CSF, the doctors found markers indicative of pyridoxine-dependent epilepsy. Their analysis of these two cases, along with seven additional cases, revealed that the mystery compound in the CSF correlated with markers of pyridoxine-dependent epilepsy, suggesting that the mystery compound was not necessary as a unique biomarker for diagnosis.

Folinic acid-responsive seizures are more complex than initially thought. The overlap with pyridoxine-dependent epilepsy is revealing, as these cases suggest that both leucovorin and pyridoxine play crucial roles in seizure control. Interestingly, there has been a reported case of a boy with cerebral folate deficiency (CFD) whose seizures could only be controlled when pyridoxine was added to the leucovorin treatment.[113] This research has significantly advanced the treatment of pyridoxine-dependent epilepsy, as current guidelines now recommend the combined use of both pyridoxine and leucovorin for optimal seizure management.

Cerebral Folate Deficiency and Epilepsy

Folinic acid-responsive seizures suggest a link between some forms of epilepsy and folate metabolism. However, they do not always align with CFD, where patients exhibit low folate (5-MTHF) levels in the brain. So, what do we know about CFD cases and their overlap with epilepsy?

Over the past few decades, several such cases have been discussed in the literature. In 2002, Dr. Ramaekers published the first series of five children with CFD, all of whom exhibited neurodevelopmental regression within the first year of life and experienced occasional seizures.[114] Subsequent reports of CFD with seizures were published by the Baylor group in 2005[115] and by doctors at Schneider Children's Medical Center of Israel in 2007.[116] In these cases, leucovorin demonstrated a significant therapeutic effect on seizure control.

In 2007, Dr. Ramaekers reported the first case of a child with CFD associated with a mitochondrial disorder.[117] The child's seizures persisted despite mitochondrial treatments and only resolved when leucovorin was added to the regimen. While most CFD cases involve children, similar cases have been reported in adults. One such case describes an adult with long-standing epilepsy who developed worsening seizure frequency later in life.[118] An overnight EEG revealed electrical status epilepticus in sleep (ESES)—a prolonged seizure that is difficult to stop occurring during sleep. A lumbar puncture confirmed the presence of CFD. The CFD was the result of the folate receptor autoantibodies (FRAAs). Leucovorin treatment significantly improved the patient's seizure burden.

More recently, Dr. Rossignol and I systematically reviewed all published cases of CFD.[119] We found that leucovorin improved seizures in 75% of children with both CFD and ASD and in 54% of children with CFD without ASD.

While more studies must be done to fully elucidate the relationship between CFD and epilepsy, knowing that many patients have already obtained full or partial seizure control from leucovorin is highly encouraging.

PATIENT STORIES

Victor

Epilepsy can be a terrifying condition for families who live in constant fear of life-threatening seizures, especially those that strike during sleep.

Victor's mother shares their journey to uncovering both the cause and a solution for her son's persistent epilepsy, which continued despite trying multiple anti-epileptic drugs and leucovorin.

This story underscores the critical role of a lumbar puncture and working with experienced physicians in cases where CFD is suspected. Thankfully, Victor's mother never gave up in her search for answers, ultimately learning that leucovorin (when dosed properly) was able to control Victor's seizures.

Victor's Story
By Honey R., Victor's Mom

During my first trimester with my twins, I was incredibly sick and lost a significant amount of weight. The boys were born a month early, but aside from their prematurity, the delivery was uneventful. Victor was born first, but he had low amniotic fluid and struggled with a weak sucking and swallowing. In his first year, Victor's development was typical, but he faced significant challenges after every "well visit." He suffered from constant ear infections, breathing issues, and croup, which led to repeated rounds of antibiotics. His illnesses seemed to follow vaccinations.

At their 18-month well visit, both twins became sick again, but this time, they didn't bounce back as they had before. Day by day, they became more delayed, and by their next checkup, they were over a year behind in development, despite previously being within the "typical" range. They stopped babbling, walking, crawling, and responding to us.

At 21 months, our pediatrician referred us for formal evaluations. We were told both boys had a reaction to the vaccines, and we held out hope for a way to "repair" their injuries. Given the severity of their regression, particularly the severe hypotonia and weakness, the doctor suspected a mitochondrial issue. He began treating them with supplements to support mitochondrial function, including leucovorin. However, the response was underwhelming, so a more experienced doctor introduced a stronger set of supplements to address the damage.

One day at school, Victor threw himself back to avoid an aide, hit his head, and suffered a concussion. A week later, he had his first grand mal seizure at school. Fortunately, the staff were trained to handle seizures and called an ambulance right away. The seizure lasted about four minutes before he was transported to the emergency department.

After that, Victor began seeing the chief of neurology at our local hospital. He was prescribed an anti-epileptic drug (AED), but it didn't work—Victor continued having breakthrough seizures.

One of the scariest moments occurred when Victor had a seizure during a hospital observation. A nurse entered his room, turned on the light, and the sudden brightness triggered a severe grand mal seizure that lasted over four minutes. His oxygen levels dropped, and the staff had to press the Code Blue button.

The on-call neurologist prescribed another AED, administering the first dose intravenously in hopes of controlling his seizures. Unfortunately, the breakthrough seizures persisted, and the new AED caused severe hyperactivity. Our primary doctor, Dr. Usman, worked closely with the neurologist to find the right AED to reduce Victor's seizures. Dr. Usman suspected a connection between his seizures and mitochondrial dysfunction, potentially leading to CFD. I was familiar with CFD, and we decided to test for folate receptor autoantibodies, but the results came back negative.

Although the test was negative, Dr. Usman remained convinced that CFD was the issue. I reached out to Dr. Edward Quadros, who invented the folate receptor autoantibody test (FRAT), to understand the reasoning. Dr. Quadros explained that Victor's dairy-free diet could have lowered his antibody levels, making them undetectable in the test.

When I asked if reintroducing dairy could improve test accuracy, Dr. Quadros strongly advised against it, fearing it could worsen Victor's condition. I felt helpless as Victor's seizures continued, unsure how to stop them without understanding their cause. If CFD was behind his seizures, why wasn't leucovorin helping? Leucovorin is supposed to treat CFD, so I expected it to control his seizures, especially alongside AEDs.

Our neurologist, part of the hospital's elite "Gold Team" for complex cases, prescribed a full-time school nurse for Victor and ensured oxygen was available due to the risk of oxygen desaturation. He also ordered a multi-specialty workup, and we consulted infectious disease specialists, immunologists, neurologists, and a mitochondrial specialist. Despite exhaustive testing, we found no answers.

Finally, our Gold Team neurologist gently told us, "Sometimes children die from seizures. Good luck, and God bless." It was heartbreaking. I loved that doctor, but we knew he had reached the limits of what he could do. We were even offered a "Make a Wish" trip to Disney, accompanied by Victor's full-time aide to manage his oxygen.

Even after the medical team had given up, I turned to Dr. Usman. She recommended we see a nationally recognized mitochondrial specialist who could perform a lumbar puncture and muscle biopsy on both boys. Our local neurologist agreed, and the procedures were scheduled. At Dr. Usman's suggestion, I also reached out to Dr. Frye and Dr. Rossignol for additional opinions. The procedures went as smoothly as possible, though both boys woke up from anesthesia with severe post-spinal tap headaches. Thankfully, the effort was worthwhile. The test results confirmed Dr. Usman's suspicions—Victor had both a mitochondrial disorder and CFD.

Dr. Usman referred us to Dr. Frye to treat both conditions. He significantly increased Victor's leucovorin dose, explaining that the lack of response was due to an insufficient dosage—a "squirt gun" approach when we needed a "firehose." After increasing the leucovorin, Victor's seizures stopped, though he experienced some hyperactivity in the first few months. Finally, we could breathe again, although the fear of another seizure never left me. After Victor's first seizure, I hadn't been able to sleep for years, constantly on edge, fearing another life-threatening episode. Watching your child turn blue during a seizure feels like watching them get hit by a bus over and over - I felt powerless to stop it.

Over time, I came to believe that CFD was indeed the cause of Victor's seizures, and leucovorin was the key to controlling them. But it wasn't until we reached 10 seizure-free years that I truly began to relax. Now, at 12 years seizure-free, I know without a doubt that Dr. Usman and Dr. Frye's treatments saved Victor's life. Had we not found a solution, I'm not sure I'd be here today. Raising twins with ASD, a constantly traveling husband, and no family support took a massive toll on my health. The correct diagnosis and treatment for Victor didn't just save him—it saved me, too.

I am forever grateful for Dr. Frye's expertise and Dr. Usman's discernment, and I praise God for leading us to the right answers.

PATIENT STORIES

Patrick

Patrick has a rare and severe form of genetic epilepsy known as Dravet syndrome. With this condition, mutations in the SCN1A gene impair the brain's sodium channels – leading to atypical neuronal activity.

Despite facing many challenges and life-threatening setbacks, Patrick is now thriving. His family's unwavering determination to navigate the complexities of his medical condition has led to his optimal treatment.

His mother's inspiring story serves as a beacon of hope for any family facing even the most extreme health challenges.

Patrick's Story

By Katherine J., Patrick's Mom

Hope. Hope is a magnificent and powerful force. Just as powerful is the belief that, with proper management, living a good quality of life is possible for those with conditions like CFD and SCN1A, the gene responsible for my son's epilepsy, known as Dravet syndrome. I want to begin by telling you where we are now, before sharing where we've been, so that you can truly feel the strength and power of hope and belief.

Today, despite the challenges, Patrick is thriving. He's a vibrant 10-year-old, about to start 5th grade. He's incredibly happy, kind, and loving, and he works harder on his health than anyone I know. Patrick enjoys Legos, Minecraft, Jeeping, and traveling—especially to Disney. Last year, he even learned to play ice hockey, and now he's learning to swim so we can take him to Hawaii. There, he hopes to visit the USS Arizona to honor America's fallen heroes and swim with dolphins.

These are moments we never thought we would experience, and with every cherished memory, I'm acutely aware of how fortunate we are to have him with us. I'm sharing this because I want you to know Patrick—before you learn about his diagnoses and the journey we've been on.

In terms of his health, Patrick has excellent seizure control (though not perfect, it's considered exceptional for Dravet syndrome). He is on just one anti-epileptic drug—a rarity in the Dravet community—along with high-dose leucovorin, subcutaneous IgG therapy, a specialized diet, and a full mitochondrial cocktail, including B12 and folinic acid injections. He has a private one-on-one teacher, and with support, he can follow a neurotypical school curriculum. Patrick can walk, run, and, as I mentioned earlier, ice skate! However, he has gait issues, leading to frequent falls and poor coordination, which is typical for Dravet syndrome. He also tires easily due to both Dravet and mitochondrial dysfunction, requiring a wheelchair for longer outings.

Patrick is immunocompromised and receives subcutaneous IgG infusions, which also help with seizure control and immune modulation, addressing both autoimmune and hyperimmune responses. He has some developmental delays and neurodivergent behaviors, particularly with executive functioning, sensory processing, a weaker sense of danger, planning, and reality perception. He also lives with severe ADHD.

Patrick's type of epilepsy is considered catastrophic and medication-resistant. Many children with his specific Dravet mutation experience seizures that leave them immobile, non-verbal, and severely delayed, often enduring frequent, life-threatening seizures. Tragically, many children with Dravet syndrome succumb to Sudden Unexpected Death in Epilepsy (SUDEP). We never take Patrick's health for granted, and his commitment to thriving is a lifelong journey.

While Patrick is doing well today, it wasn't always this way. We've come a long way from where we were when we first met Dr. Frye at the end of 2018.

This is Patrick's story...

Patrick was born a happy, healthy baby at 37 weeks. However, after receiving his 4-month vaccines, he had a severe reaction that began within hours. He experienced complex focal seizures, myoclonic seizures, frequent vomiting, a full-body rash, and an inability to sleep for more than 40 minutes at a time. This reaction, along with all these symptoms, persisted for six months.

During this time, my husband and I were so sleep-deprived that we had to rely on family support and hire caregivers just to function. Despite the seizures, his doctors dismissed them, attributing the twitching to normal baby behavior. An immunologist confirmed that Patrick had indeed reacted to the vaccines but advised us to continue vaccinating him, saying, "pour a stiff drink and let him cry."

After the reaction, Patrick was never quite the same. He no longer smiled or laughed as he once did and stopped sleeping peacefully, instead waking up screaming in terror before falling back asleep. He continued to experience random bouts of projectile vomiting and developed several food allergies. Faced with these ongoing issues, we made the difficult and frightening decision to stop vaccinating him.

After his vaccine reaction, we noticed that when Patrick got sick, he would become extremely ill. Most illnesses turned into bacterial infections in his lungs or ears and took four times longer than usual to resolve. Then, at 14 months, our lives changed forever—Patrick had his first full-body convulsive seizure. It lasted nearly 10 minutes. He was foaming at the mouth, his eyes rolled completely back, he stopped breathing, and his skin turned from blue to gray. The doctors told me it was a febrile seizure and assured us he likely wouldn't have another. Unfortunately, they were wrong.

Just two months later, Patrick fell ill again and had another seizure. I watched in horror as two men held down my 16-month-old son while they performed a spinal tap to rule out meningitis due to the seizure's duration and his elevated inflammatory markers.

From 2015 to 2017, Patrick experienced one status seizure after another—long, life-threatening events, some requiring CPR and all needing rescue medications. His triggers varied from obvious factors like illness and sleep deprivation to more subtle things like temperature changes (being too hot or too cold), visual patterns, or even playing too hard. Those years were terrifying; it felt like an invisible bullet was always looming over our child. Our local fire department and emergency response team knew us by name. They once told me that when they heard the first three digits of our home address, they immediately started heading our way.

We constantly second-guessed and analyzed everything in an attempt to stop the seizures—from Patrick's routine to what we fed him. We meticulously documented everything. I sought the help of an integrative specialist because I was concerned Patrick might be developing ASD, and traditional doctors dismissed my belief that he had mitochondrial issues and was immune-compromised. Their response was, "kids get sick." They only wanted to medicate him, but we were too afraid to agree. Instead, we controlled his triggers by severely limiting his lifestyle.

The integrative doctor promised me that if I followed everything he recommended, he could help Patrick stop seizing. Patrick's lab results showed numerous abnormalities, but nothing conclusive. On paper, he appeared to have ASD and signs of mitochondrial dysfunction. We spent tens of thousands of dollars on testing, supplements, and dietary changes. We put Patrick in total isolation to prevent illness, bought special light-filtering glasses to eliminate visual triggers, and adhered to a strict sleep routine.

Patrick would show slight improvements, only to worsen again. He'd go months without a seizure, and then they'd return, eventually becoming a weekly occurrence. The seizures also began to change—Patrick developed complex focal, non-convulsive status seizures, which were terrifying. During these episodes, his body would become lifeless, his eyes would roll back, and the only way to track the seizure was by monitoring his vital signs. He also developed facial seizures with eye fluttering and grimacing. His gait deteriorated, his sleep issues worsened, and his fine and gross motor skills became noticeably delayed.

At 2.5 years old, we decided to start him on his first anticonvulsant medication, Lamictal. Before we could reach a therapeutic dose, Patrick lost his memory, stopped talking, became extremely unstable while moving, and eventually lost the ability to use the right side of his body. Desperate, I reminded the doctor of his promise, and true to his word, he flew to a conference he hadn't planned on attending to consult with Dr. Frye about Patrick's case.

Dr. Frye recommended a Folate Receptor Alpha Autoantibody test. Four weeks later, we finally had a diagnosis for much of what Patrick was experiencing—Cerebral Folate Deficiency (CFD). For the first time since his birth, we knew one of the key enemies to his health. At that time, Dr. Frye was only treating patients with ASD, and his waitlist was a year long. Despite this, we began treatment with Leucovorin and some mitochondrial support.

The results were immediate—Leucovorin drastically improved Patrick's sleep, allowing him to sleep peacefully through the night for the first time ever. His speech, fine and gross motor skills improved overnight, and the random projectile vomiting stopped. Remarkably, he went an entire year without a seizure—during a time when seizures typically peak in young children with Dravet syndrome. My husband and I truly thought he was cured.

To celebrate Patrick going a full year without a seizure, we decided to let him start experiencing life outside the isolation he had been in for years. We enrolled him in a karate class, and he loved it! We cried as we watched him play with other children and kick his foam target. During one class, a little boy coughed in Patrick's face. I gasped and whispered to my husband, "Did you see that?" He laughed and reassured me that Patrick would be fine.

Two days later, Patrick had a seizure while eating, and I found myself desperately trying to clear the food from his mouth as he bit down on my finger. The seizure lasted over 20 minutes and triggered a cycle of illness and prolonged seizures like we had never seen. Patrick's condition worsened—his speech became slurred, his memory faltered, and his gait issues grew more pronounced.

The EMS teams that responded to his seizures often prepared for CPR due to the extreme instability of his vitals. In an effort to help, we decided to try Keppra, but it neither stopped the seizures nor prevented the frequent illnesses he contracted from being hospitalized multiple times a week. Patrick ultimately spent 21 days in the PICU, with his final stay nearly costing him his life.

Desperate, I searched for Dr. Frye on my phone while sitting in the dark, watching Patrick's vitals flashing on the monitors. I discovered he had moved to another hospital and decided to take a chance, calling to ask for an appointment. I spoke to his assistant, sobbing, as I begged for Patrick to be seen by Dr. Frye. On our way home from the hospital, she called to tell me that Dr. Frye had agreed to take our case.

It was the beginning of our new beginning.

We packed Patrick into an RV and drove to Phoenix to see Dr. Frye. Over the course of three visits in two years, Dr. Frye was able to unravel Patrick's complex medical needs and find the right treatments. During that time, we learned we had been using the wrong dose of leucovorin, the Keppra dosage was so low it was non-therapeutic, and Patrick had never undergone an epilepsy gene panel—which later revealed his SCN1A mutation and confirmed his Dravet syndrome diagnosis. His mitochondrial cocktail was incomplete, and he needed B12/folinic acid injections and IgG therapy to regulate and support his immune system.

As we introduced each treatment, step by step, I often felt overwhelmed. But I watched as Patrick began to come back to life. He went three years without a single seizure and has had only one status seizure in the past four years. While he still experiences small focal and absence seizures, they are manageable. His life is now full of promise and hope. Every year, I hold my breath when it's time for his end-of-year school testing. But as of now, he's able to complete a standard curriculum—though with some struggles—and is accomplishing far more than we ever thought possible.

I'd like to end with a cautionary tale. After Patrick was finally diagnosed with Dravet syndrome, his specialist suggested that, now having a primary diagnosis, we could put him on Depakote and remove his mitochondrial support and leucovorin. We stopped her immediately. We insisted that Patrick would remain on those treatments for life because of the dramatic improvements we had seen, both before and after he started them. We also declined Depakote, stating that Patrick would need to have many unprovoked seizures before we would consider a drug with such severe side effects, especially one known to damage mitochondria.

CFD remains poorly understood in the medical community, particularly in relation to folate receptor autoantibodies. From my experience, I have reviewed over 20 test results for children with SCN1A mutations, and the prevalence of folate receptor autoantibodies is significantly higher than in the general population. Given this, I strongly encourage anyone with an SCN1A mutation to undergo a FRAT test and determine the appropriate leucovorin dosage that best supports them.

Additionally, I have reviewed more than 20 mitochondrial function tests for children with SCN1A, and none have returned normal results—an unsurprising finding considering the medications and interventions these children undergo. For this reason, I also strongly recommend a mitochondrial cocktail for anyone with an SCN1A mutation. The remarkable stories of improvement that I have encountered are truly astounding.

The key to Patrick's success has been treating the whole child, not just the Dravet syndrome. I'm grateful that Patrick's journey has had a ripple effect in our community and that Dr. Frye answered the call of a desperate mother from the PICU.

I've shared with Dr. Frye many times that I will never find the right words to fully express my gratitude for his dedication to research, his compassion, and his unwavering commitment to helping children. How do you properly thank someone for saving your child's life? For giving a family the hope, guidance, and knowledge to overcome a devastating prognosis and defy the odds? Words simply cannot suffice. If you are reading Patrick's story, my deepest hope is that we can impact your life, even in the smallest way, just as Dr. Frye has impacted ours.

A Physician's Perspective

Like many others with CFD who respond to leucovorin, Victor was a mystery patient with no clear treatment path until he underwent a lumbar puncture. The insight and persistence of his primary physician, Dr. Usman, led to a diagnosis that transformed Victor's life and the life of his family. Many doctors consider CFD so rare that it's often dismissed as an unlikely diagnosis. However, when all other possibilities are ruled out, even the most improbable diagnosis becomes possible.

Victor's case was particularly complex, and a lumbar puncture was critical to his diagnosis. In addition to CFD, he had a mitochondrial disorder, requiring high doses of leucovorin. Since the folate receptor alpha (responsible for transporting folate into the brain) relies on energy to function, mitochondrial dysfunction severely impairs this transport mechanism. In such cases, patients may need 4-8 mg/kg/day of leucovorin, which is a very high dose. Therefore, confirming the diagnosis first is crucial, especially when the initial response to leucovorin is lackluster, but CFD is still suspected. In Victor's case, the collaboration of multiple physicians led to significant improvements in his life.

Patrick's story highlights the complexity of treating a single abnormality, while other underlying factors may worsen the disease. By identifying and addressing these additional contributors, his brain function improved significantly.

First, the presence of folate receptor autoantibodies may have hindered adequate folate transport to the brain, as evidenced by his positive response to leucovorin. Second, signs of mitochondrial dysfunction likely further disrupted folate transport and neuronal function. Third, Patrick was trapped in a vicious cycle—frequent illnesses lowered his seizure threshold, while severe seizures further weakened his body. Strengthening his immune system helped break this cycle, allowing his body to recover from chronic stress and regain stability.

Diseases are often simplified, with treatments targeting a single organ or system. However, many conditions are multifactorial, requiring a more comprehensive approach. In Patrick's case, whether the complexity of his physiological challenges arose from the SCN1A mutation, other genetic or epigenetic factors, or environmental influences remains uncertain. Nonetheless, recognizing and understanding these contributing factors is essential to advancing treatments for children with Dravet syndrome and improving their long-term outcomes.

These cases underscore the severity of drug-resistant epilepsy and the critical need to consider CFD as a potential diagnosis when evaluating patients with life-threatening seizures. CFD can be identified through a lumbar puncture, which measures 5-MTHF concentration in the cerebrospinal fluid (CSF) (see Chapter 15).

The decision to perform a lumbar puncture and the timing of investigating treatable causes of epilepsy vary among physicians and medical centers. While a lumbar puncture is an invasive procedure, it is generally safe. In cases where seizures are so refractory that they threaten a person's life, a lumbar puncture should be seriously considered. This is especially important when multiple anti-epileptic drugs fail to control seizures, as treatment resistance is a key indicator that further investigation is necessary.

Seizures associated with CFD can manifest in various, often unexpected, forms. Case reports in the medical literature describe severe and diverse manifestations across different patient populations.

One case report described a teenager with drug-resistant epilepsy since the age of five who suddenly experienced a significant increase in seizures, along with becoming mute and catatonic.[120] He developed status epilepticus, with an EEG showing continuous generalized epileptiform discharges, and he required mechanical ventilation. A CSF examination revealed CFD. Remarkably, after starting leucovorin at 25 mg twice a day and pyridoxine at 100 mg daily, he showed rapid recovery. When he later relapsed, increasing the leucovorin dose to 75 mg twice a day stabilized his condition.

In another case, an infant developed Ohtahara syndrome, a severe and difficult-to-treat form of epilepsy that starts early in life.[121] The addition of leucovorin to the treatment regimen resulted in good seizure control for the child. Additionally, two children, aged 8 and 12 years, who experienced neurodevelopmental regression and new onset myoclonic epilepsy were found to have CFD and mutations on the FOLR1 gene.[122] Both also had a history of developmental delays and were found to have atrophy on brain MRI. The epilepsy partially responded to intramuscular leucovorin.

In my practice, I frequently find that children with refractory epilepsy respond well to leucovorin. Folate receptor autoantibodies are often positive in these children, suggesting that leucovorin may be helpful. While I don't always perform a lumbar puncture, and therefore cannot confirm classic CFD in every case, leucovorin often proves beneficial when combined with standard AEDs to control seizures.

Patrick's case is a perfect example of how medicine tends to make assumptions and fit patients into predefined diagnostic boxes. While this approach makes diagnosis and treatment more efficient, the human body doesn't always conform to these categories.

Dravet syndrome, also known as Severe Myoclonic Epilepsy of Infancy, is a form of epilepsy that typically begins in the first year of life. It is often misdiagnosed or overlooked for several reasons. One key reason is that the first seizure in a child with Dravet syndrome is frequently triggered by a fever, sometimes following vaccination. In children between 6 months and 6 years old, febrile seizures—seizures caused by fever—are relatively common and are generally considered benign, often resolving on their own as the child grows. Because of this, it is not uncommon for a child with Dravet syndrome to be initially diagnosed with febrile seizures, with no further investigation, delaying the correct diagnosis.

Another reason Dravet syndrome can be missed is that seizures are a known, but usually self-limiting, adverse effect of vaccinations. As a result, the first seizure in a child with Dravet syndrome may be mistaken for a benign vaccine-related event, making it indistinguishable from other common seizure syndromes at that early stage.

Dravet syndrome is caused by a mutation in the SCN1A gene, making it a genetic disorder. Since genetic mutations are not easily fixable, Dravet syndrome is considered untreatable in terms of curing the underlying cause, though advanced research is exploring ways to address the genetic defect and potentially resolve seizures. The seizures associated with Dravet syndrome are notoriously difficult to control and usually require multiple AEDs, which are often administered aggressively due to the constant risk of status epilepticus. As such, the diagnosis of Dravet syndrome typically involves a regimen of intensive seizure management.

Recently, I have been evaluating several children with Dravet syndrome, many of whom tested positive for folate receptor alpha autoantibodies and responded positively to leucovorin. The exact reason for this is not yet fully understood. However, it is possible that frequent seizures lead to oxidative stress, mitochondrial dysfunction, and inflammation, which may disrupt neurotransmitter production. These are all key physiological processes connected to the folate cycle.

Similar to the case of DHPR deficiency mentioned earlier, epilepsy may create conditions in which higher levels of folate are required to maintain optimal brain function. Additionally, the inflammation caused by frequent seizures may trigger the production of the FRAAs, resulting in low levels of folate in the brain and further exacerbating the condition.

Another important consideration for children with epilepsy is whether their antiepileptic drugs interfere with folate metabolism. Several commonly used seizure medications—including Depakote (Valproic Acid), Dilantin (Phenytoin), Phenobarbital, Tegretol (Carbamazepine), Mysoline (Primidone), and Lamictal (Lamotrigine)—affect folate processing in different ways.

For example, Depakote inhibits dihydrofolate reductase, reducing folate availability, which is why pregnant women must exercise caution to prevent neural tube defects when taking AEDs. In contrast, Carbamazepine increases folate degradation, lowering folate levels in the blood and reducing overall folate bioavailability. Given these effects, monitoring folate levels and considering supplementation or alternative treatments, including folate in higher doses, may be crucial for optimizing neurological health in children with epilepsy.

Patrick's mother was determined to find an alternative to the treatment that wasn't working for her son. Patrick's poor response to lamictal may have been explained by his higher-than-normal need for folate due to having FRAAs, although lamictal in known to make seizures worse in Dravet's syndrome and is usually avoided as a treatment.. As his mom began to piece together the underlying abnormalities in his body with the help of the integrative specialist, she identified potential areas that could be treated. This set her on a journey to discover treatments that could improve Patrick's overall health and brain function, including leucovorin, mitochondrial support, and immunomodulation.

One thing is clear from examining the link between leucovorin and epilepsy: it has shown promising benefits in many cases of refractory epilepsy and may serve as a valuable adjunctive treatment for individuals struggling to gain seizure control, as demonstrated by Victor's and Patrick's inspiring stories.

CHAPTER 8.

Neuroinflammation

Background

Inflammation is the body's natural defense mechanism against injury and infection. It plays a critical role in recruiting immune cells to the affected area to fight pathogens and repair tissue damage. During this process, the body releases cytokines—signaling molecules that attract immune cells to the site. This response increases blood flow and makes blood vessels more permeable, resulting in swelling and warmth in the affected area. Once immune cells arrive, they work to eliminate harmful invaders and initiate tissue repair. Under normal circumstances, inflammation subsides as healing progresses.

However, different types of dysfunction in the immune system can lead to inappropriate or persistent inflammation. This can happen when the immune system fails to shut down the inflammatory response, leading to chronic inflammation. If the immune system does not effectively eliminate the threat, it may remain in a prolonged state of activation, causing further damage. Alternatively, the immune system may become overactive without a clear threat, triggering inflammation where it is not needed, as seen in autoimmune diseases.

Abnormal immune function has been implicated in various neurodevelopmental and psychiatric disorders, including two conditions known as Pediatric Autoimmune Neuropsychiatric Disorder Associated with Streptococcal Infections (PANDAS) and Pediatric Acute-onset Neuropsychiatric Syndrome (PANS).

PANDAS and PANS are both characterized by the sudden onset of neuropsychiatric symptoms, including tics, obsessive-compulsive disorder (OCD) symptoms, and/or food restriction. While the concept of infection-triggered neuropsychiatric disorders has existed for decades, the formal definition of PANDAS in 1998[123] and PANS in 2012[124] have helped expand research and clinical understanding of immune-related neuropsychiatric conditions in children. Unlike PANDAS, which specifically ties symptoms to Group A streptococcal infections, PANS encompasses a wider range of triggers, including viral infections, immune dysfunction, metabolic disturbances, and environmental factors.

Both PANS and PANDAS can fall under the category of autoimmune encephalopathy, a condition in which the immune system mistakenly attacks the brain, often leading to neuroinflammation and dysfunction. This immune response frequently involves antibodies targeting brain tissue, much like how folate receptor autoantibodies (FRAAs) bind to folate receptor alpha. While the specific autoantibodies and immune targets in these disorders may vary—and many are likely yet to be identified—the resulting brain inflammation and neurological dysfunction contribute to cognitive, behavioral, and motor impairments.

Similarly, another condition involving inflammation within the central nervous system (CNS) is Multiple Sclerosis (MS). MS is a chronic illness caused by the immune system mistakenly attacking nerve fibers. In MS, the protective covering of nerve fibers, called myelin, becomes inflamed and damaged, disrupting the transmission of nerve signals. Symptoms can vary widely but often include muscle weakness, difficulty walking, vision problems, and cognitive changes.

PANS, PANDAS, and MS are examples of conditions involving a dysregulated immune system that leads to CNS inflammation. Understanding the mechanisms behind immune system dysregulation is crucial for developing effective treatments that reduce inflammation and restore proper function in the brain and nervous system.

The Scientific Evidence

Folate plays a role in initiating and maintaining the body's inflammatory response.[125] Low folate levels are commonly found in chronic inflammatory diseases and worsening inflammation. This can lead to damage in the brain, immune system, liver, gastrointestinal tract, and blood vessels, and may also exacerbate inflammation caused by infections.[126]

Given that folate deficiency is commonly seen in chronic inflammation, some researchers have proposed that it may be involved in the pathogenesis of inflammation.[127] In fact, emerging evidence suggests a strong link between folate deficiency and inflammation, particularly within the nervous system. While the direct causal relationship between folate deficiency and neuroinflammation remains uncertain, a number of studies have linked folate deficiency to worsening neurological dysfunction.

A rodent study demonstrated that folate deficiency exacerbates inflammation and activates microglia (the brain's inflammatory cells) following brain injury caused by ischemia.[128,129] Similarly, a zebrafish model showed that folate deficiency not only reduced levels of neurotransmitters like dopamine and serotonin, affecting learning and memory, but also led to neuroinflammation.[130]

Inflammation is often assessed using biomarkers such as C-reactive protein (CRP), homocysteine, and tumor necrosis factor alpha (TNF-α). CRP is a protein produced in the liver in response to inflammation, infection, and tissue damage. Homocysteine is a key amino acid which serves as an intermediary in many biochemical processes involving methylation, control of deleterious reactive compounds, and detoxification. Both high and low levels of homocysteine are concerning for neurological health, which is why it is an important indicator neurological function. TNF-α is a proinflammatory cytokine that plays a key role in immune system regulation, inflammation, and cellular apoptosis (programmed cell death). Studies investigating the role of folate in inflammation often measure these biomarkers to understand how folate influences immune function.

Research indicates that folate and vitamin B12 supplementation may help reduce inflammation during pregnancy and could be a potential treatment for vascular disease. In individuals with type 2 diabetes, folic acid supplementation has been shown to lower levels of CRP, homocysteine, and TNF-α compared to a placebo group.[131] However, a meta-analysis on folate's impact on inflammation found that folate significantly improved only one inflammatory marker, CRP, but not others like TNF-α.[132]

Dr. Quadros and Dr. Ramaekers, two of the leading researchers credited with uncovering the pathogenesis of Cerebral Folate Deficiency (CFD), published a case report linking CFD to elevated inflammatory markers in the brain of a girl with mitochondrial disease.[133] Their findings provide further evidence of the connection between folate metabolism, mitochondrial dysfunction, and neuroinflammation.

While it remains unclear whether folate deficiency can directly cause neuroinflammation, it certainly appears to exacerbate the condition. Importantly, it also indicates that folate plays a vital role in controlling inflammation.

PATIENT STORIES

Daniel

Daniel's medical journey is highly complex, marked by rare genetic factors, unusual lab results, and atypical symptoms, including gastrointestinal issues and vision changes.

As a young child, he was diagnosed with Autism Spectrum Disorder (ASD), experiencing severe speech, cognitive, and motor delays. However, now as a teenager, many of his ASD symptoms have disappeared, and his vision has been fully restored. Today, he is a highly independent and capable high school student, excelling both academically and in extracurricular activities.

His remarkable recovery has been truly inspiring. As a unique addition to this book, Daniel shares his own first-hand account of his experiences growing up with ASD. Paired with his mother's perspective, his story offers a rare and invaluable glimpse into the world of ASD and CFD from both a patient and caregiver standpoint.

Daniel's Story
By Daniel's Mom

Our son faced some challenges from birth, including low muscle tone, reflux, and constipation. Around 7 months old, he began having difficulty breathing and seemed unusually fatigued. By the time he was a year old, we noticed he wasn't playing with toys in the typical way.

When he was 15 to 18 months old, we observed that his left eye started turning inward toward his nose. He would repetitively open and close toy bus doors or spin wheels in his hand. The doctor prescribed glasses with bifocals and recommended patching his eye. We were hopeful that this would address the issue and explain his lack of eye contact and fixations.

At his 2-year pediatrician visit, I shared my concerns about his development, including the fact that he wasn't playing with toys or walking like most children his age. However, the pediatrician reassured me to wait and give it more time. By the time he was 3 ½ years old, he was evaluated by the local early intervention team. The results showed that our son was in the 18th percentile for speech, had an IQ of 65, and was at least two years behind in gross and fine motor skills. We were told he had autism, and we immediately began intensive therapies to address his delays.

Our son experienced significant stomach pain, along with bouts of diarrhea, constipation, and gastroesophageal reflux. After seeking a second opinion, we discovered several issues, including a homozygous MTHFR polymorphism that affected his ability to metabolize folate.

He soon began a milk-free and gluten-free diet, along with methylfolate and subcutaneous B12 injections. A few weeks later, my husband called me at work to tell me that our son had found some markers and was drawing all over the carpet and walls. We were ecstatic because he had never drawn anything before. Shortly afterward, his preschool teacher called to tell us he had started drawing at school and was interacting much better with his peers.

PATIENT STORIES

Over the next few months, his occupational and physical therapists told us he was making so much progress that he would soon graduate from their program. His eye doctor also shared that his visual acuity had improved from 20/175 to 20/70 during this time. One day, while we were out for a family walk, our son pointed to the sky and asked, "What is that?" We finally realized he was pointing at the sun. He then told us he had never seen the sun before.

When our son was 5 years old, we took him to see Dr. Richard Frye, who recommended starting leucovorin and increasing his dosages of carnitine and B12. We saw significant improvements after making these changes. By the time he was 6 years of age, his vision had improved to 20/30, and his eye doctor informed us that he had developed full depth perception and peripheral vision. The possibility of our son driving a car one day, something we had never thought possible, became a real hope.

We continued seeing Dr. Frye annually and conducted follow-up testing at each visit. After one round of testing, Dr. Frye determined that our son needed an increased leucovorin dose. As his medication dosages were adjusted, his vision improved to 20/20, and his auditory processing issues, which had been a struggle, were no longer a problem. By age 8, Daniel was greeting people when they came to our home. I vividly remember the first time he greeted my mom on New Year's Day—he ran out to her car to say hello and asked if she needed help carrying anything. That same day, he came up to me and said, "I love you, Mom," for the very first time, and he gave me my first kiss. I never imagined I'd hear those words.

He also started attending a new school, and during parent-teacher conferences, we were amazed to learn that our son had become one of the most outgoing kids in the entire school. No longer the withdrawn child making unintelligible sounds, he began asking people how their day was going and even offered to help when a classmate got hurt on the playground.

At the age of 12, during the pandemic, our son used his 3D printer to make masks for first responders. He continued expanding his circle of friends, meeting virtually for Minecraft sessions or getting together in the community. He built dozens of remote-controlled planes, with wingspans ranging from 3 to 10 feet, and at age 14 years, he earned his FAA license to fly remote-controlled planes. He also started taking guitar lessons, and we began doing annual recitals several times a year. Last year, he played and sang Christmas songs for Santa at a community event, and he surprised his grandmother by singing "Merry Christmas" to shoppers at Costco. The sensory overload at Costco is immense, and it was incredibly humbling to see how far he had come—from a child who used to sit in a corner spinning wheels for hours to singing "Feliz Navidad" to a crowd of holiday shoppers.

We are deeply grateful for the blessing of Dr. Frye and his groundbreaking research, which has transformed our son's life. Without Dr. Frye, I might still have a child sitting in a corner, endlessly opening and closing a toy bus door, disconnected from the world around him.

How Leucovorin Helped Me

An essay by Daniel in his own words

Before I was cured of autism, school was impossible. I was crying every day before even leaving the house. I had no friends. Instead, during recess I would invite teachers to play train with me around the gymnasium. Impossibly enough, I couldn't follow the instructions from the teacher when she asked me to either think about the topic to write from a given instruction, or to write in general.

Writing was often difficult since I would forget how each letter of the alphabet or even numbers were supposed to be written. For example, I would often write the number nine, the letter Z, or the letter N backwards. After school hours, there was nothing fun to do when I returned home. I had zero hobbies! Instead, I would talk about what I was interested in at the time, trains.

Seeing the world was different for me. My left eye turned in which made it rather strenuous for my mom to help me look straight. In addition to that I had tunnel vision, seeing was difficult peripherally. Also, I would see weird objects sometimes looking like creatures that weren't there. They would only last for about a second per object. Most of the non-real objects were seen in my peripheral vision.

When I was much younger, about three or four years of age, I couldn't point at things or ask for what I wanted or even needed. Part of the issue with asking for what I wanted was the ability to multitask. To the average person asking for something should be rather easy since it could be something of value or something that the person wants. Even if the room was isolated from the outside world, it still was impossible for me to do. I couldn't point, speak, or even look at what I wanted. It clearly showed my inability to multitask and that I was barely able to do one simple thing. I couldn't ask for something which was a task.

Often, I wouldn't have many feelings towards anything rewarding or positive in general. The only thing that felt positive to me at the time was sitting in a corner and spinning the wheels on a toy bus all day. Why did it feel positive you may ask? Probably because there were too many things making me upset in the room like loud noises or even the lighting. Doing something that took my mind off of the things that were making me upset often helped even if it meant that I would have to constantly do that thing thousands of times, which was oddly satisfying and rewarding.

Some things that bothered me, often resulting in meltdowns or sitting in the corner, were loud places, walking on grass barefoot, all kinds of bugs with legs including butterflies, music and noises. Loud places and walking on grass often resulted in meltdowns in the beginning. Taking a shower also bothered me from the loud noise and the feeling from the small jets on the shower wand. Most of the time it would feel like I was about to fall off a cliff; sometimes I felt angry or just in general scared. The only thing that still bothers me today are bugs. When I encounter them, I felt like I am going to fall off a cliff. So far, an electric bug zapper, or bug assault gun which uses table salt to kill them, made me feel better.

My parents took me to see Dr. Frye when I was five years old. He prescribed leucovorin. After a couple of years, I started getting better. I'm now a straight A student in every subject except biology. I can write enormous paragraphs such as what you're reading right now. The biggest essay I've ever written so far is a ten-paragraph essay. I can ask for extremely specific things for my birthday. I am excellent at math, and I taught the entire algebra-one class for a day.

For extracurricular activities and hobbies, I play guitar, design, and print parts with my 3D printer, build and fly remote control planes at an airfield with fifty other men, and take care of a thirty-two-gallon aquarium. I am a member of the Capitol Area Flyers which is the airfield I go to.

I have fifteen airplanes with roughly a third of them that I built. I have 3D printed masks for first responders during the height of Covid. I have both a Minecraft server and Discord server which now has fifteen friends. In addition to the hobbies listed I can often do two to three hobbies a day on top of school! I went from nothing to five hobbies!

A Physician's Perspective

Daniel is a remarkable patient with a continually evolving medical journey, exemplifying the complexities of multisystem dysfunction. When I first met Daniel, I was intrigued by his exceptional response to treatments such as methylfolate and mitochondrial supplements, which led me to suspect CFD. To further investigate, we proceeded with a lumbar puncture to gather more information

The results confirmed that his cerebrospinal fluid (CSF) had below-normal levels of 5-MTHF, supporting a CFD diagnosis. Additionally, we identified oligoclonal bands, a marker of inflammation. The presence of these bands indicates autoantibody production within the central nervous system (CNS)—an abnormal immune response that should not occur, further highlighting the immune dysfunction underlying his condition.

The CNS is typically off-limits to the immune system, except for specialized immune cells called microglia, which are unique to the CNS. Oligoclonal bands, markers of inflammation, are often seen in conditions like multiple sclerosis, where the immune system invades the CNS and damages the brain and spinal cord.

However, Daniel did not have multiple sclerosis, as his brain's MRI scan was normal. This suggested that another inflammatory process was involved. We tested Daniel's CSF for a panel of known autoantibodies that target the brain but found no conclusive results. The cause of the inflammation in his brain remained unknown.

While Daniel responded well to leucovorin, he still exhibited many ASD symptoms, and his eyesight had not fully recovered. Given the inflammation indicated by the oligoclonal bands in his CSF, our team decided to try intravenous immunoglobulin (IVIG) therapy to modulate his immune response.

IVIG is essentially a collection of antibodies from donors that helps to calm an overactive immune system, especially when harmful autoantibodies are present. It works in two ways: first, by binding to and eliminating harmful autoantibodies, and second, by interacting with immune cells to reduce their activity. Unlike other treatments that suppress the immune system's ability to fight off infections, IVIG also provides protective antibodies, making it a safer option for managing immune-related issues.

With both leucovorin and IVIG, Daniel made remarkable progress, which continues to this day. Although we attempted to discontinue IVIG, the results were less than ideal, so it has remained part of a long-term treatment plan.

Despite his improvements, the underlying cause of his inflammation, CFD, and apparent mitochondrial dysfunction remained unclear. To investigate further, we conducted a detailed genetic analysis called trio whole exome sequencing (WES). This test examines every known gene by reading the letters in the exome, the critical part of each gene. Since humans have about 23,000 genes, and each gene contains roughly a 50,000 letters, the test analyzes an astounding 1.1 billion letters!

To improve accuracy, the test also analyzes genetic samples from both parents, allowing us to distinguish inherited variations from potentially significant mutations unique to Daniel that could help explain his condition. These spontaneous genetic changes are known as de novo mutations—a term derived from Latin, meaning "from the beginning" or "anew."

Since de novo mutations arise spontaneously, without being inherited from either parent, they can provide crucial insights into the underlying cause of a condition. In Daniel's case, one particularly notable variation was identified in a gene that plays a key role in the cell's internal transport system, potentially impacting its function in a meaningful way.

Daniel's Complicated Story Comes Together

Daniel had remained a mystery for a long time, but WES provided new insights. Working with other genetic specialists, we identified the genetic mutation that is key to his condition. This gene is responsible for making tiny "motors" within cells, which are especially important in nerve cells. These motors transport essential components, such as mitochondria, to where they are needed. In nerve cells, this process is crucial because mitochondria and other vital parts must be moved along the axon—the long "wire" that connects one nerve cell to another.

At the end of the axon is the synapse, where neurotransmitters are released to communicate with other nerve cells. Neither the axons nor the synapses can produce mitochondria on their own, so these motors must carry mitochondria from the cell body, down the axon, to the synapse. If the motors fail to do their job, worn-out mitochondria at the end of the axon cannot be replaced. As a result, the axons and synapses experience mitochondrial dysfunction—not because the mitochondria are faulty, but because they are unable to be replenished.

Figure 8.1 illustrates the internal transportation system that moves mitochondria within nerve cells. The synapse, located at the end of a neuron, sends signals to the next neuron and is connected to the neuron's body by a long structure called the axon. Since the axon and synapse have limited ability to perform cell maintenance, they rely on the neuron's body for essential tasks like producing new cellular components, including mitochondria. To maintain proper function, cellular resources must be transported from the neuron's body down the axon to the synapse through a process called anterograde transport. Meanwhile, worn-out components at the synapse are returned to the cell body via retrograde transport for recycling or disposal.

This movement occurs along a structural "track" in the axon known as the microtubule, on which small motor proteins called kinesins travel. These motors require energy in the form of ATP, which is produced by mitochondria. If mitochondrial function is compromised or the kinesin proteins are faulty, the transport system can fail, preventing the axon and synapse from receiving new cellular parts and efficiently removing waste, leading to dysfunction.

Understanding how the microtubule transport system works and how it can fail sheds light on Daniel's condition. As his mother explained, Daniel had motor delays. As he got older, he had difficulty walking and sometimes experienced such physical fatigue that he needed a wheelchair. He also struggled with vision problems. When a cell's internal transport system breaks down, the longest nerve cells are typically the most affected, as they have the greatest distance between the nerve cell body and the synapse. These include the nerves that control the legs as they are farthest from the motor cortex and require two very long neurons to transmit a neuronal signal for the legs to move.

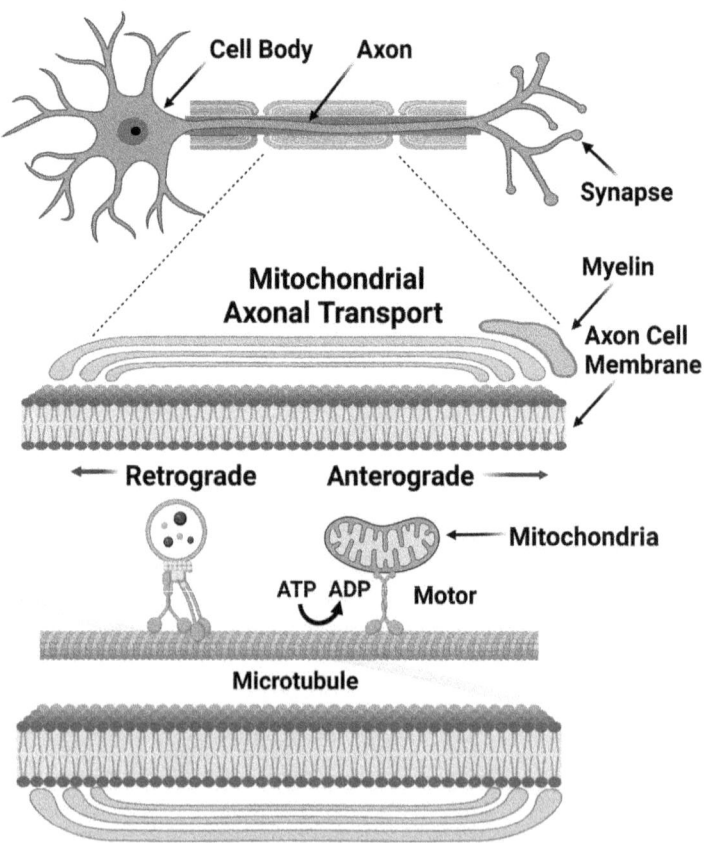

Figure 8.1 Motors of a Nerve Cell. Image created with BioRender.

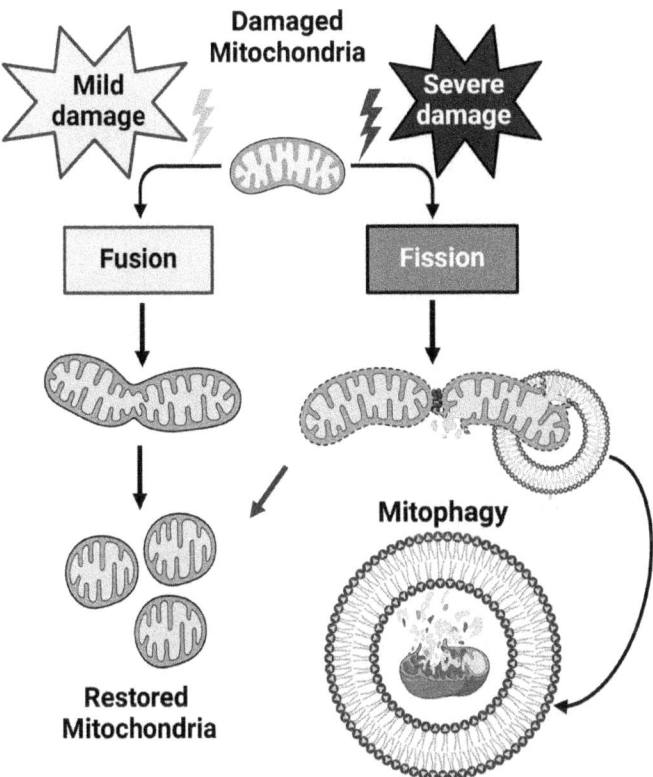

Figure 8.2 Self-restoration of mitochondrial function. Image created with BioRender.

While the optic nerves connecting the retina to the brain are not particularly long, they are constantly active, processing visual information from the environment. This high activity demands substantial energy and frequent mitochondrial repair and replacement. If damaged mitochondria at the synapses aren't replaced efficiently, the optic nerves can't function properly, which could explain Daniel's vision issues.

Cells have the ability to repair mitochondria to keep them functioning optimally. If a mitochondrion is mildly damaged (as shown on the left side of the Figure 8.2), it can fuse with a healthy mitochondrion to form a functional unit. This repaired mitochondrion can then divide to produce several fully functioning mitochondria. However, if a mitochondrion is severely damaged (as shown on the right side of Figure 8.2), it can isolate the dysfunctional portion through a process called fission. The damaged part is then targeted for removal through a process called mitophagy, where it is engulfed by a phagosome. The phagosome digests the dysfunctional portion, recycling its components. The remaining healthy part of the mitochondrion can then form a fully functional mitochondrion again.

While these repair and recycling processes are effective, they have limitations. Essentially, mildly damaged mitochondria can be repaired through fusion, or their dysfunctional parts can be removed through mitophagy. After repair, healthy mitochondria divide to form new ones. However, when no healthy mitochondria are available for fusion, or the damage is too severe, these processes are insufficient to replenish mitochondrial function.

Worn-out mitochondria generate excessive oxidative radicals, leading to damage and inflammation. This inflammation, in turn, worsens mitochondrial dysfunction, creating a vicious cycle of oxidative stress, inflammation, and further mitochondrial dysfunction.

The harmful triad of oxidative stress, mitochondrial dysfunction, and inflammation creates a self-reinforcing cycle that leads to progressive cellular damage and dysfunction. This cycle can be triggered by any one of these abnormalities. For instance, mitochondrial dysfunction can generate oxidative stress and activate immune responses through various mechanisms. When mitochondria are impaired, they release damage-associated molecular pattern molecules (DAMPs), which in turn activate inflammatory pathways.

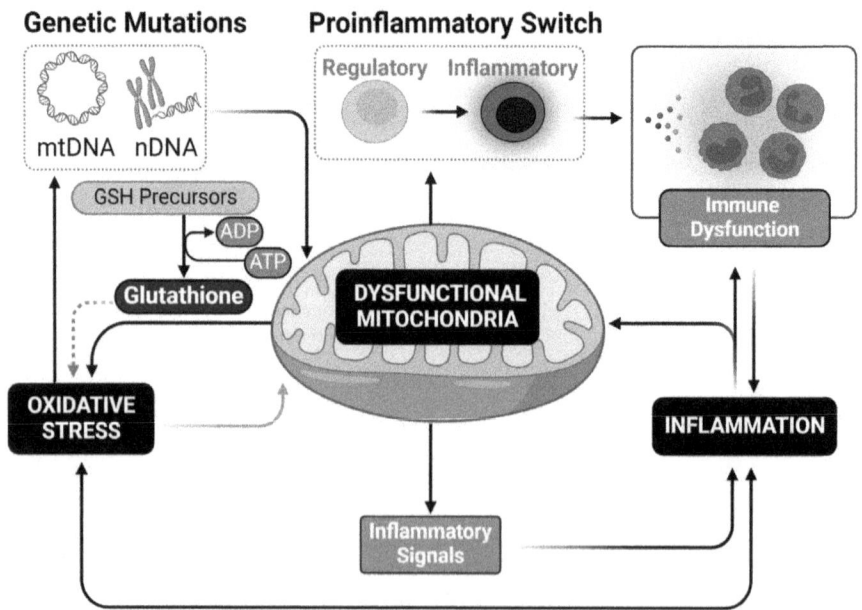

Figure 8.3 The Terrible Trio: Oxidative Stress, Inflammation, and Mitochondrial Dysfunction. Adapted from Frye et al.[138] Created with BioRender.

Because regulatory immune cells rely heavily on proper mitochondrial function, mitochondrial dysfunction can make it difficult to regulate immune responses. Inflammation further exacerbates the problem by releasing signals that suppress mitochondrial activity. Meanwhile, mitochondrial dysfunction causes oxidative stress and inflammation, which damages lipids, proteins, and genetic material. This damage not only activates more inflammatory pathways but also leads to further cellular dysfunction. To make matters worse, the molecule responsible for neutralizing reactive species that cause oxidative stress, glutathione, requires energy to be produced. As a result, mitochondrial dysfunction leads to reduced glutathione production, leaving the cell with less capacity to control damaging reactive species and worsening the vicious cycle.

Recall that Daniel's CSF and laboratory tests also indicated that he was experiencing inflammation, and he responded well to leucovorin, which treated his CNS folate deficiency.

Cerebral Folate Deficiency and Neuroinflammation

Recall the earlier studies cited in this chapter linking folate to neuroinflammation. Daniel was another example of this phenomenon by testing positive for both CFD and oligoclonal bands in his CSF.

Many patients come to my clinic seeking treatment for PANS, often because they have not fully responded to standard, immune-based treatments. A significant number of these patients test positive for folate receptor autoantibodies (FRAAs) and show improvement with leucovorin therapy.

In a recent study, we found that approximately 63% of children with PANS, as well as its related condition PANDAS, tested positive for FRAAs.[134] Like PANS and PANDAS, CFD can also present abruptly and may involve movement disorders such as tics. In cases where CFD leads to ASD, repetitive, OCD-like behaviors may also occur. The reason for the overlap between these conditions is not entirely clear, but it is believed that the production of FRAAs stems from an immune system abnormality.

Additional evidence comes from other inflammatory conditions as well. As explained earlier in the chapter, MS is an inflammatory disease of the central nervous system caused by the demyelination of nerve fibers. When the condition worsens, then subsides, and later reappears in episodes known as "flare-ups," it is referred to as Relapsing-Remitting Multiple Sclerosis (RRMS).

Interestingly, a 2024 Iranian study found that approximately 85% of adults with RRMS tested positive for folate receptor alpha autoantibodies (FRAAs) — a significantly higher percentage compared to a healthy control population.[135]

Like with PANS and PANDAS, it is not known why individuals with these inflammatory conditions test positive for FRAAs at such a high rate; however, in the case of MS, it is thought that folate deficiencies in the CNS may play a role in the breakdown of myelin integrity.

Daniel's case, along with many of the PANS and PANDAS cases I encounter, as well as other neuroinflammatory conditions, often show significant overlap with CFD when fully evaluated.

One condition that illustrates this connection is Acute Cerebellar Ataxia, a childhood disorder characterized by unsteadiness, slurred speech, and abnormal eye movements (nystagmus). It most commonly follows a viral illness, such as chickenpox (varicella). In most cases, the condition is benign, with children making a quick and complete recovery within a few weeks. A CSF examination may show mild inflammation, and brain MRI scans can reveal slight cerebellar inflammation.

Although typically self-limiting, I have encountered two cases where patients did not recover as expected. In both instances, CSF analysis revealed below-normal levels of 5-MTHF, indicating CFD. One case was particularly severe: a child who had been developmentally typical before illness experienced dramatic regression, becoming mute and losing the ability to move their arms and legs.

After spending several weeks in a rehabilitation unit with minimal progress, an LP confirmed low 5-MTHF levels in the CSF, leading to a trial of leucovorin treatment. The response was remarkable—the child began improving rapidly in therapy, and within a few months, they were running, talking, and engaging as a typical child once again.

CFD has been linked to other inflammatory syndromes as well. Aicardi-Goutières syndrome, a genetic neurodegenerative disorder of childhood, triggers immune system activation and leads to neuroinflammation. Diagnostic findings for this disorder often include elevated inflammatory markers and low 5-MTHF concentrations in the CSF.[136]

Additionally, non-neurological inflammatory conditions, such as juvenile rheumatoid arthritis, have also been associated with CFD.[137] This is particularly intriguing because in a published case, a young patient with juvenile arthritis exhibited cognitive and motor difficulties, which are not typically seen in arthritis.

Many inflammatory conditions, such as lupus, are well-documented to have neurological and psychiatric manifestations. Given the link between CFD and inflammation, testing for FRAAs or low 5-MTHF levels in the CSF when cognitive symptoms arise alongside non-neurological autoimmune conditions could help uncover a broader role for CFD in inflammatory disorders. This is also a promising area of research, as both published case reports and my own clinical experience suggest that leucovorin treatment has led to remarkable improvements in many patients with primary inflammatory disorders. Further investigation into this connection could open new therapeutic possibilities for individuals with neuroinflammatory complications of autoimmune diseases and inflammatory disorders.

CHAPTER 9.
GENETIC DISORDERS

Background

The idea that living organisms inherit traits across generations has fascinated people for centuries. However, it wasn't until 1865 that Gregor Mendel, an Austrian monk, conducted scientific studies on pea plants to understand the mathematical principles of inheritance. By cross-breeding plants with different characteristics, Mendel uncovered that traits can be dominant or recessive, and he calculated the likelihood of these traits appearing in future generations. The principles he discovered, known as Mendelian inheritance, remain foundational in genetics today. Mendelian inheritance is based on the idea that a single gene controls each trait.

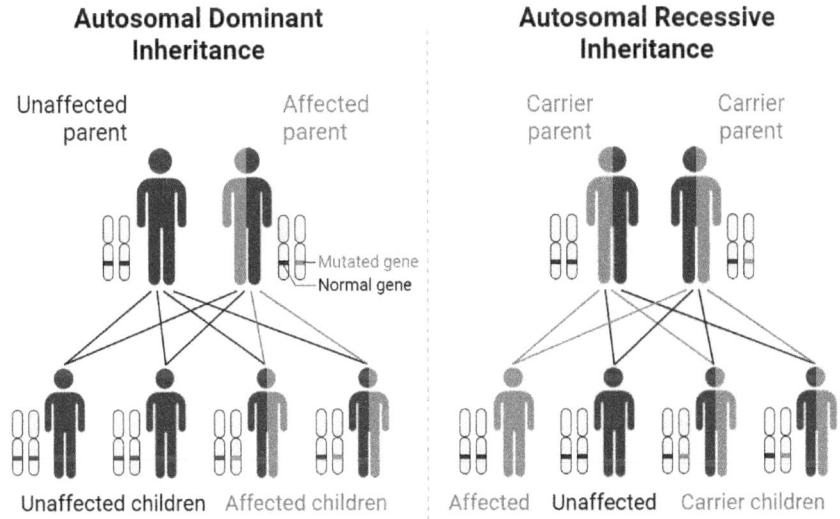

Figure 9.1 Inheriting a disorder through Mendelian Inheritance. Image created with BioRender.

Humans have 22 pairs of chromosomes and one pair of sex chromosomes, all of which carry our genes. Each chromosome has one copy of a gene, so most genes are present in two copies—one from each parent. An exception occurs in males, whose sex chromosomes (X and Y) are different and do not always carry the same genes. In the case of a dominant disorder, only one copy of the gene is needed to express the trait. This means that an affected parent has a 50% chance of passing the gene to each child since each parent randomly contributes one of their two chromosomes. Children who do not inherit the dominant gene will neither display the trait nor be carriers. It is rare for severe diseases to be inherited in a dominant manner because individuals with severe conditions are less likely to reproduce, limiting the disease's transmission over time.

Conversely, a recessive disorder requires two copies of the gene for the trait to manifest. In recessive inheritance, both parents are carriers and may be unaware they possess the gene, especially if it's a rare trait in the population. In such cases, there is a 25% chance that a child will inherit the disorder, a 50% chance they will be carriers, and a 25% chance they will be unaffected and non-carriers. Many inherited disorders are recessive because carriers often do not show symptoms, allowing the gene to persist silently within the population. There are also unique patterns of inheritance for disorders linked to genes on the sex chromosomes, which will not be covered here.

While the mathematics of inheritance began to be elucidated by Mendel, the exact mechanisms of genetic information storage remained a mystery until 1953, when James Watson and Francis Crick discovered the double-helix structure of DNA at the University of Cambridge. A decade later, scientists began to understand how DNA's four chemical bases work together to encode genetic information. The field of genetics took a monumental step forward in the 1990s with the launch of the Human Genome Project, an international effort to map the entire human genome. Completed in 2003, the project not only mapped the genome but also spurred the creation of technology that could read the genome with higher fidelity and speed. Today, genetic research has advanced to the point where a person's entire genome can be mapped in just a few weeks (or days if needed urgently).

This process is now commonly used to investigate disorders with unclear origins, including many neurodevelopmental disorders. In the past, many genetic disorders were identified by distinct physical features. However, as more genetic disorders are discovered, we are finding that many lack obvious physical characteristics, making genetic testing increasingly vital for an accurate diagnosis.

When a gene is identified, one of the key questions is understanding its role in the body. A gene provides the code for a specific protein, which in turn has a unique function. However, this function is not always immediately clear. While many genes associated with neurodevelopmental disorders might be expected to code for brain-specific proteins, this isn't always the case.

For instance, the neurological symptoms seen in CFD can stem from mutations in the FOLR1 gene, which is involved in folate transport rather than being specific to brain function. Often, it takes extensive research to determine the exact function of a gene and how it contributes to the associated disorder.

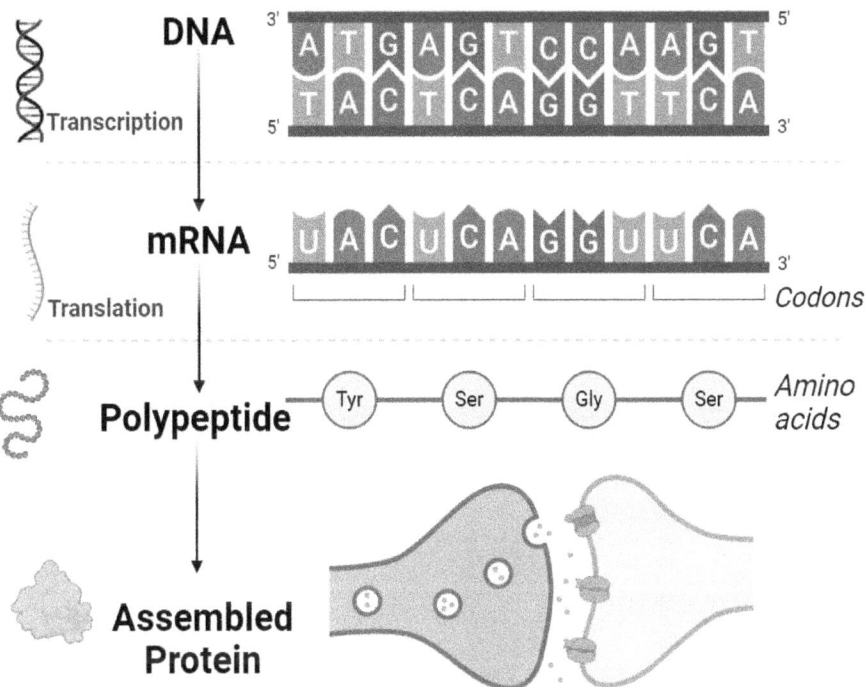

Figure 9.2 The genetic code functions as the body's instruction manual, stored in the form of DNA on our chromosomes. DNA consists of four chemical bases—Adenine (A), Thymine (T), Guanine (G) and Cytosine (C)—that pair up (A with T, and G with C). As shown in the figure, this pairing allows two DNA strands to fit together in a complementary way, which enhances the stability of the DNA molecule.

When the body needs specific instructions, the DNA strands separate, creating an intermediate messenger called RNA that carries a copy of the genetic code. In RNA, the bases A, T, G, and C from DNA are transcribed as A, U, G, and C, where Thymine (T) is replaced by Uracil (U).

This code is organized into sequences of three-letter groups called codons, with each codon representing one of the 20 amino acids the body uses. During the process of translation, the RNA sequence is decoded to assemble a long chain of amino acids, known as a polypeptide. This chain folds into a three-dimensional structure to form a protein, which can serve various functions, such as acting as an enzyme or as a receptor on a neuron for neurotransmitters. Image created with BioRender.

Numerous genetic disorders have been linked to CFD. For example, early research into CFD found an association with Rett syndrome, a neurodevelopmental disorder that primarily affects girls, despite no direct connection between the syndrome's genetic mutation. Throughout this section, several stories feature children with genetic disorders who are found to have CFD. Many other neurodevelopmental disorders also appear to be associated with CFD, which are explored in the following review.

The Scientific Evidence

Rett syndrome was one of the first genetic syndromes to be associated with CFD. It is caused by a mutation in the MECP2 gene, located on the X chromosome. While Rett syndrome is most commonly diagnosed in females, males can also have this gene mutation. However, because males have only one X chromosome, the presentation of the condition is typically much more severe and often fatal in early life. In females, who have two X chromosomes, the impact of the MECP2 mutation is more variable due to X-inactivation, which affects the level of expression of the mutated gene versus the normal MECP2 gene on the other X chromosome.

Infants with Rett syndrome typically develop normally during the first months of life, but after the first year, they begin to lose previously acquired skills. For example, a young child with Rett syndrome may lose speech and motor abilities, with the loss of purposeful hand movements being one of the hallmark symptoms of the condition.

The link between Rett syndrome and CFD was initially reported in a few isolated cases in Europe.[139] A case series from Spain involving 16 Rett syndrome patients found that most exhibited low 5-MTHF concentrations in their CSF, and many responded well to leucovorin treatment.[140] This study suggested that CFD may be a problem in a majority of patients wtih Rett syndrome.

But the relationship between Rett and CFD became less clear as more studies were published. A group of physicians in the United States published a report indicating that only two out of 76 females with Rett syndrome had low 5-MTHF levels in their CSF.[141] Three years later, Dr. Ramaekers in Europe reported on a series of 33 Rett syndrome patients, with 42% showing low 5-MTHF concentrations in their CSF and 24% testing positive for FRAAs.[142]

Two years after that, researchers in Portugal found that 32% of 25 patients with Rett syndrome had low 5-MTHF levels in their CSF; however, they observed no clinical improvement with leucovorin treatment.[143] To explain the wide variation in results, Dr. Ramaekers suggested that higher folate levels in the CSF of Rett syndrome patients in the United States might be due to food folate fortification in

North America (discussed in Chapter 2). Since the 1990s, the FDA has required that grain products produced in the U.S. (such as bread, pasta, rice, and cereal) be fortified with 140 mcg of folic acid per 100 grams of grain.[144]

Another genetic syndrome associated with CFD is STXBP1. Mutations in this gene can disrupt neurotransmitter regulation at synapses in the brain. The first story in this book introduced Caroline, a young girl with this mutation. Caroline experienced severe seizures and developmental delays, which are common among children with this genetic disorder. For many years, Caroline responded well to high-dose leucovorin, which helped her overcome many motor and cognitive challenges during treatment. While leucovorin did not control her seizures, it did improve her quality of life.

Caroline is not alone in benefiting from leucovorin. Other children with STXBP1 mutations have also reported symptom improvement with this treatment. For example, doctors in Hong Kong reported a case of an infant with an STXBP1 mutation and Ohtahara syndrome, a severe seizure disorder, who similarly responded well to leucovorin treatment.[145]

While the STXBP1 gene is not directly involved in folate metabolism, other genetic disorders have a more direct link to CFD. The first reported case of a child with a SLC46A1 gene mutation occurred in China. This mutation impacts the proton-coupled folate transporter (PCFT) which is responsible for transporting folate from the gut into the body and across the blood-brain barrier. The child began experiencing seizures at three years old, followed by neurodevelopmental regression, muscle weakness, and sleep problems by age five.[146] Examination of the child's CSF revealed undetectable levels of 5-MTHF. Treatment with leucovorin led to rapid improvement. Similar cases involving PCFT-related mutations were reported in India[147] and the United States.[148]

Another case of a folate-related genetic mutation involved 14-year-old who developed progressive myoclonic epilepsy, neurodevelopmental regression, intractable seizures, weakness, and ataxia who was found to have compound heterozygous mutations in the MTHFR gene.[149] These mutations lead to a reduced ability to produce 5-MTHF in the folate cycle, potentially contributing to decreased folate levels in the central nervous system. Treatment with leucovorin, betaine, and methionine resulted in significant clinical improvement, as well as improvement on the EEG.

It is important to note that this patient had genetic mutations in her MTHFR gene, which is different than having polymorphisms. (Polymorphisms of MTHFR are discussed in Chapter 3). Mutations, which are rare, tend to cause permanent alternation in the genetic sequence that may cause significant disruptions in the enzyme function, leading to much more dramatic presentations than what is typically seen with polymorphisms.

We are learning that many patients with CFD have underlying genetic mutations. Examples include those with mitochondrial disorders such as Alpers syndrome, Kearns-Sayre syndrome (KSS), Leigh syndrome, Neuropathy-Ataxia-Retinitis Pigmentosa (NARP) syndrome, and Mitochondrial Encephalomyopathy Lactic Acidosis and Stroke-like episodes (MELAS). These conditions have been associated with both ASD and CFD, and many patients with these disorders have responded to leucovorin treatment.[150, 151]

The following chart describes some of the other genetic conditions that have been associated with CFD. This is not an exhaustive list, but rather a representation of the diverse genetic conditions in which patients have presented with CFD. Unraveling how genetic mutations affect the human body is a highly complex process, as mutations often do not exhibit a direct, linear connection to the symptoms observed.

Some Genetic Conditions Associated with CFD	Symptoms
Alpers syndrome Also known as Alpers-Huttenlocher syndrome. Often caused by mutations in the POLG gene, which is crucial for mitochondrial DNA replication.	A progressive neurodegenerative disorder that typically appears in infancy or early childhood. Alpers syndrome is characterized by severe seizures, developmental regression, liver dysfunction, and psychomotor retardation. Symptoms can include ataxia (loss of coordination), muscle weakness, and loss of cognitive function.
CASK-Related Disorders Typically caused by mutations in the calcium/calmodulin-dependent serine protein kinase (CASK) gene located on the X chromosome.	A mutation the impacts brain development and function. Symptoms include microcephaly, underdevelopment of the brainstem, developmental delays and movement disorders, seizures, nystagmus or other vision problems, and sensorineural hearing loss.
Dravet syndrome Typically caused by mutations in the SCN1A gene, which provides instructions for producing a sodium channel protein necessary for proper neuron function.	A progressive and severe form of epilepsy that generally begins in infancy, triggered by a fever. It affects cognitive, motor, and behavioral development leading to ASD-like traits. Ataxia, gait abnormalities, poor growth, sleep disturbances and scoliosis impact some children.
Kearns-Sayre Syndrome (KSS) Typically caused by large deletions in mitochondrial DNA.	A mitochondrial disorder that often presents before age 20 and affects multiple systems in the body, particularly the eyes and muscles. Symptoms include progressive external ophthalmoplegia (paralysis of the eye muscles), ptosis (drooping eyelids), retinal degeneration, cardiac conduction defects, and muscle weakness. Other symptoms can include hearing loss, kidney problems, and endocrine issues like diabetes.

Leigh syndrome (LS) Also known as Leigh disease or subacute necrotizing encephalomyelopathy. Caused by mutations in either mitochondrial DNA or nuclear DNA that impair mitochondrial energy production. A common gene associated with Leigh syndrome is SURF1.	A severe neurological disorder that usually presents in infancy or early childhood. Symptoms often begin with developmental delays, poor muscle tone, vomiting, and irritability. As the disease progresses, symptoms may include ataxia (loss of coordination), seizures, difficulty swallowing, breathing problems, and involuntary eye movements. LS primarily affects the brainstem and basal ganglia, causing progressive neurological decline.
Mitochondrial Encephalomyopathy Lactic Acidosis and Stroke-like episodes (MELAS) Commonly caused by mutations in the maternally inherited MT-TL1 gene in mitochondrial DNA, which affects mitochondrial protein synthesis and energy production.	Elevated lactic acid levels can lead to symptoms such as nausea, vomiting, muscle pain, fatigue, and shortness of breath. Common symptoms include seizures, headaches, difficulty with motor skills, and progressive cognitive decline. As the disease progresses, it can lead to significant neurological impairments. Stroke-like episodes can cause sudden muscle weakness, vision loss, severe headaches, seizures, and altered consciousness. Rate of progression and severity varies.
Neuropathy, Ataxia, and Retinitis Pigmentosa (NARP) Associated with a mutation in the MT-ATP6 gene in mDNA, which affects the production of ATP, the cell's main energy molecule.	A mitochondrial disorder that primarily affects the nervous system and retina. Symptoms typically appear in adolescence or early adulthood and include peripheral neuropathy (nerve damage), ataxia, and retinitis pigmentosa, muscle weakness, learning disabilities, and hearing loss.
Rett Syndrome Caused by a mutation in the MECP2 gene. MECP2 is on the X chromosome and makes a protein critical for the development and function of the brain and nervous system.	Generally recognized between 6 to 18 months of life when impairments in the child's ability to speak, walk, eat, or breathe become pronounced. Rett syndrome has a hallmark trait of constant, repetitive hand movements and the loss of purposeful hand use.
SATB2-Associated Syndrome (SAS) A rare genetic disorder caused by mutations or deletions in the SATB2 gene. The SATB2 gene plays a crucial role in early development, particularly in the formation of the brain, bones, and facial structures.	SAS primarily affects neurological function and development, and can affect bone development, potentially leading to issues such as low bone density (osteopenia), distinctive facial features, or other skeletal and dental anomalies. Symptoms include speech and language delays, intellectual and developmental delays, ASD features, and feeding or growth issues.
STXBP1-Related Disorders Also known as STXBP1 Encephalopathy. The STXBP1 (syntaxin-binding protein 1) is a gene essential for neurotransmitter release and communication between neurons.	Individuals with STXBP1 mutations experience severe seizure disorders that can start in infancy and are often resistant to treatment. STXBP1 mutations are frequently associated with significant developmental delays, movement disorders, intellectual disabilities, ASD features, and motor skills (talking, walking, sitting).

PATIENT STORIES

Leland

Leland's story teaches us that children with genetic disorders are not doomed to the fate dictated by their condition. Leland has a rare congenital gene mutation that is associated with challenging symptoms such as speech delays and cognitive impairments, with many of the impacted children remaining non-verbal for life.

Thanks to the proactive approach of his mother, Leland's condition was explored more deeply, and leucovorin was introduced as a means of addressing his speech delays. He responded wonderfully and is now able to engage more fully in his community due to his new-found verbal abilities.

Leland's Story
By Katie, Leland's Mom

Leland is a bright and kind-hearted, 10 year-old boy who was born following a challenging pregnancy. During the first trimester, I experienced a subchorionic hemorrhage and illness involving the flu, accompanied by a fever. At 39 weeks, I developed HELLP syndrome, a severe pregnancy complication affecting the liver and blood, necessitating an emergency cesarean delivery. Thankfully, Leland was unaffected at birth, but I was separated from him for four days while recovering in the ICU.

From the start, Leland had feeding difficulties due to a weak latch and suckle. We supplemented breast milk the first four months, eventually transitioning fully to organic formula. He experienced colic and sleep disturbances during his first three months, but introducing a probiotic helped settle the colic and improve his sleep. By five months, he was a happy boy sleeping through the night. He was seldom ill but did experience adverse reactions to immunizations, including 106°F fever after each Pneumococcal vaccine.

Leland interacted well as an infant but babbled less than expected and met many milestones at the later-end of typical developmental stages. He favored his right hand, often clenching his left and repetitively rotated his wrists side-to-side like an orchestra conductor. When he began crawling, he used the back of his left hand instead of his palm. The lack of babbling and unusual inchworm-crawl were my first concerns about his development. Despite this, our pediatrician advised us not to worry.

By 18 months, he had acquired roughly 10 words but still did not point. Following a high fever from his last Pneumococcal vaccination at 19 months, Leland lost all speech, ceased making eye contact, and began displaying behavioral problems. Yet, our concerns remained dismissed, so we found a new pediatrician who referred us to a developmental specialist. Over the course of two years, Leland was evaluated for ASD but the specialist suspected a different condition and subsequently referred us to a neurologist.

PATIENT STORIES

By age three, Leland occasionally approximated a word but then did not use it again for months. He was unable to retain words until age four and consistent verbal communication only began around 5½ years old. The neurologist ordered an MRI, a 24-hour EEG, and whole exome sequencing. The MRI was normal, but the EEG detected seizures during sleep, and genetic testing revealed SATB2-Associated Syndrome (SAS).

In 2018, information on SAS was limited but we were able to enroll Leland in a clinical research registry. This confirmed his developmental and language delays were consistent with SAS, though the underlying mechanisms were unclear.

Throughout this time, we were proactive in seeking ways to support Leland. Since age two, he had been under the care of a holistic practitioner, who prescribed nutritional supplements, including folate, B12, and CBD, with noticeable improvements. Genetic testing also showed a heterozygous C677T MTHFR polymorphism, suggesting he could benefit from folate. This led me to research correlations between nutritional deficiencies and language delays, eventually discovering Dr. Frye's work with leucovorin.

With guidance from our holistic practitioner, we started Leland on a low dose of leucovorin. After two years of supplementation with some benefits, we suspected that a higher dose might yield better results. So we decided to consult Dr. Frye, a specialist in this area.

Once meeting with Dr. Frye, he ordered additional tests. Though Leland tested negative for folate receptor autoantibodies (FRAA), Dr. Frye suggested leucovorin to address seizure-like activity observed during a 72-hour EEG in the left temporal lobe, an area of the brain important in language processing. Leland began with 25 mg of leucovorin twice daily, gradually increasing the dosage. However, the evening dose caused insomnia, so we only kept the morning dose. Leucovorin was well tolerated, and we continued with his other supplements, including mitochondrial support and CBD.

Upon starting the higher dose of leucovorin, we saw immediate, significant improvements in Leland's spoken and written language, suggesting a possible link to CFD. Both school and private speech therapists reported his extraordinary progress initiating conversation, sharing personal stories, engagement and eye contact. Although he still struggled with tenses, word order, and pronunciation, he begun self-correcting and required less prompting.

In the classroom, his general education teacher also noted improvements in language, reading comprehension, and confidence. Leland began raising his hand to eagerly answer questions, participating in peer discussions, reading aloud, and completing assignments more accurately and timely.

At home, Leland was holding back-and-forth conversation with family, singing, and vocalizing pretend play with his stuffed animals—something we once thought we would never see!

After almost two years of leucovorin treatment and some adjustment to dosing, Leland continues to blossom and surpass all expectations. He is excelling academically and has been accepted into his school's gifted and talented program. After more than 8 years of speech therapy, Leland is finally approaching the completion of his therapy plan. He has also gained the confidence to participate in extracurricular activities, like soccer, swimming, piano, performing arts and ministry. Most importantly, he has become more independent and can better advocate for himself.

Leland is a smart, diligent, and happy child who expresses gratitude for everyone who has helped him. He says, "I like Dr. Frye because he is so kind and very helpful, too." We are all grateful for this journey and optimistic about the future, as leucovorin has greatly improved Leland's quality of life and that of our entire family.

A Physician's Perspective

Leland and other children with mutations in the SATB2 gene have a condition called SATB2-Associated Syndrome (SAS), also known as Glass syndrome. This rare genetic disorder causes a range of symptoms, including speech and language delays, as well as impairments in cognitive and motor skills.

SATB2 is a gene that is involved in the formation of the brain, head and face during prenatal development. Although it is generally believed that these congenital abnormalities are unchangeable, Leland's case suggests otherwise. Within a few months of starting leucovorin, he showed remarkable improvement. In my practice, I have treated other patients with SATB2 mutations who have responded positively to leucovorin.

Many patients with low 5-MTHF levels in their CSF have underlying genetic disorders. In one study examining patients with various reported encephalopathies and detailed CSF measurements, 71 out of 584 individuals were found to have a 5-MTHF deficiency.[152] Further analysis revealed that CFD was present in many patients with known genetic disorders, including Kearns-Sayre syndrome, Rett syndrome, Glutaric aciduria type 1, Williams syndrome, and other rare genetic conditions (some of these findings are illustrated in Figure 15.2 in Chapter 15). As previously discussed, many individuals with CFD have underlying genetic mutations that do not directly involve the folate pathway. This study supported that conclusion, demonstrating that certain genetic disorders can lead to a secondary CFD.

For this reason, I often recommend whole genome sequencing (WGS) for my patients. WGS can help identify rare mutations that may be causative or contributory to the patient's symptoms. This is especially important if CFD has been diagnosed without a clear cause or the patient has unusual symptoms.

WGS provides a comprehensive analysis of the entire genome, including both coding and non-coding regions, offering a broader view but at a higher cost. In contrast, whole exome sequencing (WES) focuses specifically on the exons, the regions directly involved in protein production. Since exons make up only about 1-2% of the genome, WES can be more efficient and cost-effective, although it may miss variants that impact gene regulation. In addition, WGS sequences the mitochondrial genome, examines trinucleotide repeat disorders like Fragile X and small copy number variations.

In some cases, mitochondrial DNA testing may be appropriate. Mitochondrial point mutations, deletions, and duplications are sometimes linked to mitochondrial diseases associated with CFD. If a classic mitochondrial disease is not present, but mitochondrial dysfunction is suspected, a non-invasive buccal (cheek) swab enzymology is available commercially or enzymology can be obtained from fibroblasts or muscle, although these require invasive procedures. Enzymology evaluates mitochondrial function based on enzyme activity within the mitochondria.

Understanding the genetic and mitochondrial factors underlying the patient's CFD can inform the dosage and method of leucovorin treatment necessary for an optimal response.

I frequently evaluate children with genetic mutations, and I almost always test for FRAAs. If the test is positive, I initiate a trial of leucovorin. To date, I have had many successes with this approach. I often receive referrals for cases where CFD was diagnosed but subsequently dismissed. In one case, a child with a congenital disorder of glycosylation was evaluated at a major U.S. clinical research center and diagnosed with CFD, yet no treatment was offered to the family.

The risk associated with leucovorin treatment is low, while the potential benefit is high. The risk-benefit ratio for leucovorin is considerably better than for most other prescription medications.

Given that treatments for genetic disorders are typically limited, as they are often considered unchangeable, exploring a treatable associated condition like CFD has minimal downsides. It also holds substantial potential for improving both the child's short- and long-term development, as well as the overall quality of life for the child, as it did for Leland and his family.

CHAPTER 10.

So What About Vaccines?

I hesitate to mutter the "V" word as it rarely leads to a productive conversation. However, since so many stories in this book mention vaccines, medications, and medical procedures as potential contributors to the child's illness, I think it's important to address the elephant in the room.

Notably, I did not select these stories because they mentioned vaccines. In fact, it was quite the opposite: parents were invited to share their compelling stories about Cerebral Folate Deficiency and/or leucovorin treatment without any consideration of their views on vaccines or other aspects of medical care.

So why do so many parents associate vaccines and other medical treatments with their child's illness?

As a scientist, I approach this by listening to all perspectives and trying to understand the underlying factors. Here, I will offer my thoughts on this phenomenon.

Horror Vacui

Aristotle proposed that "Nature abhors a vacuum." *Horror vacui* is the Latin term that translates to "fear of empty space." Consequently, any empty space gets quickly filled. Despite decades of research, medical science has made little progress in understanding the causes of neurodevelopmental disorders like Autism Spectrum Disorder (ASD). This area of medical science remains a black hole, where countless ideas are being sucked in as possible explanations.

The human mind is a correlation machine: we instinctively link coinciding events and associate facts in an effort to understand the world better– that's simply how our brains work. Neurodevelopmental disorders often begin in early childhood, a time when doctor's visits for vaccinations are common and memorable. Sometimes by coincidence, changes in a child's development occur contemporaneously with a vaccination event. Moreover, medical procedures can feel unnatural, making them easy targets to blame when something unusual happens, especially if no other explanation is readily available.

"We Know Autism is Genetic"

A common response to parents' concerns is a familiar rebuttal: "we know autism is genetic." I must challenge this perspective. Autism is highly heritable, and some scientists and doctors mistakenly equate heritability solely with genetic disorders. I've encountered numerous lectures that perpetuate this misconception, often with titles like: "Heritability = Genetics."

This is just wrong. Genetics is one way of passing on traits through generations, but it is not the only way. For example, mothers who experience severe malnutrition or smoke heavily during pregnancy can affect their children's health through environmental exposures and epigenetic changes—modifications that influence gene expression without altering the underlying genetic code. Similarly, cultural and behavioral factors that are not encoded in DNA can be passed down between generations and may impact risk factors for certain conditions.

Beyond the common conflation of heritability with genetics, this concept is wrong because it is not supported by science. Empirical studies show that a minority of ASD cases can be attributed to genetics,[153, 154, 155] and when an explanatory gene is found, it is most often a *de novo* mutation, meaning that it is not inherited. Studies have also shown that when siblings have genetic causes for their ASD, more than 60% of the time, the causative genes differ between the siblings, again, indicating that ASD is not passed down from the parents.[156]

Over the years, I have organized many introductory ASD conferences for primary care physicians, and I always include a lecture by a geneticist. After the lecture, I often ask my primary care colleagues whether they "drank the Kool-Aid." Most genetic lectures begin by claiming that ASD is genetic due to its high heritability and conclude by asserting that a variant found through whole exome sequencing is likely the cause of ASD because it is *de novo* (not inherited). That reasoning is contradictory and defies logic!

One may conclude that I have an aversion to genetics or that I do not find it useful in the investigation of ASD; however, it is quite the opposite. In addition to publishing several papers on the genetics of ASD, I am currently leading a Special Issue for the journal *Gene*. Along with my colleagues, I have published research papers demonstrating that the yield of identifying *de novo* variants can be doubled through whole genome sequencing—compared to standard bioinformatics pipelines—when these variants are carefully reviewed by an experienced physician.[157] Whenever possible, I perform whole genome sequencing on my patients and personally examine every identified variant (typically over 100 per patient).

The bottom line is that genetics has not lived up to the hype, and parents are often disappointed by the results. When I order a genetic test, I prepare my patients to manage their expectations. While I do recommend genetic testing—because any findings can provide valuable insights—it's essential to be honest with patients and parents about its limitations. We need to put genetic testing into perspective and broaden our focus to include other factors that may contribute to the development of neurodevelopmental disorders like ASD, especially gene-environmental interactions.[158]

"Vaccines are Absolutely Safe"

This is another misleading claim, that when repeated as a mantra, makes the already polarized vaccine conversation worse. "Absolute safety" requires the complete eradication of all risks, an unattainable standard for any medical intervention. Vaccines do exactly what they are supposed to do: they help more than they harm. This makes their use no different than that of prescription medications where the risks of adverse effects are lower than the likely benefits offered to the patient.

Most people agree that vaccines have been a significant medical achievement, but doctors must be honest with families and patients about their risks and limitations. A complete conversation called "informed consent" must include pros, cons, and alternatives. Informed consent is a fundamental, ethical, and legal requirement in healthcare, and yet when it comes to vaccines, it is seldom carried out.

As a neurologist, I have regularly seen the adverse effects of vaccines. While an attending physician at different children's hospitals, I treated patients presenting with Guillain–Barré syndrome, Transverse myelitis or Acute Disseminated Encephalomyelitis (ADEM) that followed a vaccination event. While these are acknowledged as "rare" side effects, at least one of these cases came through my doors every other month, if not more often.

Having worked in some of the largest children's hospitals where complex cases are often referred, my exposure to these cases is likely over-represented compared to the average physician. That said, these events do happen, and when they do, the parents were rarely informed ahead of time that the outcomes were potential adverse effects of the vaccines. Luckily, most of the time these neurologic disorders are self-limiting with an excellent prognosis, but this is not always the case.

Vaccines have also been linked to some of the disorders discussed in this book.

It is well known that the first seizure in children with Dravet syndrome is often triggered by a vaccine-induced fever.[159] Such a fever would be benign for most children but could be very serious for a child with a genetic mutation lowering their seizure threshold. This is only one example of a genetic vulnerability. Another study looking at children with underlying mitochondrial disease who experienced neurodevelopmental regression into ASD following fevers found that the fevers were not uncommonly caused by vaccines.[160]

In such cases, some argue that the fever, not the vaccine, was the trigger. While such an argument is "technically" true, exonerating the vaccine is disingenuous. Clearly the vaccination was an iatrogenic trigger for the disorder—caused unintentionally by the medical intervention. These cases alert us to the fact that some patients may be more predisposed to adverse events. It also identifies an opportunity for better screening so that at-risk children can be more accurately identified to prevent unintended consequences of vaccinations.

Given that fevers are potential triggers for both seizures and other neurological adverse events, it is surprising that most parents and doctors are unaware that specific vaccine choices may increase those risks. For example, children who are 12-47-months of age can either receive the quadrivalent MMRV (measles, mumps, rubella, and varicella) vaccine or the trivalent MMR and single varicella vaccines administered separately.

Children who receive the MMRV combination vaccine respond with fevers of 102°F or higher more frequently than those who receive the separate shots (22% versus 15%). Additionally, the children who receive the combination MMRV have double the risk for febrile seizures in the 7 to 10 days following the vaccine administration.[161]

Upon hearing such information, some may disregard it, assuming that it came from an "anti-vax" publication. Such skeptics would be surprised to learn that this information was actually discovered through a carefully conducted study by Kaiser Permanente involving over 459,000 children. These findings and warning are references on the CDC website, where it states: "Children who have a personal or family (sibling or parent) history of seizures should generally be vaccinated with MMR and varicella vaccines separately instead of MMRV vaccine."[162]

"The Debate is Finally Over"

In 1998, Dr. Andrew Wakefield, a British physician became widely known for his controversial paper linking the MMR to ASD in *The Lancet*, a highly regarded medical journal.[163] Soon after his paper's publication, both his research and his career were heavily criticized by the medical community. Many scientists and doctors blamed Andy Wakefield for making parents believe that vaccines cause ASD.

In 2010, I was working at a large medical center when the UK's General Medical Council (GMC) removed Dr. Wakefield's medical license and *The Lancet* retracted his infamous paper.[164] All of my colleagues remarked "aren't you glad that the vaccine debate is now over?" So many medical providers believed that he was the primary cause of all of the vaccine controversy, a sentiment echoed in many subsequent medical publications.[165]

Going forward, when parents shared concerns about vaccinating their children, I would ask them, "Are you asking me this because of Dr. Wakefield?" Almost every parent responded the same way: "Who is Dr. Wakefield?"

Despite his perceived notoriety and being credited with fueling all vaccine skepticism, among the parents I consulted, Dr. Wakefield and his work were not well-known. As my discussions with parents unfolded, I learned that most just felt uncomfortable giving their tiny infants 20+ vaccine doses before the age of one. It just didn't seem right for a small child to have all those injections.

In most of these conversations, parents just want to discuss their concerns. Very often I hear stories about pediatricians who have dismissed their questions, or worse, pediatricians who have threatened to throw them out of the practice if they do not vaccinate their child exactly on schedule. In my opinion, that is just bad doctoring.

Medicine is both an art and a science. Historically, the art of medicine involved making a unique and positive connection with the patient to provide them with individualized and optimal care. When it comes to vaccines, most parents just want to know more. When a doctor refuses to provide additional information, it builds a mistrust that undermines the relationship. In this way, the denial of honest information about vaccines has fueled the anti-vax movement, not made it better. Studies underscore the importance of personalized communication to address vaccine hesitancy among parents of children with ASD.[166]

Then Came COVID

As if the vaccine conversation was not contentious enough, the COVID pandemic opened a new Pandora's box of vaccine skepticism. It's important to recognize that the pandemic was an exceptionally challenging period in history—a time when a highly lethal virus, about which we knew little, was devastating many cities. I believe everyone was doing their best under these chaotic circumstances. Whether we could have managed things better to minimize the damage is something that we will never fully know.

COVID vaccines were widely administered under the pretense of being the risk-free solution for a population who was eager to return to normalcy. Little to no discussion about vaccine safety took place, yet the public became increasingly aware of adverse effects through first-hand experiences.

Unlike childhood vaccine side effects where the patients are often too young or incapable of describing their experiences, COVID vaccines were given en masse to adults who could articulate their personal reactions. The strategy of claiming vaccines were "perfectly safe" backfired and resulted in widespread distrust of the medical system. Consequently, many people are now reluctant to receive further vaccinations of any kind.

Compassion as a Subversive Activity

Dr. David K. Urion, one of my mentors at Harvard, wrote a remarkable book titled *Compassion as a Subversive Activity*.[167] It explores the healing power of compassion in a rigid system of medicine, particularly in the care of children with disabilities. The book's foundation is based on the Gospel of Mark, though its message extends to those of any faith. Dr. Urion shares stories of families facing incredibly difficult situations, emphasizing that instead of criticizing their choices, mistakes, or tough questions, physicians should respond with compassion.

Compassion enables doctors to guide patients through their unique journeys. Recognizing that every patient follows a different path, it is crucial for physicians to listen, offer guidance (rather than commands), and walk alongside their patients. In these challenging circumstances, the physician's role is to partner with the family to find the best path forward. Thus, the tendency to remove detailed information from conversation with the family has heavily damaged the doctor-patient relationship.

As someone whose practice is heavily biased towards children with complex, life-threatening, and rare genetic conditions, I am often exposed to families who live in the numerator of "1 in 1,000," "1 in 10,000" and even "1 in 1,000,000" risk ratios. Sadly, for ASD, the risk ratio in the United States is now "1 in 36." Until science can provide these families with more concrete explanations for their children's conditions, specifically ASD, their stories deserve to be heard without judgement.

The painfully slow pace of research into the causes of neurodevelopmental disorders unfortunately leaves fertile ground for a growing mistrust of vaccines. The way to combat vaccine skepticism is through informed consent and a prioritization of ASD research. From where I sit, the lack of urgency, acknowledgement, and funding for these efforts (not Andy Wakefield) have led to our current circumstances.

PART III.
FOLATE IN PSYCHIATRIC CONDITIONS

Thus far, this book has focused on the role of folate in neurological disorders, with a strong emphasis on neurodevelopmental disorders affecting infants and children. However, folate abnormalities may also play a significant role in many psychiatric conditions, including those more commonly recognized in adults.

Many people confuse neurological and psychiatric disorders because both involve the brain. While there is overlap, these disorders are generally distinguished by their underlying causes and how they are studied and classified in medicine.

Neurological disorders are often linked to observable abnormalities in the brain or nervous system, such as structural changes seen on an MRI, electrical activity measured by an EEG, or genetic mutations identified through genome sequencing, as discussed in Chapter 9.

In contrast, psychiatric disorders are primarily characterized by behavioral, emotional, and cognitive symptoms, which may not always have clear, observable biological markers. These conditions are often diagnosed through clinical evaluations and behavioral assessments.

Some conditions exhibit both neurological and psychiatric features—such as autism spectrum disorder (ASD) in children and Alzheimer's disease in adults—where a combination of biological abnormalities and behavioral symptoms may contribute to the diagnosis. As research advances, many psychiatric conditions are increasingly being linked to measurable biological markers.

Part III of this book will explore recent research highlighting the emerging role of folate in psychiatric disorders of adulthood.

CHAPTER 11.

Psychiatric Disorders

Background

Psychiatric diseases are distinct from many other medical disorders. Generally, most medical conditions are diagnosed through blood tests or other objective measurements. Alternatively, psychiatric disorders are based on a collection of symptoms.

The DSM, discussed in Chapter 5, is a manual that categorizes psychiatric disorders by listing specific symptoms that, when combined together, form various diagnoses. Given the subjective nature of these symptoms, it can often be challenging to assign one specific diagnosis, and many individuals receive multiple psychiatric diagnoses. The absence of objective tests also complicates the personalization of treatment.

In this chapter, we describe several psychiatric disorders that have been associated with CFD. Thus, CFD may represent the first testable and treatable condition linked to psychiatric disorders, at least in some cases, opening the possibility of substantially improving symptoms with a simple, safe treatment.

Depression

There are several types of depression, but the most commonly recognized form is Major Depressive Disorder (MDD). For a diagnosis of MDD, symptoms must include either a persistently depressed mood or a loss of interest or pleasure in activities for most of the day, nearly every day, for at least two consecutive weeks. These symptoms must also cause significant distress or impair daily functioning.

Additionally, an MDD diagnosis requires a combination of other symptoms, such as increased or decreased activity levels; feelings of worthlessness or inappropriate guilt; diminished ability to think, concentrate, or make decisions; and recurrent thoughts of death, suicidal ideations, or suicide attempts. Somatic symptoms such as weight loss or gain, sleep disturbance, and fatigue are also included as possible indicators.

Bipolar Disorder

If a person with MDD experiences manic or hypomanic episodes, they might fall into the diagnosis of Bipolar Disorder. A manic episode is characterized by a significantly elevated, expansive, or irritable mood and increased goal-directed activity or energy, present most of the day, nearly every day, for at least one week.

Additional symptoms often include inflated self-esteem or grandiosity, decreased need for sleep, excessive talkativeness, racing thoughts, distractibility, agitation, and involvement in activities with a high potential for negative consequences. Hypomanic episodes are similar to manic episodes but can be less severe and do not result in significant impairment of daily functioning. Individuals with Bipolar Disorder typically cycle between episodes of Major Depression and Manic or Hypomanic episodes.

Suicidal Behavior

A serious consequence of MDD is suicide. Suicidal behavior can range in severity. The least severe is suicidal ideation, where a person has thoughts about suicide. This doesn't necessarily mean they have a plan, but it becomes more serious if they do. The most severe form is a suicide attempt, where the individual takes action to carry out their plan.

It is important to distinguish suicidal behavior from non-suicidal self-injurious behavior, which is often seen in children with neurodevelopmental disorders and is not intended as a suicide attempt.

Schizophrenia

Schizophrenia is a severe mental disorder characterized by episodes of psychosis, delusions, hallucinations, and disorganized thinking or speech. These symptoms must be present for a significant part of a one-month period and persist for at least six months to confirm a diagnosis. Schizophrenia symptoms are generally categorized into positive and negative symptoms. Positive symptoms include delusions, hallucinations, disorganized thinking or speech, and movement disorders including repetitive movements or catatonia (lack of movement). Negative symptoms involve a reduced emotional expression (flattened affect), social withdrawal, lack of pleasure in activities, decreased speech, and difficulties completing everyday tasks. Together, these symptoms can profoundly affect an individual's ability to function.

Eating Disorders

Another set of psychiatric disorders is eating disorders. While conditions like schizophrenia and depression are easily recognized as mental disorders, eating disorders are sometimes, incorrectly, viewed as lifestyle choices. Eating Disorders come in many varieties and are classified by the DSM, just like other mental disorders. They can range from eating too much (Binge Eating) to refusing to eat (Anorexia Nervosa) or having restrictions in which food that you eat (Avoidant/Restrictive Food Intake Disorder).

Psychiatric Disorders and CFD

Several psychiatric syndromes have been linked to CFD. In Part II, Chapter 8 describes how many children with PANS and PANDAS tested positive for FRAAs and had a positive response to leucovorin.[168] PANS and PANDAS are associated with many psychiatric symptoms including OCD-like behavior, irritability, anxiety and depression. These cases imply a relationship between psychiatric symptoms and folate metabolism.

Similarly, a link between depression and CFD was uncovered by Dr. Lisa Pan, a psychiatrist, who demonstrated that adults with treatment-resistant major depressive disorder, especially those with suicidal ideations, had CFD.[169] Her research also showed that both depression and suicidal ideations significantly improved with folate treatment in many cases.

Dr. Pan's research aligns with findings from an earlier double-blind, placebo-controlled study from 1990. In this study, patients with major depression or schizophrenia who had red-cell folate levels below 200 µg/L (considered deficient) were treated with 15 mg of L-methylfolate daily for six months. The treatment group showed significant improvements in clinical symptoms and social interaction compared to the placebo group, with the differences between the groups increasing over time.[170]

Other studies have explored the use of folates as an adjunctive treatment for psychiatric disorders, many of which are commonly treated with selective serotonin reuptake inhibitors (SSRIs). SSRIs like Prozac (Fluoxetine), Zoloft (Sertraline), Lexapro (Escitalopram), Paxil (Paroxetine), and Celexa (Citalopram) are prescribed for psychiatric conditions believed to involve imbalanced or low levels of serotonin, a neurotransmitter that regulates mood, emotions, and behavior.

As their name suggests, SSRIs work by inhibiting the reuptake of serotonin in the brain, thereby increasing the amount of serotonin available in the synaptic cleft (the space between neurons). By blocking the reabsorption of serotonin into the releasing neuron after it transmits a signal, SSRIs enhance neural communication and help alleviate symptoms associated with mood and anxiety disorders.

Researchers at the Center for Treatment-Resistant Depression at Massachusetts General Hospital in Boston conducted a series of clinical trials to examine the effects of L-methylfolate in patients who were resistant to the standard treatment of SSRIs. In the initial double-blind, placebo-controlled trials, they found that adding 15 mg of L-methylfolate daily to the SSRI for 60 days resulted in a significant improvement in depression symptoms compared to adding a placebo to the SSRI.[171]

In the second double-blind, placebo-controlled trial, the researchers found that 15 mg of L-methylfolate added to the SSRI daily for 30 or 60 days significantly lessened the overall severity of the depression. Additionally, they found the levels of improvement were dependent on genetic variations, biomarkers of inflammation, and folate metabolism.[172] In the last clinical trial, the participants who completed the earlier trials were offered 12 months of 15 mg of L-methylfolate daily. Many of the patients continued to improve and some even made a full recovery.[173]

One year after that study, another publication showed similarly promising findings. In an open-label trial of 10 patients with bipolar depression, taking 15 mg of L-methylfolate daily for six weeks resulted in a significant improvement in symptoms of depression but not mania.[174]

Dr. Ramaekers (introduced in Chapter 4) examined patients with another psychiatric disorder, schizophrenia. He found that 83% of 18 adolescents and adults with schizophrenia who were unresponsive to conventional treatment tested positive for FRAAs.[175] Among the seven patients whose 5-MTHF levels were measured from a lumbar puncture, six showed low concentrations. These low 5-MTHF concentrations were associated with neurotransmitter disturbances, and treatment with leucovorin for at least six months resulted in significant clinical improvement in symptoms.

Dr. Ramaekers' research aligned with previous studies. Researchers at Massachusetts General Hospital conducted two randomized, double-blind, placebo-controlled trials examining the therapeutic effect of B-vitamins on schizophrenia. In the first study, treatment with 2 mg of leucovorin and 400 μg of vitamin B12 daily for 16 weeks significantly improved negative but not positive symptoms.[176] Notably, this therapeutic effect was linked to genetic variations in the FOLH1 gene, which is responsible for producing an enzyme in the intestine that facilitates the absorption of folate molecules.

In the second study, 55 patients with schizophrenia were treated with 15 mg of L-methylfolate daily for 12 weeks.[177] This treatment led to improvements in negative symptoms and overall scores on the Positive and Negative Syndrome Scale. Neuroimaging studies also demonstrated increased brain activation and greater cortical thickness, indicating that the treatment resulted in both behavioral improvements and structural changes in the brain.

Folate treatment may have therapeutic potential for a wide range of psychiatric disorders, including eating disorders. This was demonstrated in a randomized, double-blind, placebo-controlled study of 24 patients with eating disorders and low folate intake, who received 10 mg of folic acid daily for six months. The treatment resulted in significant improvements in cognitive function and depressive symptoms.[178]

Implications

These studies present intriguing evidence suggesting that folate supplementation can improve symptoms in patients with various psychiatric disorders that are resistant to conventional treatments. At least two studies have shown that treatment-resistant psychiatric patients may have a high rate of CFD, which could explain the beneficial effects of folate supplementation.

It is important to point out that only one study, the study by Dr. Ramaekers, measured FRAAs in psychiatric disorders. This is unfortunate because FRAAs can be easily measured, and their presence can inform whether leucovorin or other reduced forms of folate might be effective treatments.

Similar to recent findings showing that individuals with PANS or PANDAS may have FRAAs and respond well to leucovorin, it could be highly beneficial to test treatment-resistant psychiatric patients for FRAAs. Leucovorin offers a favorable safety profile compared to many psychiatric medications, making it a promising option for those unresponsive to standard treatments.

Most importantly, for psychiatric patients who have not found relief from SSRIs and other conventional treatments, the serious consequences of untreated psychiatric illness—such as worsening symptoms, impaired daily functioning, self-harm, and an increased risk of suicide—underscore the need for alternative interventions. A treatment like leucovorin, which has already demonstrated success in numerous patients, including some achieving full recovery, highlight the importance of exploring folate deficiencies, particularly CFD, as a potentially life-saving step in the management of psychiatric conditions.

CHAPTER 12.
Neurocognitive Disorders of Older Age

Background

Many older adults and elderly individuals unfortunately suffer from neurodegenerative disorders. These conditions are invariably progressive and have proven challenging to treat effectively.

Neurodegenerative disorders lie at the intersection of neurology and psychiatry, as they often involve cognitive decline, behavioral changes, neurological symptoms, and altered brain function. In psychiatry, they are referred to as neurocognitive disorders.

Dementia

Dementia is a common neurodegenerative disorder primarily affecting older adults. It refers to the progressive loss of cognitive abilities, including memory, thinking, reasoning, and social functioning.

Dementia is an umbrella term often accompanied by a descriptor indicating its cause. For example, vascular dementia is a common type caused by reduced blood flow to the brain, often due to cardiovascular disease, including hypertension and diabetes.

Alzheimer's Disease

Alzheimer's Disease (AD) is one of the most well-known types of dementia and neurodegenerative disorders. It is a progressive and irreversible condition that accounts for 60-80% of dementia cases.

Early symptoms often begin with memory loss, followed by more debilitating signs such as confusion, disorientation, mood swings, difficulty with speech or walking, and eventually, an inability to perform basic daily functions. AD generally progresses through four stages that include:

1. Mild cognitive impairment (MCI)
2. Early-stage Alzheimer's (mild)
3. Middle-stage Alzheimer's (moderate)
4. Late-stage Alzheimer's (severe)

Currently, Alzheimer's disease affects approximately seven million people in the United States.

In addition to AD, dementia is also seen in other neurodegenerative disorders such as Parkinson disease (PD). Parkinson's disease is a progressive neurodegenerative disorder caused by the degeneration of dopamine-producing neurons in the substantia nigra, a region of the brain responsible for motor control.

Because dopamine is essential for smooth and controlled muscle movement, many primary symptoms of Parkinson's include: tremors (involuntary shaking), bradykinesia (slowness of movement), muscle rigidity, and postural instability (balance problems, leading to falls).

Beyond motor symptoms, PD is also associated with non-motor symptoms, including cognitive changes and mood disorders, which can overlap with other forms of dementia. Many times, before a more specific diagnosis can be made, dementia is preceded by subtle memory and cognitive changes, which may serve as warning signs of MCI or may simply be part of normal aging and therefore benign.

Neurocognitive Disorders and CFD

Over the past decade, the role of folate in cognitive changes associated with aging has gained recognition, leading to therapeutic implications. Several studies have looked at the role of folate in the development and progression of different forms of dimentia and AD. One systematic review and meta-analysis found that low dietary folate is a risk factor for MCI.[179]

In a large study of older adults (ages 60-75) who had been free of dementia symptoms for the previous 10 years, folate deficiency (low folate) was linked to an increased risk of developing dementia, as well as higher mortality, as the adults aged.[180] Additionally, a Japanese study that followed patients over 20 years found that serum folate levels at the start of the study were associated with the risk of disabling dementia later in life, such that lower folate concentrations at the beginning of the study were associated with an increased risk of dementia and higher folate concentrations at the beginning of the study were associated with a decreased risk of dementia.[181]

A systematic review and meta-analysis from China with several thousand participants indicated that B-vitamin supplementation, when initiated early and maintained over extended periods (at least 12 months), slowed cognitive decline.[182] Also the meta-analysis showed that in a population without dimentia, lower folate and higher homocysteine levels (but not B12 or B6 deficiency) were associated with a higher risk of dimentia. Higher folate intake (but not higher B12 or B6 intake) was associated with a lower risk of dimentia.

Several studies have examined dementia risk within specific elderly subgroups, revealing a striking relationship between low folate levels and the likelihood of developing cognitive impairment. For example, a large study of elderly Latinos found that low red blood cell (RBC) folate concentrations were linked to lower scores on the Modified Mini-Mental State Examination—a standard cognitive assessment for dementia—and an increased risk of dementia.[183]

The Women's Health Initiative Memory Study, a large, female-focused study, looked at postmenopausal women with no prior history of dementia or MCI. This study found that women with a folate intake below the Recommended Daily Allowance were more likely to develop MCI or probable dementia.[184]

Another substantial study followed a group of dementia-free elderly patients for 2.4 years and discovered that dementia and Alzheimer's disease were associated with a significant decline in folate and a marked rise in homocysteine.[185] Recall from Chapter 8 that both low folate and elevated homocysteine are often found in neuroinflammatory conditions. Among patients with Alzheimer's and vascular dementia, folate was correlated with cerebral blood flow, a factor crucial to preventing disability, such that lower folate was associated with more compromised blood flow and higher folate levels was associated with better cerebral blood flow, possibly hinting at a mechanism for this observation.[186]

In a randomized trial involving newly diagnosed Alzheimer's patients taking donepezil (a neurotransmitter medication), participants were divided into two groups. One group received donepezil along with a daily dose of 1.25 mg folic acid for six months, while the other group took donepezil only. Those who received the folate supplement showed several improvements, including better scores on the Mental State Examination, an improved SAM/SAH ratio (indicating better metabolic health), and improved inflammatory markers.[187]

Notably, the lowered inflammatory markers included measures commonly associated with Alzheimer's severity, such as amyloid-beta 40 levels and presenilin, markers of disease progression, the 42/40 ratio, a marker indicating the potential for plaque formation in the brain, and mRNA expression of tumor necrosis factor-α, a marker of chronic brain inflammation.

Implications

These studies, including several large-scale investigations, provide compelling evidence that inadequate folate levels may contribute to the development of dementia. Collectively, they suggest that folate supplementation may help alleviate certain dementia symptoms and reduce inflammatory markers.

Similar to the pediatric neuroinflammatory cases described in Chapter 8, brain inflammation is increasingly recognized as a contributing factor to cognitive impairments in the elderly. While none of the dementia or AD studies measured folate levels in the cerebrospinal fluid, the observed lower folate levels in the blood likely correlate with reduced folate levels in the brain, making these cases not unlike the folate deficiencies found in the brain during malnutrition. Markers such as elevated homocysteine and cognitive decline are found in both, and can be improved by the simple act of increasing folate intake (along with B12).

The surprising results of some of these studies—where patients with AD showed improved cognitive scores following folate treatment—challenge the long-standing belief that AD is a progressive and irreversible condition.

Given the limited treatment options for dementia and the profound emotional and economic burden it places on families and society, a relatively simple intervention like folate supplementation could offer significant relief, helping elderly individuals maintain a better quality of life in their later years.

Part IV.

Working Your Way Through CFD

Cerebral Folate Deficiency (CFD) syndrome presents with a variety of symptoms, though none are specific to CFD alone. This is why CFD is classified as a syndrome—a collection of symptoms shared by many, but not all, affected individuals, making precise diagnosis challenging. While some syndromes have hallmark features, the symptoms of CFD are often nonspecific and may resemble those of other disorders. As a result, further testing is often necessary to confirm the diagnosis or rule out other conditions.

This section of the book provides practical guidance for managing suspected cases of CFD. It outlines the key symptoms, diagnostic testing, treatment protocols, dosing strategies, and ongoing management, serving as a valuable resource for both clinicians and families. There is also a recommended sequence for diagnosing and treating CFD. For those beginning the book with this section, it is helpful to review the patient stories in Part II, which illustrate the complexity and multifaceted presentation of this condition. Children with CFD often have comorbid conditions which can complicate and delay the diagnosis.

Additionally, real-life patient stories highlight that treatment success is not always immediate. Adjusting doses and exploring combination therapies may be necessary to achieve optimal outcomes. While this book features patients who have responded well to treatment, it is important to acknowledge that some patients do not experience significant improvement. As research into the causes and mechanisms underlying autism spectrum disorder (ASD) and CFD continues, we remain hopeful that future discoveries will enhance treatment options and help individuals with these conditions reach their full potential.

CHAPTER 13.
Who Should Be Tested?

Diagnosing Cerebral Folate Deficiency (CFD) is particularly challenging because its symptoms vary depending on the age at which it manifests and the severity of the disorder (See Figure 13.1). These factors influence the presentation of symptoms, further complicating the diagnostic process.

CFD has been associated with severe epilepsy arising in the neonatal period.[188] Therefore, neonates with severe, treatment-resistant epilepsy that cannot be explained by other causes, such as hypoxic-ischemic encephalopathy, should be screened for CFD.

When CFD begins in the first year of life, it often results in severe neurological and developmental symptoms, including significant irritability, abnormal involuntary movements, and muscle spasticity similar to that seen in cerebral palsy.[189] If left untreated, symptoms of CFD can progress. Later in the first year of life, a loss of previously acquired skills and a stagnation in head growth may occur.

While these symptoms are not specific to CFD and can be seen in other genetic and metabolic disorders, CFD should be strongly considered when these signs are not explained by a confirmed diagnosis or appear as new symptoms after birth. For instance, cerebral palsy is typically detected at birth and is usually associated with abnormal brain neuroimaging. Therefore, in children with new onset symptoms and relatively normal brain scans, CFD should be considered as a possible diagnosis.

In later childhood, typically around the second year of life, symptoms of CFD may include epilepsy and/or autism spectrum disorder (ASD). CFD is often considered in children with epilepsy who also present with other neurodevelopmental or neurological symptoms, particularly if their epilepsy is difficult to control and unresponsive to standard antiepileptic treatments. In such cases, CFD should be investigated as a possible underlying cause.[190]

For children with ASD, there are not any specific symptoms unique to CFD. Therefore, in my practice, I screen all ASD patients for CFD if they are not making the expected progress in their therapies.[191] Although not extensively studied, I have observed that many patients referred to me with PANS or PANDAS test positive for folate receptor alpha antibodies (FRAAs) and respond well to leucovorin treatment—sometimes even more effectively than to standard treatments for these conditions, such as antibiotics or intravenous immunoglobulin. PANS is characterized by the sudden onset of OCD-like behaviors, and in PANDAS, tics are also common. These symptoms align with movement disorders that have frequently been linked to CFD. A recent study that our group conducted found that the prevalence of FRAAs in PANS/PANDAS is 63%.[192]

In my practice, I have also observed that some children with neuroinflammatory disorders who experienced poor recovery from acute inflammatory episodes were found to have CFD and responded remarkably well to treatment. There is one case-report of a child with CFD presenting with severe self-injurious behavior,[193] a symptoms also reported in some cases of ASD, PANS, and PANDAS.

As discussed in Chapter 12, several researchers have published an intriguing case series suggesting that certain adult-onset psychiatric disorders may be linked to abnormalities in cerebral folate metabolism. For example, Dr. Vincent Ramaekers, the original discoverer of CFD, recently published a case series involving adolescents and adults with treatment-resistant schizophrenia who had low folate concentrations in their CSF and responded positively to leucovorin treatment.[194] Interestingly, there has been a case report of an adolescent with CFD presenting with catatonic schizophrenia.[195] Additionally, Dr. Lisa Pan published a case series on adults with treatment-resistant major depressive disorder and suicidal ideation who also had low folate concentrations in their cerebrospinal fluid (CSF) and showed improvement with folate treatment.[196]

Another study which examined CSF 5-MTHF in various neurological conditions in adults found that 69 of 224 (31%) had CFD with 25 (36%) of those with severe CFD.[197] The patients with severe CFD had neurological symptoms associated with mitochondrial diseases, hepatic encephalopathy and primary brain calcifications or had an unknown etiology. Although symptoms were not distinct, these patients tended to have pyramidal signs, movement disorders, cerebellar syndrome and intellectual disability (See explanations of symptoms in Chapter 14). One distinctive feature is that the CFD patients tended to have more neurological symptoms than those without CFD.

Age	Symptoms
Near Birth (1st Month)	Treatment-Resistant Myoclonic Epilepsy
Infancy (Year 1)	Developmental Regression New Onset Cerebral Palsy Movement Disorder Acquired Microcephaly
Toddler (Years 2-3)	Autism Spectrum Disorder (ASD) Epilepsy Vision Loss Hearing Loss
Childhood (Years 4-12)	Sudden Onset Obsessive Compulsive Disorder Self-Injurious Behavior Tics Ataxia
Adolescence (Years 13-18)	Sudden Onset Obsessive Compulsive Disorder Tics Ataxia Catatonia Schizophrenia
Adulthood (Years 19-40)	Complex Neurological Disorder Treatment Resistant Schizophrenia Multiple Sclerosis Major Depressive Disorder with Suicidal Ideations Electrical Status Epilepticus in Sleep (ESES)
Middle to Older Age	Dementia Parkinsons Disease Enlarged Ventricles Intracranial Hypertension Normal-Pressure Hydrocephalus

Figure 13.1 Chart showing how CFD symptoms manifest for different age groups. (See symptoms descriptions in Chapter 14).

Another study examined 5-MTHF and the folate receptor alpha (FRα) and folate-dependent hydroxymethyltransferase (FDH) protein concentrations in the CSF of adults with various neurological and psychiatric conditions derived from several brain banks. Brain bank samples from those including epilepsy, schizophrenia, bipolar disorder, Parkinson's disease, multiple sclerosis, mild traumatic brain injury and moderate and severe Alzheimer's disease as well as control samples were analyzed.[198]

CSF from living patients with dementia, intracranial hypertension and normal-pressure hydrocephalus were also obtained. 5-MTHF concentrations were non-significantly lower in schizophrenia, bipolar disorder and Parkinson's disease and were statistically significantly depressed in multiple sclerosis, moderate and severe Alzheimer's disease, as well as living patients with intracranial hypertension, normal-pressure hydrocephalus and Alzheimer's disease. 5-MTHF concentrations were markedly depressed in these patients, including those with intracranial hypertension and normal-pressure hydrocephalus. Interestingly, after 24 hours of CSF removal through a lumbar drain, the 5-MTHF concentration increased in the patient with normal-pressure hydrocephalus.

Along with the decrease in 5-MTHF concentration, certain conditions also demonstrated a reduction in FRα and/or FDH proteins—two proteins essential for the transport of 5-MTHF into neurons and astrocytes. Based on rat studies, the authors hypothesize that ventricular enlargement is associated with a loss of FDH and/or FRα release into the CSF, resulting in a 5-MTHF deficiency.

Although not all conditions presented with statistically significant decreases in folate, the lower levels of 5-MTHF in CSF observed in many of these conditions may explain the findings discussed in Chapters 11 and 12, where patients with psychiatric and neurocognitive disorders in older age experienced improvement with folate supplementation.

While few studies have examined CFD in adult populations, the symptom profile of CFD and the established link between folate and dementia suggest that some patients with dementia could potentially have CFD. Therefore, individuals of all ages presenting with neurological and psychiatric symptoms—particularly those who do not respond to standard treatments—may benefit from being evaluated for CFD.

CHAPTER 14.
The Symptoms of CFD

Cerebral Folate Deficiency (CFD) is associated with a broad spectrum of neurological, developmental, and psychiatric symptoms. As noted in earlier chapters, many symptoms of CFD are not unique to this condition and are often attributed to more commonly diagnosed disorders.

However, when symptoms persist or worsen despite treatment for other suspected conditions, they may serve as important indicators of an underlying folate deficiency. In addition to the symptoms themselves, the timing of their onset, their progression, and their severity can provide valuable insights for differential diagnosis. For instance, seizures that do not respond to standard anti-epileptic medications may suggest the presence of CFD.

Many patients with CFD also have comorbid conditions such as autism spectrum disorder (ASD), epilepsy, or dementia. As a result, symptoms of CFD are often mistakenly attributed to these broader diagnoses. This is particularly unfortunate because many of these conditions have limited biomedical treatment options. In contrast, CFD is treatable, and appropriate intervention often leads to significant symptom improvement. Therefore, thoroughly investigating the origin of all symptoms can provide an opportunity for much-needed relief for patients who are often suffering.

The following section provides a comprehensive list of symptoms associated with CFD, which can be used to track symptom progression over time. After the worksheet, a detailed description of each symptom is included to help readers better understand and recognize them.

Cerebral Folate Deficiency Checklist			
	Present	When Started	Severity
Neurological Signs			
Microcephaly			
Ataxia (Poor Coordination)			
Pyramidal Signs			
Movement Disorders			
Epilepsy or Seizures			
Electrical Status Epilepticus in Sleep (ESES)			
Neurodevelopmental Regression (NDR)			
Enlarged Ventricles			
Developmental Disorders			
Intellectual Disability			
Autism Spectrum Disorder (ASD)			
Communication Disorder			
Repetitive / Restrictive Behavior			
Self-Injurious Behavior			
Psychiatric Signs			
Irritability			
Obsessive Compulsive Disorder (OCD)			
Depression			
Suicidal Ideation			
Schizophrenia			
Catatonia			
Other Symptoms			
Vision Changes			
Hearing Loss			

Figure 14.1 The CFD Symptoms Checklist

Microcephaly

Microcephaly is defined by a smaller than expected size of the upper skull where the brain is located. This measurement is known as the occipital-frontal circumference and is made by assessing the circumference from the forehead to the back of the skull where the occipital portion of the skull is. This represents the maximum circumference of the head. During infancy and early childhood, skull growth is driven by the growth of the brain, so when the brain does not grow the skull does not grow (see Figure 14.2).

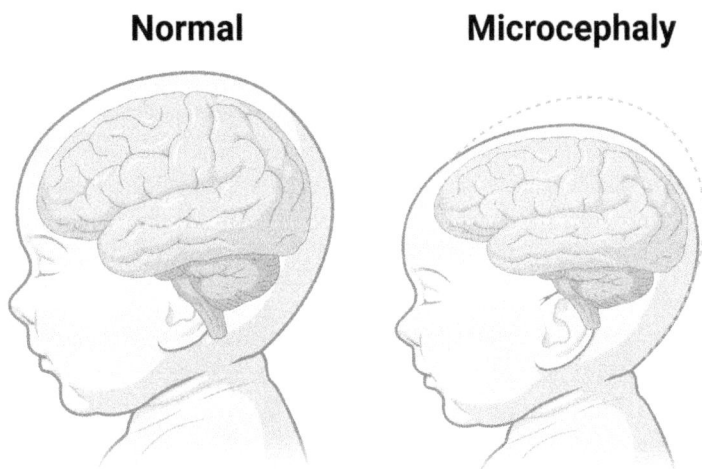

Figure 14.2 Microcephaly is typically diagnosed by measuring the head circumference and comparing it to standardized growth charts. Image created with BioRender.

There are two types of microcephaly, congenital and acquired. Congenital microcephaly is defined as below normal head size at birth and suggests that brain growth was inadequate during fetal development. Acquired microcephaly occurs when the head size is normal at birth but then stops growing early in life. This suggests that some underlying disorders are preventing the brain from developing normally. Children with known medical conditions, such as prematurity or Down syndrome, often exhibit altered patterns of head growth and are typically assessed using specialized head growth charts. Acquired microcephaly is a concerning condition that requires immediate investigation, as it can result from various underlying disorders, including serious genetic, metabolic, or infectious conditions.

Some, but not all, children with severe CFD in the first year of life have acquired microcephaly, so this symptom is a red flag for possible CFD but does not rule out CFD if it is not present.

Ataxia

Ataxia, a symptom often associated with CFD, is defined as poorly coordinated muscle movements that typically manifest as clumsiness. It is most noticeable when walking, where it looks like balance difficulties, but it can also affect speech, hand and eye coordination, and swallowing.

Ataxia results from dysfunction in the cerebellum, a part of the brain located at the back of the skull responsible for coordinating movement. However, other conditions can also cause incoordination, including muscle weakness, hypotonia (poor muscle tone), spasticity (muscle stiffness), and apraxia (difficulty with motor planning). Therefore, it is essential for a specialist to conduct a thorough examination to determine the underlying cause of any coordination difficulties.

Because ataxia does not typically appear until a person is able to walk, speak, or demonstrate controlled motor skills, it may go unnoticed until developmental delays become apparent or when a patient experiences neurodevelopmental regression. Although infants can have ataxia, it may be clinically indistinguishable from other movement disorders due to the limited motor control expected during this early developmental period.

If a child or adult who previously performed motor tasks without difficulty suddenly develops ataxia, and other potential causes such as genetic conditions, stroke, or alcohol abuse have been ruled out, CFD should be considered as a possible underlying cause.

Pyramidal Signs

Pyramidal signs indicate dysfunction in the pyramidal tract, a network of neurons that connect the brain's motor control areas to regions in the spinal cord responsible for directing the neurons that control muscle movement. Damage to this part of the central nervous system results in reduced control over muscle movement.

This dysfunction typically presents as spasticity, where muscles become overly tense, stiff, and unable to relax. Reflexes are often hyperresponsive, meaning they can be triggered easily. In some cases, however, muscle tone may be reduced, resulting in hypotonia, where muscles are excessively floppy.

When pyramidal abnormalities are present at birth, they often indicate cerebral palsy. Pyramidal signs have also been observed in cases of CFD, particularly in severe instances that begin during the first year of life. If pyramidal signs are not present at birth but develop or worsen throughout the first year, it should raise suspicion for CFD as a potential cause.

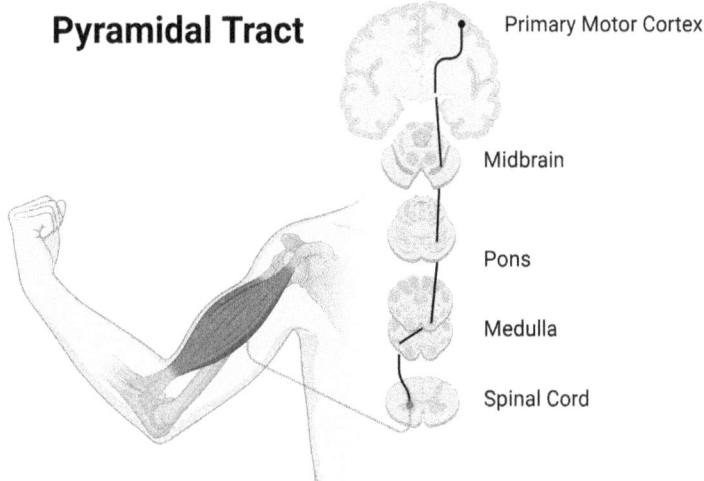

Figure 14.3 The pyramidal tract is a major pathway in the central nervous system that transmits signals from the brain to the spinal cord, which then directs voluntary muscle movements throughout the body. Image created with BioRender.

Movement Disorders

Movement disorders encompass a wide range of involuntary, atypical muscle movements, which may involve excessive movement, reduced movement, or abnormal muscle tone. In cases of CFD, most movement disorders are hyperkinetic, characterized by rapid, repetitive, and purposeless choreoathetoid movements. Choreoathetoid movements combine two distinct types of motor dysfunction. Firstly, chorea, which is described as involuntary, "dance-like" motions that flow from one body part to another; and secondly, athetosis, which is described as slow, writhing movements that typically affect the hands, feet, face, or tongue.

Individuals with CFD may exhibit sudden, jerky movements interspersed with slower, twisting motions. These movements are often purposeless and difficult to control, sometimes presenting as quick, flailing movements of the arms or legs, which can be profoundly debilitating for those affected.

While choreoathetoid movements are most common in CFD, other movement disorders associated with CFD include dystonia (sustained muscle contractions causing abnormal postures or twisting movements), myoclonus (sudden, brief, involuntary muscle jerks or twitches), and tremors (rhythmic shaking of a body part).

Patients with CFD may experience multiple movement disorders simultaneously, with symptoms that can fluctuate in severity, appear intermittently, or worsen over time, further complicating diagnosis and management.

Neurodevelopmental Regression

As previously discussed, neurodevelopmental regression (NDR) is typically diagnosed when a child who was developing normally suddenly loses previously acquired skills. This regression is often triggered by an illness or seizure, though in some cases, the loss of skills occurs gradually over several months.

NDR can also occur in individuals with developmental delays or ASD. Approximately one-third of children with ASD experience NDR between one and two years of age, though it can also occur outside of this age range.

Examples of NDR include the loss of motor skills, language abilities, and cognitive functions. For instance, a child who previously demonstrated the ability to self-feed, crawl or walk independently, and speak may lose these skills over time. Children who once used words may revert to babbling or become mute. Motor regression may manifest as a more clumsy and uncoordinated gait, often accompanied by frequent falls. Parents may report that children seem to have forgotten how to perform tasks they once completed with ease, such as operating toys, using the toilet, reading, counting, or dressing themselves. NDR can also present as a loss of interest in previously enjoyable activities or decreased social engagement.

When NDR is atypical—such as when multiple regressions occur or when regression leads to severe neurological symptoms—it is often linked to an underlying metabolic disorder, such as CFD or mitochondrial disorders, or an immune-related condition.

Electrical Status Epilepticus in Sleep

Electrical status epilepticus in sleep (ESES) is a pattern of epilepsy characterized by electrographic seizures occurring during deep sleep. ESES is defined by the presence of electrographic seizures during 80% or more of slow wave sleep; however, studies suggest that even lower percentages of slow wave sleep with electrographic seizures can result in similar symptoms. Clinical seizures may or may not be present with ESES.

ESES is observed in several neurological conditions, most of which are associated with daytime cognitive and behavioral changes. In young children, this condition can lead to behavioral and cognitive symptoms consistent with ASD. ESES has also been documented in adults with CFD.[199]

Diagnosing ESES requires an electroencephalogram (EEG) performed during slow wave sleep, necessitating an overnight EEG study. (See Chapter 7 for explanation of EEGs). ESES, if found, is both rare and serious, as it can cause lasting neurodevelopmental impairment, which is why it is critical to explore CFD as a potential treatable cause.

Enlarged Ventricles

The brain is surrounded by cerebrospinal fluid (CSF), which cushions it from sudden movements and plays other critical roles. Within the brain itself, there are spaces called ventricles that also contain CSF. Under normal conditions, this fluid flows in and out of the ventricles into the surrounding CSF through a series of specialized canals. Additionally, new CSF is continually produced by the choroid plexus, located inside the lateral ventricles, while old CSF is reabsorbed by arachnoid granulations—structures within the arachnoid mater, one of the brain's protective linings.

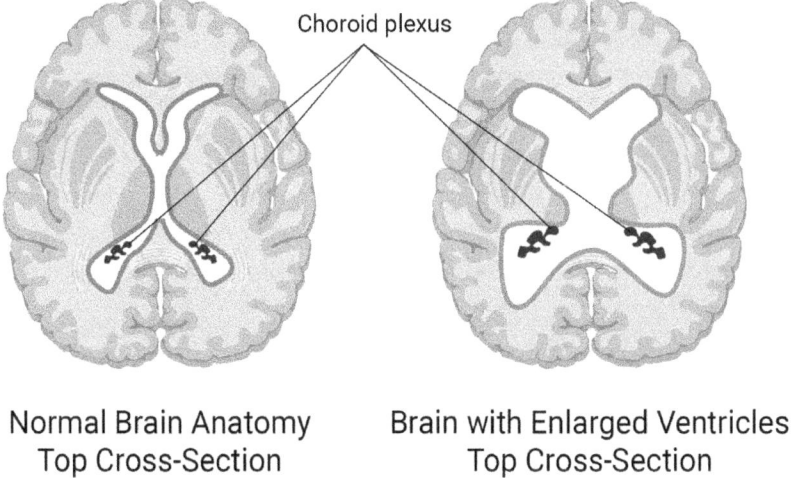

Figure 14.4 Enlarged ventricles in the brain

Several conditions can disrupt this delicate balance of CSF production, flow, and absorption, leading to neurological symptoms. The dynamic equilibrium of CSF regulates the pressure within the brain. Rarely, a leak can reduce CSF volume and pressure, causing the brain to sag within the skull, often resulting in severe headaches. More commonly, an increase in CSF pressure or volume occurs, which can compress the brain, leading to neuronal dysfunction and, in severe cases, cell death.

There are numerous causes of elevated CSF pressure or volume. For example, very preterm newborns may experience brain bleeds that leak blood into the CSF and ventricles. This can block the arachnoid granulations responsible for reabsorbing and recycling CSF, leading to a significant enlargement of the ventricles. Similarly, genetic conditions may obstruct the cerebral aqueduct—a canal connecting the ventricles inside the brain to the surrounding CSF spaces. Such blockages result in fluid buildup in the lateral ventricles.

Enlarged lateral ventricles are also observed in conditions more common in older adults, such as intracranial hypertension and normal pressure hydrocephalus. Research has demonstrated that these fluid buildup conditions are associated with impaired folate transport into the brain. This includes CFD and reduced activity of key folate transport proteins, such as folate receptor alpha (FRα) and folate-dependent hydroxymethyltransferase (FDH).[200] These findings highlight the complex interplay between CSF dynamics and critical metabolic processes within the brain.

Intellectual Disability

Intellectual disability was historically defined solely by an IQ score significantly below the population norm (below the 1st percentile), with classifications ranging from mild to severe. However, contemporary diagnostic criteria also consider an individual's adaptive functioning in daily life when determining the severity of intellectual disability.

While IQ tests remain the primary tool for assessing intellectual disability, it is essential to acknowledge their limitations and potential testing biases. Most standardized IQ tests place a heavy emphasis on language, which can disadvantage individuals with severe language impairments, leading to artificially low scores due to difficulties in comprehending instructions or verbally expressing responses.

To mitigate this, non-verbal IQ tests have been developed, relying solely on gestures for instruction. Research indicates that individuals with language impairment may score 10 to 20 points lower on traditional IQ tests compared to non-verbal assessments.

Additionally, factors such as attentional difficulties, hyperactivity, and anxiety can influence IQ test performance. Therefore, a comprehensive evaluation that considers these contributing factors is critical when interpreting IQ scores.

Communication Disorder

When most people think of communication, they often associate it with language. However, the earliest form of communication that infants develop is non-verbal. This is why the acquisition of skills such as pointing is a critical milestone in infancy. Communication encompasses both verbal and non-verbal interactions used to convey information and engage with others.

This distinction is essential in differentiating a communication disorder, often observed in individuals with ASD, from a language disorder, in which language abilities are impaired, but the overall capacity to communicate may remain intact.

The Importance of Pointing

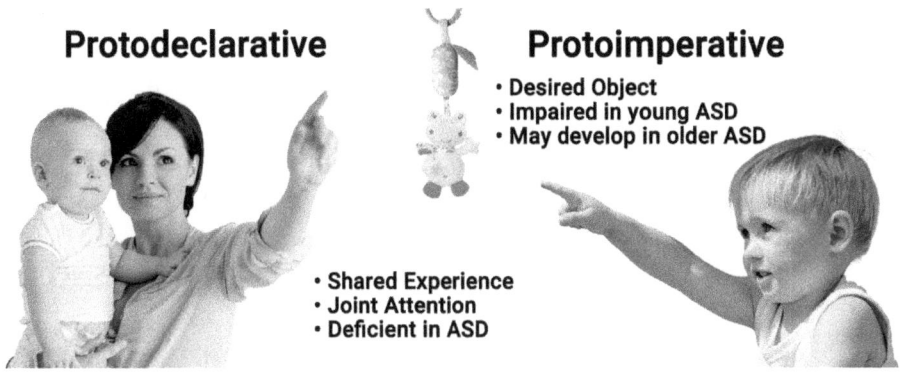

Figure 14.5 Pointing is an important form of communication and a sign of appropriate development. The purpose of protodeclarative pointing is to share an experience and establish joint attention with another person. Protoimperative pointing is when a child points at an object with the intention of obtaining it or as a way of making a demand. Both forms of pointing may be deficient in children with ASD.

Repetitive and Restrictive Behavior

Repetitive and restrictive behaviors are common features in many psychiatric disorders. Repetitive behaviors involve stereotyped movements that are performed repeatedly and can be triggered by emotional states such as distress or excitement. These behaviors are often categorized into two types:

- **Lower-order repetitive behaviors:** Simple, seemingly involuntary actions such as hand-flapping, rocking, or finger-tapping
- **Higher-order repetitive behaviors:** More complex, non-functional routines or rituals that are consciously planned and rigidly adhered to

Restrictive behaviors refer to inflexible routines or intensely focused interests. Individuals may feel compelled to perform certain actions in a specific manner to avoid distress. Their interests may be highly narrow, often focusing exclusively on a single topic, object, or activity for extended periods.

A defining characteristic of both repetitive and restrictive behaviors is the significant distress experienced when these behaviors are interrupted or prevented. For example, a child may become extremely upset if the route to school is altered, insisting on taking the exact same route each day to maintain a sense of routine and predictability.

Irritability

Irritability is characterized by a severe negative reaction to seemingly mild stimuli, which may lead to anger, outbursts, aggression, or self-injurious behavior. It is often associated with a low frustration threshold and a short temper. In some cases, it can describe individuals who are frequently in a bad mood or easily upset.

This behavior is defined by the aberrant behavior checklist (ABC) which defines irritability as self-injurious behavior, aggression, temper tantrums and outbursts, slamming doors and stamping feet, mood instability, demanding, screaming, yelling, crying and whiny.

Self-Injurious Behavior

Defined by behavior that hurts oneself, self-injurious behavior is not uncommon in intellectual disability, behavioral disorders and psychiatric conditions. Common behaviors include head-hitting, head-banging and biting, which, when severe, can cause physical injury. In many cases, biting results in swelling and scaring of the area that is constantly being bitten. Head banging can become so severe that it causes vision loss because of retina detachment. Self-injurious behavior should be differentiated from suicide attempts where an individual is trying to injury themselves to end their life.

Obsessive Compulsive Disorder

Obsessive-Compulsive Disorder (OCD) involves an overwhelming need to perform specific routines—sometimes repeatedly—to alleviate intense feelings of distress (compulsions). It is also marked by persistent, often unwanted thoughts or mental fixations on particular subjects, or a need to control the environment to adhere to a specific set of rules (obsessions). Mental obsessions may center on a particular interest to the exclusion of all others, or they can involve distressing thoughts, such as fears of contamination or beliefs that one's actions are sinful, known as scrupulosity.

Catatonia

Catatonia is characterized by a significant reduction in movement without an identifiable neurological or muscular cause. Individuals with catatonia may remain immobile or maintain a single position for hours, often with noticeable muscle stiffness. This state is frequently described as "waxy flexibility", where an examiner can move the individual's limbs, and they will remain in the new position as if molded from wax.

Catatonia can also present with mutism, where the individual has little to no speech despite being physically capable of speaking. In some cases, if speech is present, the individual may exhibit echolalia, a condition where they repetitively echo words or phrases spoken by others.

Additionally, individuals with catatonia may refuse to eat or communicate and may appear unaware of their surroundings. They may also exhibit a state of stupor, characterized by unresponsiveness and minimal to no interaction with the environment.

Vision Changes

Due to its impact on the central nervous system, CFD can be associated with a number of changes in vision. These visual changes generally occur in childhood and include:

- **Optic atrophy** - generally causes blurred vision, reduced visual acuity, and color vision abnormalities
- **Nystagmus** - causes blurred or shaky vision when focusing on objects
- **Visual field defects** - includes blind spots or tunnel vision
- **Photophobia** - causes discomfort or pain in bright environments
- **Cortical visual impairments (CVI)** - results in a difficulty recognizing objects, poor visual attention, or inconsistent visual responses
- **Strabismus** - may cause double vision or limited depth perception

While not as frequently mentioned in the literature and sometimes considered a psychiatric condition, hallucinations are also a symptom of CFD that I have frequently encountered in my clinical practice. Parents may report that their child appears to be responding to people, objects, or lights that are not present.

Evaluating vision changes in non-verbal patients can be challenging. Parents may observe that their child has lost interest in activities, become more socially withdrawn, or is stumbling more frequently. While these behaviors can indicate motor or behavioral issues, they may also be signs of visual changes, such as impaired depth perception or difficulty focusing. Children experiencing vision loss may also show regression in reading skills or complain of headaches, often due to increased strain on their visual system from changes in eyesight.

It is essential to ask parents about recent optometric evaluations and any vision assessments conducted at school or in clinical settings. Deterioration or worsening of vision is a significant symptom of CFD that, with appropriate treatment, can potentially be reversed, improving the patient's quality of life.

Hearing Loss

Like vision loss, hearing loss is also a less common, but significant symptom of CFD that generally happens in childhood, particularly if CFD is progressive. The loss of hearing due to CFD may manifest in different ways:

- **Sensorineural Hearing Loss** - caused by damage to the inner ear (cochlea) or auditory nerve pathways
- **Auditory Processing Deficits** - hearing thresholds may be normal, but the patient may have trouble processing and interpreting sounds or speech

Similar to vision changes, hearing loss can be challenging to diagnose in a non-verbal child. Caregivers may describe the resulting behaviors rather than recognizing the hearing loss itself. For example, they may report that the child no longer responds to their name or fails to follow directions. Clinical assessments of hearing such as Auditory Brainstem Response (ABR), Otoacoustic Emissions (OAE), and tympanometry are particularly valuable when evaluating symptoms potentially related to CFD. These tests objectively measure the function of the eardrum, cochlea, and brainstem in response to auditory stimuli, which helps overcome language and communication barriers that can complicate the accuracy of hearing assessments in infants, young children, or non-verbal individuals with intellectual disabilities.

While this is not an exhaustive list of symptoms associated with CFD, it represents a comprehensive overview of the most commonly reported symptoms in the literature, as well as those I have observed in my clinical practice.

Parents and patients who report symptoms to clinicians may describe them using different words than those listed in this chapter. For example, they may report urinary retention, loss of hand function, choking, and tripping, which may represent alternative descriptions of core symptoms. For example, urinary retention may be a manifestation of catatonia, while choking and tripping may result from ataxia. As previously stated, many of these symptoms are attributed to other diagnoses; however, that does not always eliminate CFD as contributing cause. For example, OCD is frequently considered a hallmark or PANS and PANDAS. However, attributing OCD to PANS or PANDAS does not exclude the possibility of CFD as an underlying etiology—particularly when standard treatments for these conditions have been administered without symptom resolution.

Lastly, when evaluating symptoms, it is essential not only to consider potential underlying conditions but also to review all medications the patient is taking, as many of these symptoms can also be side effects of medications taken for comorbid conditions.

CHAPTER 15.
Diagnosing CFD

Chapters 13 and 14 outline symptoms that may raise concerns for CFD at various developmental stages or ages, particularly when these symptoms cannot be explained by another diagnosis or fail to respond to conventional treatments. This chapter expands on these concepts to explain how specific testing procedures can confirm, support, or help rule out a diagnosis of CFD.

To Lumbar Puncture or Not to Lumbar Puncture: That is the Question

An absolute diagnosis of CFD can be made by measuring 5-MTHF levels in cerebrospinal fluid (CSF), which is obtained through a lumbar puncture (LP). Although the LP procedure is relatively simple, it can cause some discomfort. Many adults tolerate the procedure well with the use of a local anesthetic to numb the skin and soft tissue in the lower back. However, most children, as well as some adults with cognitive or communication impairments, may require sedation, which involves additional risks.

When collecting CSF for the analysis of critical metabolites, such as folate, it is essential that the physician performing the LP has experience with these specialized tests. CSF metabolite analysis requires precise collection and handling protocols to ensure accurate results, as many of these compounds are highly sensitive to degradation.

It is common for multiple samples to be collected during a single LP to test for various conditions. Each sample may be allocated to different laboratory assays, necessitating proper handling.

An opening pressure measurement should be performed at the start of the LP, before any fluid is drained. This measurement provides valuable information about intracranial pressure (ICP), which can aid in diagnosing conditions such as intracranial hypertension or cerebrospinal fluid leaks.

Samples taken for metabolites must remain uncontaminated. Unfortunately, it is common for the needle to miss the target on the first or second attempt, necessitating repositioning. This can lead to blood contamination in the CSF sample. To minimize this risk, it is recommended to perform the procedure under radiological fluoroscopy guidance, which ensures precise needle placement. (See Chapter 4 for a diagram explaining the LP procedure).

CSF samples for CFD must be immediately put on ice to preserve the stability of neurotransmitters and metabolites, which degrade rapidly at room temperature. Additionally, samples should be protected from light during storage to prevent degradation of light-sensitive compounds. For transport, samples must be shipped on dry ice, ensuring they remain frozen while also being shielded from light exposure to maintain sample integrity.

Undergoing an LP can be a significant experience for a child, so simpler, non-invasive testing methods (described in the next sections) are often considered as alternatives to a CFD workup. In many cases, these less invasive methods are favored when CFD is highly suspected and the patient is at high risk for having adverse effects from the LP procedure. However, if the patient presents with non-specific symptoms that require a differential diagnosis between multiple possibilities—such as infections in the CNS, increased intracranial pressure, or autoimmune encephalitis—an LP may be necessary. While alternative methods can assess the likelihood of CFD, certain serious conditions may still warrant an LP to investigate the presence of bacteria, specific antibodies, inflammatory markers, or elevated CNS pressure as part of a comprehensive neurological evaluation.

As noted earlier, children and some adults may require sedation for an LP. In these situations, it is essential to consider the risks associated with sedation, which can vary depending on the type of anesthesia used. Key considerations include, but are not limited to, metabolic conditions such as mitochondrial disease or dysfunction, the patient's risk of seizures, respiratory issues (such as asthma or sleep apnea), cardiac conditions, allergies, potential drug interactions, fasting requirements, and any behavioral disorders that may complicate post-LP monitoring and recovery.

The decision to proceed with an LP for diagnosis should involve consultation with a medical professional who is well-acquainted with the patient's health history and experienced in diagnosing CFD. This ensures the best decision for that individual.

In addition to procedural risks of an LP, there are other, less obvious risks. One significant danger is that the results may sometimes be falsely reassuring. For instance, a 5-MTHF concentration of 45 nmol/L, which is just above the lower limit of the normal range, might lead some physicians to rule out CFD as a cause of the patient's symptoms. However, in my experience, interpreting CSF 5-MTHF levels requires careful consideration of multiple factors. Even "normal" results can be clinically significant for some patients. Individual variability, symptom presentation, current supplementation, and underlying conditions must all be taken into account when assessing whether the reported levels are truly adequate for proper neurological function.

What is a Normal CSF Folate Level?

In our initial study on children with ASD who tested positive for folate receptor autoantibodies (FRAAs), we offered LPs to measure CSF 5-MTHF levels.[201] We observed a correlation between blocking FRAAs and 5-MTHF concentrations; however, none of the children had levels that were frankly below normal. Instead, their levels ranged between the lower limit of normal and the average for the general population. In other words, their 5-MTHF concentrations were within the lowest 50% of the normal range. Despite none of the children having a below normal concentration of CSF 5-MTHF, many of them responded positively to leucovorin treatment.

How can this be explained? As discussed in several chapters of this book, disease processes such as inflammation, oxidative stress, and/or methylation abnormalities can increase the body's demand for cofactors like folate. This situation is referred to as an *insufficiency* rather than a deficiency. Specifically, a deficiency occurs when vitamin levels are below the normal range, while an insufficiency means there isn't enough of the vitamin to meet the body's increased metabolic needs during disease.

The key issue is that standard "normal" ranges are established for healthy individuals, but these may not be suitable benchmarks for those with ongoing illness. For instance, research suggests that individuals with ASD may require higher folate levels than typically developing individuals. Consequently, even a low-normal CSF concentration of 5-MTHF might be insufficient for those with ASD or other conditions, as their bodies may need more folate than usual to support optimal brain function. Additionally, some medications—such as those prescribed for epilepsy and autoimmune conditions—can disrupt folate metabolism. As a result, patients may have an increased demand for folate while taking these drugs.

While an LP is a valuable tool for diagnosing CFD, it carries certain risks and requires careful evaluation by an experienced clinician. Interpreting 5-MTHF levels within the broader context of the patient's clinical picture is crucial. Figure 15.1 presents data points from three separate studies that established an inverse relationship between CSF 5-MTHF levels and blocking folate receptor autoantibodies (FRAAs). This suggests that higher FRAA levels are associated with lower concentrations of 5-MTHF in the cerebrospinal fluid. Figure 15.2 (two-page spread on the next page) summarizes data from multiple studies in which subjects underwent lumbar punctures to measure CSF 5-MTHF levels. Many of these studies involved specific subgroups defined by study inclusion criteria, often with limited sample sizes.

While definitive conclusions cannot be drawn from this dataset alone, the findings suggest that certain high-risk groups tend to fall within the low-normal range, which means they would not meet the criteria for a frank CFD diagnosis. Relying solely on strict cutoff values may incorrectly rule out CFD, potentially advising against folate treatment, which could otherwise be highly beneficial for the patient.

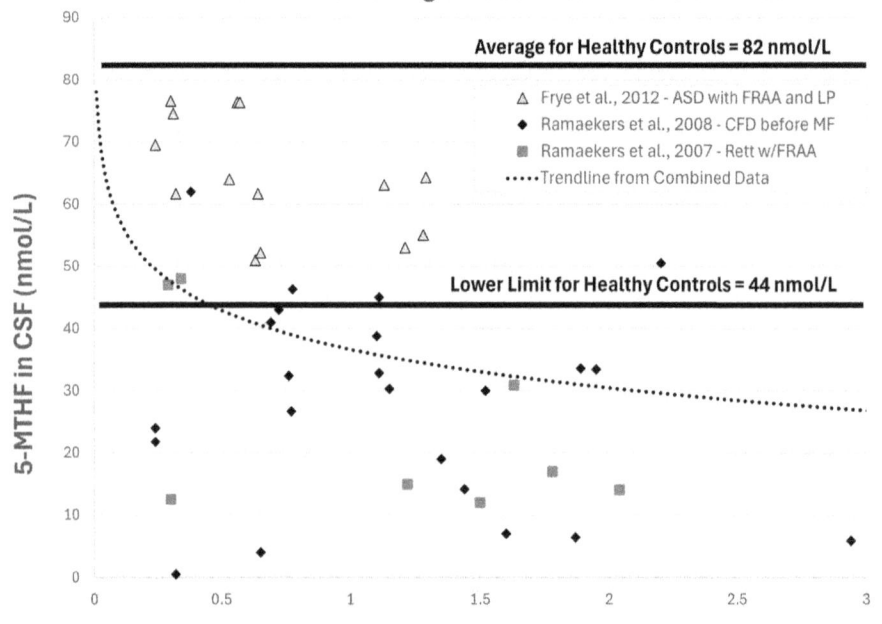

Figure 15.1 illustrates the inverse relationship between FRAAs and CSF 5-MTHF levels, using data from three separate studies. (1) The "ASD with FRAA and LP" group consists of individuals with ASD who tested positive for FRAAs and underwent a lumbar puncture to assess CSF 5-MTHF levels. (2) The "CFD before MF" group includes patients diagnosed with CFD prior to starting a milk-free (MF) diet. (Chapter 16 explores the effects of dairy consumption on CFD). (3) The "Rett w/FRAA" group represents patients with Rett syndrome (discussed in Chapter 9) who also tested positive for FRAAs.

The Folate Fix - 226

Non-Invasive Testing for Cerebral Folate Deficiency

Most commonly, CFD is caused by three problems that are not mutually exclusive: folate receptor autoantibodies (FRAAs), mitochondrial disease or dysfunction, and genetic mutations. While genetic mutations causing CFD are rare, with only a few documented cases, FRAAs and mitochondrial issues appear more frequently, as illustrated in the parent stories shared in this book.

Currently, an LP is the only method to definitively confirm a CFD diagnosis. Alternatively, the testing procedures described in this section do not measure the concentration of 5-MTHF in the CNS but rather focus on identifying the underlying causes of CFD. While these tests cannot directly confirm CFD, identifying one or more of these contributing factors significantly increases the likelihood of a CFD diagnosis.

Specific Genetic Testing

Initially, the FOLR1 gene played a crucial role in the discovery and early understanding of CFD. This gene encodes the folate receptor alpha (FRα), which is essential for transporting folate into the brain. Patients with mutations in this gene played a pivotal role in establishing the connection between low CSF folate levels and the clinical symptoms now recognized as characteristics of CFD. Early publications on CFD focused on FOLR1 gene mutations as a primary cause, leading some practitioners to mistakenly believe that patients without such mutations cannot have CFD. However, this assumption is outdated.

Mutations in the FOLR1 gene are exceedingly rare, with only about 50 cases reported worldwide. While the presence of these mutations strongly supports a CFD diagnosis, solely considering FOLR1 mutations as the cause of CFD will not correctly identify most CFD patients. Other factors such as FRAAs and mitochondrial dysfunction are more common contributors to CFD and should be considered in the diagnostic process.

As genetic testing continues to advance and become more widely accessible, focusing on a single gene mutation is becoming less desirable. Instead, comprehensive approaches—such as large gene panels, whole exome sequencing (WES), and whole genome sequencing (WGS)—offer a broader and more cost-effective means of identifying the underlying genetic causes of CFD compared to a single-gene test.

This broader approach is particularly important because, as discussed in Chapter 9, multiple genetic disorders have been associated with CFD, and few of them are directly linked to the folate receptor proteins. Limiting testing to a single gene increases the risk of overlooking other genetic contributors, reducing the likelihood of an accurate diagnosis.

CSF 5-MTHF Values in Different Cohorts

5-MTHF (nmol/L)

Healthy Controls (n = 1586)[e] — range ~40–150, mean 76

Healthy Controls (n = 63)[j] — range ~45–125, mean 73

Rett no FRAA (n = 25)[e] — range ~27–93, mean 52

Rett (n = 7)[j] — range ~20–47, mean 32

Rett with FRAAs (n = 8)[e] — range ~11–46, mean 25

Aicardi-Goutières (n = 3)[b] — range ~22–47

Kearns-Sayre (n = 8)[f] — mean 7

FOLR1 Mutations (n = 3)[a]

Specific Genetic Syndromes

Figure 15.2 presents data from studies reporting CSF 5-MTHF levels across various patient cohorts. The values within the squares represent the mean 5-MTHF concentration for each cohort, when values could be calculated. Most studies included small sample sizes, as indicated by the n = value, which denotes the number of patients in each group.

The Folate Fix

Referenced Studies Reporting 5-MTHF Values in CSF

[a]Steinfeld et al. Folate Receptor Alpha Defect Causes Cerebral Folate Transport Deficiency: A Treatable Neurodegenerative Disorder Associated with Disturbed Myelin Metabolism. The American Journal of Human Genetics. 2009 Sep;85 (3):354-363.
[b]Blau et al. Cerebrospinal fluid pterins and folates in Aicardi-Goutières syndrome: a new phenotype. Neurology. 2003 Sep 9;61(5):642-7.
[c]Ramaekers et al. A milk-free diet downregulates folate receptor autoimmunity in cerebral folate deficiency syndrome. Dev Med Child Neurol. 2008 May;50(5):346-52.
[d]Frye et al. Cerebral folate receptor autoantibodies in autism spectrum disorder. Mol Psychiatry. 2013 Mar;18(3):369-81.
[e]Ramaekers et al. Folate receptor autoantibodies and spinal fluid 5-methyltetrahydrofolate deficiency in Rett syndrome. Neuropediatric. 2007 Aug;38(4):179-83.
[f]Serrano et al. Kearns-Sayre syndrome: cerebral folate deficiency, MRI findings and new cerebrospinal fluid biochemical features. Mitochondrion. 2010 Aug;10(5):429-32.
[g]Shoffner et al. CSF concentrations of 5-methyltetrahydrofolate in a cohort of young children with autism. Neurology. 2016 Jun 14;86(24):2258-63.
[h]Ramaekers et al. Folate receptor autoimmunity and cerebral folate deficiency in low-functioning autism with neurological deficits. Neuropediatrics. 2007 Dec;38(6):276-81.
[i]Ormazabal et al. Determination of 5-methyltetrahydrofolate in cerebrospinal fluid of paediatric patients: reference values for a paediatric population. Clin Chim Acta. 2006 Sep;371(1-2):159-62.
[j]Pérez-Dueñas et al. Cerebral Folate Deficiency Syndromes in ChildhoodClinical, Analytical, and Etiologic Aspects. Arch Neurol. 2011 May;68(5):615-21.

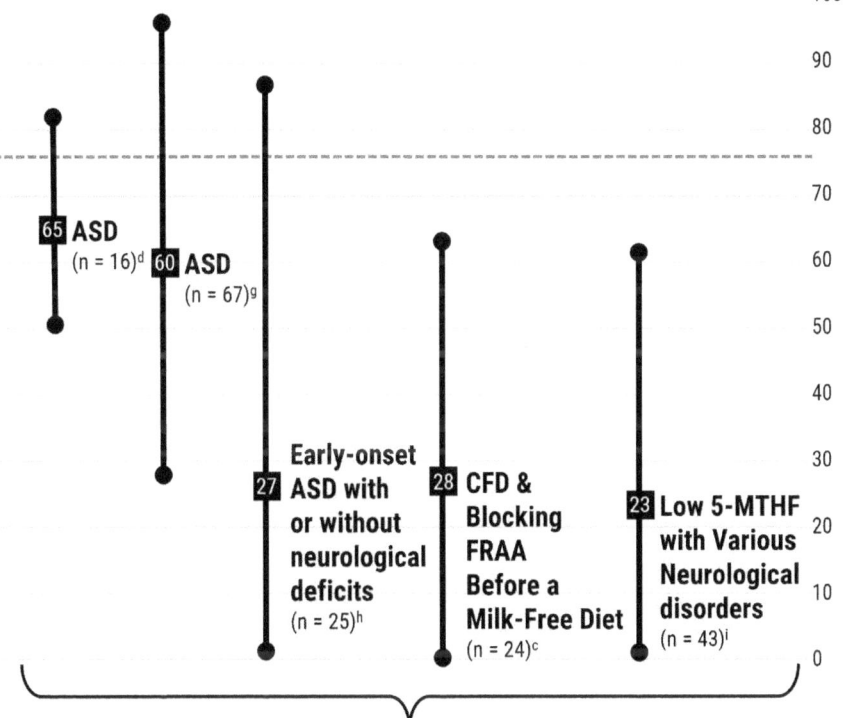

Various Neurological/Neurodevelopmental Disorders

The largest study, which included 1,586 healthy controls, reported an average CSF 5-MTHF concentration of 76 nmol/L—a value nearly double the lower threshold of the "normal" reference range (40 nmol/L). A second study summarizing 63 healthy pediatric controls showed an average CSF 5-MTHF concentration of 73 nmol/L.

Folate Receptor Autoantibodies

Folate Receptor Autoantibodies (FRAAs) are typically the first potential cause of CFD to be investigated. These autoantibodies bind to FRα, impairing its function and reducing folate transport into the central nervous system. FRAAs can be detected through a simple blood test, making them a widely accessible and practical diagnostic tool for most patients.

Two types of FRAAs have been described in literature: blocking and binding (see Chapter 4). The blocking FRAA binds specifically to the portion of FRα where folate would typically bind, thereby directly interfering with folate attachment. In contrast, binding FRAAs can attach anywhere on FRα, triggering an inflammatory response that disrupts the receptor's normal function and impairs folate transport.

The results of an FRAA test will indicate whether binding and/or blocking antibodies are present, along with the titer levels of each antibody type. In some cases, test results may be inconclusive due to factors affecting sample quality. In such instances, it may be recommended to repeat the test after addressing the confounding factors. FRAA titers indicate the quantity of these antibodies present in the patient's blood, providing insight into the extent of interference with folate transport.

Many parents and even doctors often wonder how to interpret FRAA findings. While three studies have demonstrated that the blocking FRAA correlates with CSF concentrations of 5-MTHF—suggesting that it may predict treatment response and the severity of CFD—a recent study found that the binding FRAA correlated with response to leucovorin treatment and ASD severity.[202]

While FRAA titer levels provide numerical values, the binary classification of "positive" or "negative" is often more clinically informative. Historically, most treatment studies have not specifically analyzed FRAA titers but have instead classified results as either positive or negative. In our double-blind, placebo-controlled study, FRAA positivity was associated with a favorable response to leucovorin treatment.[203] Consequently, FRAA testing is typically interpreted as positive or negative, with exact antibody titers often considered less relevant in clinical decision-making.

Another reason why FRAA positivity or negativity is more clinically significant than specific titer levels is that titers can fluctuate, particularly when their production is triggered by external stimuli such as milk protein exposure (see Chapter 16). For example, children with initially low FRAA levels may exhibit higher titers after consuming milk, while those who have eliminated milk from their diet may show lower titers over time. As a result, the most critical factor is whether the body is producing FRAAs, as this has greater implications for diagnosis and treatment than the specific titer value at the time of testing.

After receiving a positive FRAA test, a common follow-up question is whether an LP should be performed to confirm the CFD diagnosis. As discussed previously, there are pros and cons to this approach. In our initial study, we found that most parents preferred to try leucovorin when their child tested positive for FRAAs, rather than proceeding with an LP. Due to the excellent safety profile of leucovorin, most parents are comfortable initiating a trial period of the medication rather than opting for an invasive procedure. If a patient demonstrates a positive response to leucovorin, CFD can be considered a probable diagnosis (see Figure 15.3) without the need for an LP.

However, FRAA testing may yield a negative result even when CFD is present, in which case a LP could confirm the diagnosis. If the FRAA test is negative but CFD is strongly suspected, it's possible that antibody levels were too low for detection at the time of testing or that the CFD may be caused by other mechanisms such as mitochondrial dysfunction. In such cases, the test could be repeated at a later date. Alternatively, if symptoms are severe and an LP is not a feasible option, a trial of leucovorin may be a practical approach.

Beyond the Folate Autoantibody

Recently, another important folate-binding protein that interacts with the blocking FRAA has been identified in the blood of some patients. Known as the soluble folate-binding protein (sFBP), this protein binds to folate. When sFBP is present, the blocking FRAA titer may not be accurate. The presence of sFBP is detected during the FRAA analysis, and if it is found, this information is typically included in the laboratory's written report.

Although the exact nature of the sFBP has not been extensively studied, some researchers believe it may be FRα proteins that have detached from the cell membrane—potentially due to inflammation—and are now circulating in the blood, binding to folate. This protein can be thought of as a "folate sponge" in the blood, reducing the available folate.

We examined the presence of sFBP in two of our studies. In the first study, a series of patients with detectable sFBP was reported, all of whom were severely affected by both ASD symptoms and comorbidities. These patients required higher-than-normal doses of leucovorin to achieve a response. Remarkably, some of these individuals had not responded to multiple treatments, some for over a decade, yet showed improvement when leucovorin was administered at higher-than-typical doses.[204]

Our second study investigated the predictive value of folate biomarkers in a large series of individuals with ASD. This study confirmed that the presence of sFBP was associated with more severe ASD symptoms.[205]

More research is needed on sFBP to further develop its role as a reliable biomarker. Although still in the early stages of investigation, sFBP does appear to be associated with more severe cases. Individuals who test positive for sFBP may require higher doses of leucovorin than those typically needed to achieve a clinical response in the treatment of CFD.

Mitochondrial Disorders

In many of the patient stories in this book, families mention the need to address mitochondrial dysfunction in their children, which is not uncommon. Chapter 4 explains that folate transport into the brain is an energy-dependent process. To meet the brain's high metabolic demands, CSF requires much higher concentrations of folate than those found in the blood. Maintaining this concentration gradient relies on ATP production by the mitochondria, which facilitates the active transport of folate into the CSF. Diseased or dysfunctional mitochondria may be unable to produce sufficient ATP for this process, contributing to the development of CFD.

When CFD is suspected, I typically order laboratory tests to assess mitochondrial function alongside the FRAA test. Evaluating both FRAAs and mitochondrial function simultaneously provides a more comprehensive assessment as both can be abnormal. While there is not a simple way to confirm that a patient has mitochondrial dysfunction from a single test, common blood and urine tests can assess biomarkers related to energy production. These can collectively serve as a proxy for mitochondrial function. A mitochondrial workup often includes first morning fasting laboratory tests for lactate and pyruvate, amino acids, acylcarnitine, coenzyme Q10 (CoQ10), creatine kinase, alanine, oxidative stress markers, and an organic acid test (OAT).

As explained in Chapter 1, mitochondria are complex organelles that utilize, convert, and produce several biochemical intermediates to make energy. Looking at levels and ratios between these intermediaries, as well as the biochemical pathways upstream and downstream of the mitochondria can often reveal an underlying dysfunction. Mitochondria contain five major complexes within the electron transport chain (ETC) and also play a crucial role in fatty acid oxidation. Under normal conditions, mitochondria primarily produce energy through aerobic respiration in the presence of oxygen.

However, when mitochondrial energy production is insufficient to meet the body's needs, cells compensate by shifting to anaerobic metabolism in the cytoplasm. This alternative pathway is less efficient and generates different metabolic byproducts, such as lactate, which can accumulate and contribute to metabolic disturbances.

Assessing lactate levels and other metabolic markers provides insight into whether mitochondria are generating adequate energy. However, timing and collection techniques are critical for accurate interpretation. Physical activity before testing can increase lactate levels, potentially mimicking mitochondrial dysfunction. For that reason, I typically recommend drawing labs in the morning after both resting and fasting. Additionally, prolonged tourniquet application during blood collection can artificially elevate lactate levels, leading to misinterpretation of results. While not exhaustive, the following results may indicate abnormal mitochondrial function:

- Elevated lactate levels
- Elevated pyruvate levels
- Elevated lactate-to-pyruvate ratio
- Elevated alanine levels
- Elevated fatty acids
- Low carnitine
- Low CoQ10
- Elevated Creatine Kinase (CK)
- Decreased Glutathione (oxidative stress)
- Elevated fumarate, malate, or dicarboxylic acids in the urine

If these clinical tests suggest mitochondrial dysfunction, the least invasive way to further evaluate mitochondrial function is through a buccal (cheek) swab, which is a completely painless procedure that takes a few minutes. A cotton swab is used to collect epithelial cells from the inside of the cheek. The sample in placed in a sealed container and sent to a laboratory. The swabbed cells contain mitochondria that can be tested enzymatically to evaluate their functional performance. The resulting report provides an analysis of mitochondrial complex activity compared to standard reference ranges.

The buccal swab has significant limitations, with limited validation studies regarding its accuracy for diagnosis. Thus, if the buccal swab is inconclusive, further workup with skin or muscle biopsy may be needed.

Patients who have mitochondrial disease, rather than mitochondrial dysfunction, typically have severe syptoms. In fact, the diagnosis for mitochondrial disease is often established long before a CFD workup is considered. Mitochondrial diseases typically present with distinctive clinical features, prompting early genetic testing, often preceding the suspicion of CFD.

As mentioned in Chapter 9, genetic sequencing may be appropriate for a comprehensive workup. Whole genome sequencing (WGS) is generally preferred when mitochondrial issues are strongly suspected, as it sequences both nuclear DNA and the mitochondrial genome. In contrast, whole exome sequencing (WES) typically focuses on exons within nuclear DNA only. Importantly, mutations in the FOLR1 gene would be identified by either WES or WGS, making both of these sequencing methods more useful than a single FOLR1 gene test.

Evaluating mitochondrial function in patients with ASD is essential, as abnormalities can guide more targeted care and treatment. My team recently published a comprehensive review on mitochondrial abnormalities in ASD, which includes guidelines for diagnosis and treatment.[206] To optimize CFD treatment, it is crucial to address mitochondrial issues either prior to or concurrently with leucovorin therapy. This is discussed more in Chapter 17.

Other Testing

Two additional neurological tests that can identify abnormalities in individuals with CFD are brain MRI and EEG. Brain MRI may reveal structural changes while EEG can detect epileptic activity or abnormal brain wave patterns, which are common in CFD patients with seizures or neurodevelopmental symptoms.

One study followed patients with genetic abnormalities in the FRα using advanced neuroimaging techniques, including MR-spectroscopy (MRS), magnetization transfer imaging (MTI), and diffusion tensor imaging (DTI).[207] MRS normalized immediately after the initiation of therapy, while MTI and DTI—both sensitive to changes in myelin—correlated with gradual clinical improvement. This suggests that improvements were linked to the restoration of myelination.

Another study found that severe CFD patients had a lower choline to creatine ratio on MRS than non-CFD patients, with this ratio having a good sensitivity (71%) and excellent specificity (92%) for diagnosis.[208] However, it is important to realize that this latter study was only based on 7 patients, making it an interesting findings but far from a diagnostic test.

Scientists have also developed a radioactive labeled positron emission tomography (PET) folate compound which binds to the folate receptor.[209] This can be used to image the concentration of folate receptors in the body. Although this was developed for detecting tumors that overexpress the folate receptor, it is possible that it could also be used to measure the available (non-blocked) folate receptors on the choroid plexus.

More research is required to confirm these findings on the newer neuroimaging techniques, and while promising, in practice, most centers do not have access to these specialized and specific tests, and few practionners have the experience necessary to interpret the results in context of CFD.

For this reason, I often recommend the more common and accessible tests, which are MRI and EEG. Not only can they provide clues in a CFD diagnosis, they are equally important for ruling out other conditions that can be explanatory for the observed symptoms.

Changes in white matter development seen on a regular MRI have been associated with CFD and may provide diagnostic clues. However, the absence of these changes on imaging does not rule out CFD. Many patients with LP-confirmed CFD have had completely normal MRI results.

The EEG can sometimes be abnormal in cases of CFD. Since CFD is associated with seizures, seizure-like activity may be observed. Most commonly, the EEG in CFD shows generalized slowing, which is indicative of metabolic encephalopathy. While this finding is very non-specific, it can support the suspicion of CFD but is not definitive enough to rule it out.

CFD or CFD-like: What is the Diagnosis?

Throughout this book, various diagnostic methods for CFD have been discussed. While a LP remains the gold standard for a definitive CFD diagnosis, supporting evidence can justify a qualified diagnosis.

The level of diagnostic certainty may range from definite to probable, possible, or unlikely, depending on the strength of the available data (see Figure 15.3).

Certainty	Definition
Definite	• Symptoms consistent with CFD and • CSF 5-MTHF Level Below Normal (Normal is typically defined as 40 nmol/L)
Probable	• Symptoms consistent with CFD and • Known cause of CFD identified and • Positive response to Leucovorin
Possible	• Symptoms consistent with CFD and • Positive response to Leucovorin and • No other cause of Leucovorin response identified
Unlikely	• No known cause of CFD identified and • No response to Leucovorin

Figure 15.3 Framework for qualifying the strength of a CFD diagnosis

As mentioned previously, a definite diagnosis requires a below-normal 5-MTHF level in the CSF, along with symptoms associated with CFD. Without a CSF 5-MTHF measurement, a probable diagnosis can be made if a known mechanistic cause of CFD is identified (for example, a positive FRAA test), symptoms align with CFD, and there is a positive response to leucovorin. If a specific biological cause for CFD cannot be confirmed but the patient presents with symptoms and responds to leucovorin, a possible diagnosis is appropriate. In such cases, alternative diagnoses that could also respond to leucovorin should be ruled out. Finally, if no biological cause for CFD is identified and there is no response to leucovorin, then the diagnosis is considered unlikely.

This framework provides a structured yet flexible approach, allowing clinicians to classify CFD cases based on evidence while guiding appropriate diagnostic and treatment decisions.

The path to a CFD diagnosis can vary significantly from patient to patient. Some individuals with mitochondrial or genetic disorders may undergo proactive evaluation for CFD due to its known associations with these conditions. Others may only reach a CFD diagnosis after treatment-resistant comorbidities prompt further investigation.

Notably, some patients experience significant improvement with leucovorin therapy despite never obtaining a definitive CFD diagnosis. Given its excellent safety profile, leucovorin provides many patients with the confidence to proceed with treatment, even in cases where there is only a possible diagnosis.

CHAPTER 16.
Milk and CFD

Milk: It Does the Body Good?

Chapters 13 and 14 explored the symptoms of Cerebral Folate Deficiency (CFD), while Chapter 15 covered diagnostic testing, and the following chapters focus on treatment options and ongoing management of CFD. So why interrupt this logical progression with a chapter about milk?

Because in some cases, the first step in treatment isn't medication—it's lifestyle modification, particularly dietary changes. Understanding how and why milk can exacerbate CFD symptoms empowers families and clinicians to make informed choices that can have a meaningful impact on outcomes.

Milk is so deeply ingrained in daily life that we often overlook its unique properties. It is widely viewed as a nutritional staple, an essential grocery item, or a necessary part of a balanced diet. However, much of this perception is shaped by marketing and cultural norms, rather than actual biological facts. Taking a moment to examine what milk is and remembering whom it is designed for offers a new perspective—one that focuses on its biochemical properties and potential effects on health, specifically autoimmune conditions.

Many parents report that their children with autism spectrum disorder (ASD) show improvement on a milk-free diet. To understand how milk may influence both CFD and ASD, it is essential to explore the interactions between dairy consumption, the gut, and folate metabolism.

This relationship may play a key role in the diagnosis and management of CFD, helping explain why dietary modifications lead to symptom improvement in some patients with CFD and ASD. The connection between diet, immune function, and folate transport is an emerging area of research, with the potential to shape more effective treatment strategies for both conditions.

Breastmilk: A Bioactive, Adaptive Fluid

Before discussing milk as a food product, it is essential to first differentiate breastfeeding from the consumption of milk from other animals.

A human infant nursing from its mother is a natural and biologically optimal practice, strongly encouraged for all newborns. The U.S. Department of Health and Human Services (HHS) recommends exclusive breastfeeding for the first six months, with continued breastfeeding through at least the first year of life as solid foods are introduced.[210]

Breastfeeding offers well-documented benefits, ranging from nutritional to emotional, with new advantages still being discovered. In fact, a recent meta-analysis examining the potential impact of breastfeeding on Autism Spectrum Disorder (ASD) development found that six months of breastfeeding was associated with a 54% reduction in ASD risk.[211]

Human milk is a bioactive and living fluid, uniquely tailored for infant consumption. It contains an intricate balance of macronutrients, micronutrients, proteins, fats, and immunological components. Its composition is dynamic, constantly adapting to meet a baby's evolving nutritional and developmental needs in ways that science has yet to fully elucidate.

A mother's milk production adjusts in both quantity and composition to support her growing child. The earliest postpartum milk, known as colostrum, is low in lactose but rich in immunoglobulins, leukocytes, lactoferrin, cytokines, and other immunological components—providing critical protection and nutrients for newborns. Mature milk (produced a few weeks postpartum) is higher in fat, lower in protein, and lower in immunological components than colostrum.

Remarkably, changes in breastmilk occur not only over months but also throughout the day and even within a single feeding session—afternoon and evening feedings have higher fat content, and within a feeding session, the hindmilk (at the end of feeding session) has two to three times the amount of fat as the foremilk (at the start of the feeding session).[212] Additionally, studies have shown that other factors—such as left versus right breast, maternal diet, and overnight feedings—can also influence milk production and composition.[213]

Suffice it to say that human breastmilk is extremely complex and sometimes referred to as "liquid gold" because of its rich composition, which cannot be duplicated. Beyond the essential nutrients and immunological components, it also contains: stem cells, growth factors, enzymes, hormones, and natural antibiotics. Breastmilk is truly a one-of-a-kind, bioactive fluid—a perfectly designed food that can fully sustain a growing infant in ways that cannot be replicated.

The History of Human Milk Drinking Practices

Like humans, all baby mammals drink milk, but it is important to recognize that milk is biologically designed to be consumed within a species, passed from mother to offspring. In terms of milk consumption, humans are unique in two ways. Firstly, humans regularly consume the milk of other species, and secondly, humans consume milk beyond infancy and early childhood—two practices uncommon in the natural world.

The human practice of consuming milk from other species dates back thousands of years, though its exact origins remain debated depending on whether archaeological, genetic, or biochemical evidence is considered. Analysis of lipid residues in pottery suggests that milk consumption began over 5,000 years ago, possibly with nomadic populations of the Eurasian Steppes who relied on horse milk for calories during periods of migration.[214] However, proteomic analysis of dental calculus (hardened plaque) from ancient humans suggests that drinking milk may have originated even earlier—nearly 6,000 years ago in Africa, predating its emergence in the Eurasian Steppes by roughly 1,000 years.[215] Regardless of its precise origins, milk consumption has long been linked to the domestication of animals, including cattle, sheep, and goats, marking a significant shift in human dietary habits and agricultural practices.

Today in the United States, cow's milk is the most commonly consumed type of milk, while milk from other animals, such as goats and camels, is consumed to a much lesser extent. Cow milk is made of several components: 5% carbohydrate, 4% protein, 4% fat and 1% minerals, the rest is water. Compared to human milk, cow milk has higher protein and mineral contents, which can influence how it is digested and tolerated.

Milk Allergies and Intolerances

Many people are unable to drink milk due to various issues, ranging from mild discomfort and food sensitivities to severe anaphylaxis. Lactose intolerance and milk allergies are often confused and sometimes assumed to be part of a spectrum of reactions, but they are fundamentally different conditions caused by distinct components of milk.

Lactose intolerance is the inability to break down lactose, the primary carbohydrate in milk. Lactose serves as a crucial fuel for the growth of *Lactobacillus* bacteria in the digestive tract. During infancy, the intestine produces the enzyme lactase, which breaks down lactose, allowing it to be absorbed. After infancy, the body is not generally equipped to digest milk efficiently. For most people (around 68%), lactase decreases early in childhood and may become completely inactive by adulthood. If the gut lacks sufficient *Lactobacillus* to break down the lactose, it remains in the digestive tract and is fermented by other bacteria, leading to the gas, bloating, and discomfort associated with lactose intolerance.

Interestingly, although many Steppe populations today lack the lactase gene, they continue to consume large amounts of dairy. This is likely due to adaptations in their gut microbiome, where *Lactobacillus* bacteria play a key role in breaking down lactose instead of relying on the lactase enzyme.

Unlike lactose intolerance, which is a digestive issue, milk allergies result from an inappropriate immune response to proteins in milk. The two primary proteins in milk are casein and whey, with casein being the most common allergen. Human breast milk contains about 40% casein and 60% whey, whereas cow's milk has 80% casein and 20% whey. While whey is less concentrated in cow's than human milk, this does not mean that cow's milk contains only a subset of human milk proteins. In fact, one of the major whey proteins, β-lactoglobulin (which makes up about half of whey protein in cow's milk), is completely absent in human milk. These protein variations between human and cow milk contribute to the increased allergenicity of cow's milk for some individuals.[216]

Between lactose intolerance and milk allergies, it is unsurprising that there is a booming 11 billion-dollar industry dedicated to producing milk substitutes.[217] Some products aim to remove the triggering component (such as lactose-free milk), while others use completely different products derived from plants to mimic the look, texture, and flavor of milk. Another category of products includes supplements designed to improve milk tolerance, such as digestive enzymes, probiotics, and prebiotics, which work in different ways to support lactose digestion and gut health. Digestive enzyme supplements, such as lactase, directly aid in breaking down lactose, making dairy products easier to digest for individuals with lactose intolerance. Probiotics, particularly strains like *Lactobacillus* and *Bifidobacterium*, help improve gut flora and naturally produce lactase, aiding in lactose digestion. Meanwhile, prebiotics serve as food for beneficial gut bacteria, promoting a healthier gut environment that may indirectly support lactose metabolism.

How Milk Differs from Other Dairy Products

It is often assumed that individuals who cannot tolerate drinking milk must also avoid all dairy products, but this is not necessarily true. The ability to tolerate dairy depends on the underlying reason for milk intolerance, whether it is lactose intolerance, a milk protein allergy, or another sensitivity.

Dairy products differ from milk in several key ways, particularly in their composition and how they are processed. Fermented dairy products like yogurt and cheese undergo bacterial transformation, which alters the milk's original components. In yogurt, live bacteria continue breaking down lactose after consumption, aiding digestion and contributing beneficial microbes to the gut microbiome. *Lactobacillus* is one of the primary bacteria found in yogurt, making yogurt more tolerable than milk for those with lactose intolerance.

Cheese production further modifies milk's structure. The process begins with the addition of rennet, an enzyme that breaks down proteins, causing curdling of casein and the separation of whey, which is removed in most cheeses. Cheeses are then aged with specific microorganisms, which vary by type, converting lactose into lactic acid or other sugars while also breaking down fats and proteins. These transformations significantly change the composition of cheese, often reducing its irritating content.

Products like butter, ghee, and cream are primarily composed of milk fat, containing minimal amounts of lactose and protein. For example, butter is about 82% fat and 17% water, making it much lower in lactose than milk. Because of their composition, these fat-rich dairy products are often well tolerated by individuals with lactose intolerance, though those with milk protein allergies may still react to residual proteins.

Heating and pH changes during the production of milk products cause significant modifications to their underlying components, which can impact both their physical properties and tolerability. These alterations often lead to the denaturation (unfolding) of proteins, exposing previously buried hydrophobic regions. As a result, the proteins aggregate and form new interactions, altering the consistency, texture, and functionality of the final product. This process plays a key role in the thickening of yogurt, the curdling of cheese, and changes in milk's solubility and stability, ultimately affecting how these products are digested and tolerated by different individuals.

By understanding how different dairy products are processed, it becomes clear that not all dairy is equally problematic, and some forms may be tolerated even by those who cannot drink milk.

Biological Components of Milk

Even though problematic for some, casein and whey serve important functions in milk and even have medicinal properties, especially for infants who have immature immune systems.[218] For instance, proteins like lactoferrin, k-casein, casein-phosphopeptides, kappacin, caseicidin, caseicins, and glycomacropeptide all exhibit antibacterial and antiviral activities.[219] In fact, some cow milk proteins and peptides were explored as possible treatments during the COVID pandemic due to promising *in silico* (modeled simulations) and *in vitro* (petri dish) experiments targeting SARS-COV-2.[220]

In addition to having antimicrobial properties, milk also contains immunoglobulins (antibodies), which help protect the gut from infections. Similar to human milk, cow's colostrum is richer in immunological components than mature milk. Cow colostrum and milk contains immunoglobulins primarily in the form of IgG, whereas human colostrum and milk predominantly contain IgA, which plays a crucial role in mucosal immunity. While these immunoglobulins differ, bovine IgG may still provide protective benefits to humans, particularly against pathogens that infect the gastrointestinal tract.[221] However, because milk contains a wide range of immune-modulating compounds, isolating and identifying the specific components responsible for each observed immune effect is a complex challenge for researchers.

Importantly, in the context of CFD, milk also contains soluble folate binding proteins (sFBPs).[222] Given folate's crucial role in DNA synthesis and cell growth and the extremely high demand for folate in newborns, it is not surprising that milk contains specialized proteins that sequester folate, facilitating its transfer from mother to infant. Laboratory studies have demonstrated that these sFBPs are highly effective at binding folate, with some experiments indicating that more folate was bound than could be accounted for by known binding sites; however, subsequent research conducted under lower pH conditions failed to replicate this effect.[223,224] Despite this variability, sFBPs are present in cow's milk and may have important implications, which will be explored next.

Milk and Folate Receptor Autoantibodies

We have gained significant insight into the structure, function, and binding activity of folate receptors through research in both the food industry and medicine.

In the food industry, sFBPs in milk—specifically the soluble folate receptor alpha (FRα)—have been extensively studied to understand how pasteurization, ultra-high temperature (UHT) processing, and fermentation affect folate concentration. These investigations have revealed that FRα is highly concentrated in cow's milk, raising questions about its potential impact on human folate metabolism.[225]

In medicine, FRα has been a key focus in cancer research because rapidly proliferating cancer cells, like growing infants, have high folate demands. As discussed in previous chapters, folate is essential for DNA synthesis and cell division. Understanding how folate is bound and transported into cancer cells has led to the development of targeted cancer therapies.

Some chemotherapy drugs like methotrexate work by blocking folate uptake, thereby inhibiting the growth of cancer cells. Other approaches use folate as a carrier to deliver drugs selectively into cancer cells, taking advantage of the fact that many tumors overexpress folate receptors on their surfaces.[226] Oncology research has also revealed that FRα structure is well-conserved across species, allowing folate-related human cancer therapies to be tested in animal models.[227]

The high degree of homology between bovine and human FRα (91%) has made cow's milk consumption a focus of CFD research. Early in their investigations of CFD, Dr. Edward Quadros and Dr. Vincent Ramaekers (introduced in Chapter 4) hypothesized that consuming milk could influence FRAA levels in affected children due to the high content of FRα in milk.

They theorized that bovine FRα might be recognized as a foreign protein by the immune system, potentially triggering the development of antibodies against bovine folate receptors. These antibodies could then cross-react with human FRα, interfering with folate transport and leading to CFD.

To test this hypothesis, their team conducted a 2008 study measuring blocking FRAA titers in 12 patients. Over several months, milk was withheld and then reintroduced into their diets. The results showed that a milk-free diet led to a decrease in blocking FRAA titers, whereas reintroducing milk caused the titers to rise again, supporting the hypothesis that exposure to bovine FRα could influence FRAA levels.[228]

This raised new questions: Does an immune reaction to bovine FRα qualify as a milk allergy? and Why don't all individuals react to milk in this way?

One possible explanation lies in comorbid conditions commonly observed in individuals with neurodevelopmental disorders. Many of these children exhibit altered gut microbiomes and signs of gut inflammation, where the gut-associated lymphoid tissue (GALT) plays a critical role in immune defense.

GALT contains plasma cells, which produce antibodies against foreign proteins. In individuals with an overactive gut immune response, bovine milk proteins like casein and whey may be misidentified as foreign invaders, triggering inflammation and the production of antibodies that cross-react with human proteins. This could contribute to both autoimmune responses and neurological symptoms observed in CFD.

Because cow's milk has been associated with inflammation and other health concerns, there is growing interest in alternative dairy sources such as goat and camel milk. Camel milk, in particular, is high in vitamin C, unsaturated fatty acids, and B vitamins and is often marketed for its anti-inflammatory properties and nutrient-dense profile.

Interestingly, a 2021 study conducted by Dr. Ramaekers' team compared the FRα content and immunoreactivity of human, bovine, camel, and goat milk. The results revealed unexpected findings: goat's milk had a higher soluble FRα concentration than cow's milk, while camel's milk exhibited the highest immunoreactivity with folate receptors.[229]

This suggests that for CFD patients with FRAAs, most animal milks—including goat and camel milk—are likely to trigger the same autoimmune response observed with cow's milk, potentially exacerbating symptoms. These findings highlight the importance of carefully considering dairy alternatives for individuals affected by CFD-related autoimmunity.

The Role of Milk in CFD

While milk has recognized nutritional benefits, many people cannot tolerate it due to lactose intolerance or milk allergies. For individuals with autoimmune CFD caused by FRAAs, consuming non-human animal milk is more likely to be harmful than beneficial. Due to cross-reactivity with FRα, milk consumption can increase FRAA titers, potentially exacerbating symptoms. While milk exposure is not responsible for all cases of CFD, it highlights how diet can influence complex medical conditions, and for these patients, avoiding animal milk may be a crucial component of treatment. In fact, in my practice, many parents have reported improvements in their children's symptoms after removing non-human animal milk as they awaited their FRAA test results.

When evaluating patients for CFD, inquiring about animal milk consumption can help interpret FRAA test results, especially if blocking antibody levels are unusually high. Conversely, long-term avoidance of animal milk may result in lower or even negative FRAA titers, despite strong clinical suspicion of CFD.

It is important to recognize that the harm of milk on CFD patients' health stands in contrast to recent systematic reviews and meta-analyses, which suggest that milk provides more overall health benefits than harms for most people.[230] Milk's greatest benefits occur during infancy, when its unique nutritional composition supports growth and immune development. However, as people age, certain milk components—such as lactose and specific proteins—can become digestive irritants or immune triggers for sensitive individuals.

In conclusion, milk is a highly unique food product, possessing both beneficial and potentially harmful properties, which can vary significantly between individuals. While processing and fermentation alter its composition, it is essential to remember that milk is fundamentally a bioactive liquid, designed by nature for infant consumption. Its core composition is tailored to meet the nutritional, immunological, and caloric needs of rapidly growing babies. This evolutionary purpose shapes the proteins, fats, carbohydrates, hormones, and immune factors present in milk, distinguishing it from other food sources in both function and effect. In CFD, these nuanced properties of milk become particularly significant in diagnosis, treatment, and ongoing management.

CHAPTER 17.
Treating CFD

As discussed throughout this book, the standard treatment for Cerebral Folate Deficiency (CFD) is leucovorin (folinic acid). Although leucovorin has been used in oncology for decades, its classification as a "cancer drug" has unfortunately led to hesitation among both patients and physicians when considering it as a treatment for CFD. For many, the term "cancer drug" evokes images of hair loss, weight loss, nausea, mouth sores, and other severe side effects associated with chemotherapy, causing understandable concern. However, leucovorin's role in cancer therapy is fundamentally different from that of chemotherapy drugs.

Chemotherapy agents like methotrexate and 5-fluorouracil work by inhibiting folate metabolism, which helps kill cancer cells but can also harm healthy cells. Leucovorin, on the other hand, serves as a rescue drug, supplying folate to protect healthy cells from chemotherapy-induced damage while still allowing the treatment to target cancer cells. Similarly, leucovorin is also used in rheumatology to counteract the folate-depleting effects of methotrexate-based treatments for autoimmune diseases.

Because leucovorin (folinic acid) and folic acid can both act as folate rescue agents in oncology and rheumatology, some medical professionals have mistakenly assumed they are interchangeable in treating CFD. However, as explained in Chapter 3, folic acid and folinic acid are biochemically distinct, and leucovorin is the preferred treatment for CFD. CFD patients are often highly sensitive to the form of folate they receive, and while leucovorin effectively bypasses the folate transport issue, folic acid can have limited effectiveness. In high doses, unmetabolized folic acid (UMFA) may even interfere with the folate cycle, potentially worsening symptoms rather than improving them.

By addressing these common misconceptions about leucovorin, we clarify that it is not a harmful "cancer drug," but rather a powerful and distinctive folate medication that plays an indispensable role in the treatment of CFD.

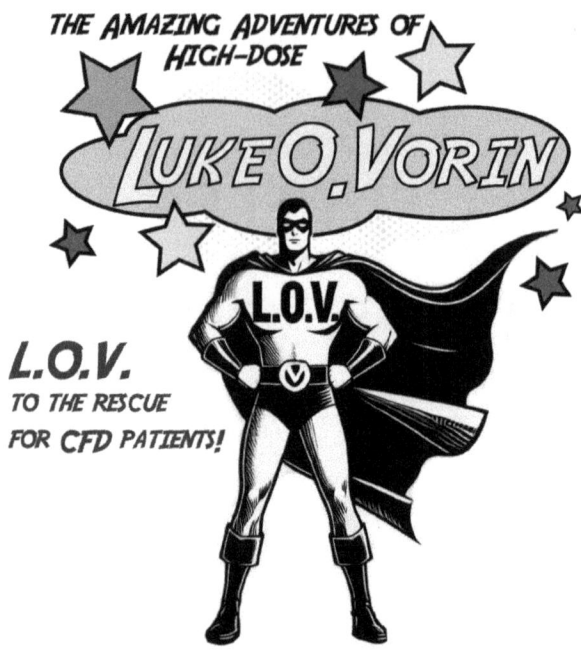

Why Leucovorin

The rationale for using leucovorin in CFD treatment is supported by several key factors. Firstly, its extensive use in oncology and rheumatology has generated a wealth of scientific data on dosing regimens, administration methods, efficacy, and safety. This established knowledge base is particularly valuable when treating a relatively novel disorder like CFD, where not all clinical variables are fully understood. Using a medication with a well-characterized profile helps minimize some of the uncertainties involved in treatment.

Secondly, oral leucovorin, the most commonly used form, is metabolized through the liver and microbiome, where it is partially converted into 5-methyltetrahydrofolate (5-MTHF) by the MTHFR enzyme and gut bacteria. This effectively delivers two forms of folate in a single treatment, maximizing its therapeutic impact. 5-MTHF directly supports methylation, a key process in gene expression, and detoxification pathways.

Additionally, since approximately half of leucovorin is converted into 5-MTHF, it directly contributes to the methylation cycle, a critical process involved in gene expression, neurotransmitter synthesis, and detoxification pathways. By providing two active folate forms in a single treatment, leucovorin not only corrects folate deficiencies but also offers broad biochemical support. Finally, leucovorin is available in multiple formulations, allowing for various routes of administration, making it adaptable to the individual needs of different patients.

Dosing

Leucovorin is typically prescribed as "leucovorin calcium" because it must be manufactured as a salt (ionic mixture) to ensure stability and solubility in the bloodstream. While folinic acid is the active component, a balancing ion is required to stabilize the compound. Calcium is the most commonly used ion, but in some cases, sodium is used instead, in which case the drug is labeled "leucovorin sodium."

The standard oral dosing regimen is 2 mg/kg/day, with a maximum of 50 mg daily, divided into two equal doses. For example, the calculated dose for a 25-kilogram (55-pound) child would be:

> 2 mg x 25 kg x 1 day = 50 mg per day divided into two 25 mg doses

In most cases, this weight-based calculation serves as the initial target dose. However, because B vitamins, including folate, can have an activating effect, which may cause increased excitement or restlessness, it is generally recommended to start with a lower dose and gradually increase over a few weeks.

A typical dose titration schedule involves starting at half the target dose for two weeks before increasing to the full dose, if well-tolerated. Using the example above, the starting dose would be:

> 50 mg x 0.5 = 25 mg per day divided into two 12.5 mg doses for 2 weeks

Although twice-daily dosing is recommended, it is commonly administered in the morning and afternoon rather than strictly every 12 hours. This is because leucovorin can have an energizing effect, which may interfere with sleep if taken too close to bedtime. Administering leucovorin during waking hours ensures that folate is available when the body needs it most for cognitive and physical activity.

Some individuals are particularly sensitive to leucovorin and may only tolerate a single morning dose. In such cases, agitation, insomnia, or increased energy are common initial side effects, but these typically subside within a few weeks of continued use. However, in a small subset of highly sensitive individuals, a slower titration schedule may be required, with some patients needing to remain at a lower dose for an extended period before increasing gradually. In rare cases, intolerance to the oral route may necessitate alternative administration methods (discussed later in this chapter). Clinical experience suggests that higher doses of leucovorin are often necessary for adolescents, adults, and individuals with mitochondrial disorders. Additionally, as discussed in Chapter 5, patients with soluble folate-binding proteins (sFBP) may require dose adjustments beyond the standard regimen to maintain a sustained clinical response. For patients who exhibit a suboptimal response to typical doses, clinicians may empirically increase the dose to assess whether a higher amount provides additional benefits. In some cases, doses up to 4–8 mg/kg/day may be required. If no recognizable improvement is observed at these higher levels, the dose can be gradually reduced back down to a lower, more optimal level.

Figure 17.2 shows the bioavailability of different doses, reflecting that availability of folate in the blood is not linearly correleated with dosage, meaning that there is a diminishing increase of bioavailability as the dose increases. For this reason, patients taking higher doses may opt to divide the doses further throughout the day. Like many drugs, administering leucovorin three times a day can maintain higher blood levels, which may enhance its effectiveness. This approach may contribute to a more consistent therapeutic blood level throughout the day, with reduced peaks and smaller troughs. Figure 17.3 shows the corresponding blood folate levels through a 24-hour period based upon different divisions of 100mg. For many patients, twice per day achieves the desired results. For others, it takes some time to find the right dosing frequency that achieves the clinical response, minimizes side effects like aggitation, and works withing their daily schedule.

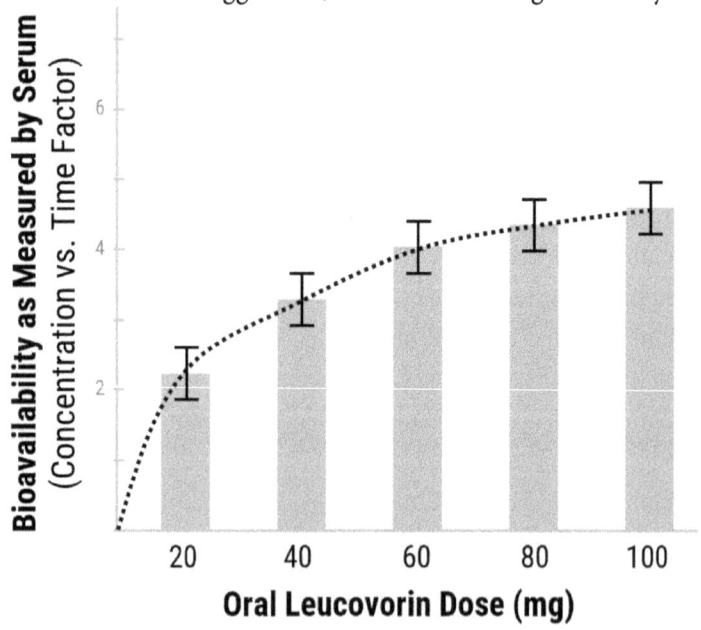

Based on Leucovorin Pharmacokinetics, Professional Service Lederle Laboratories, 1987.

Figure 17.2 Bioavailability of oral leucovorin based on different dosages

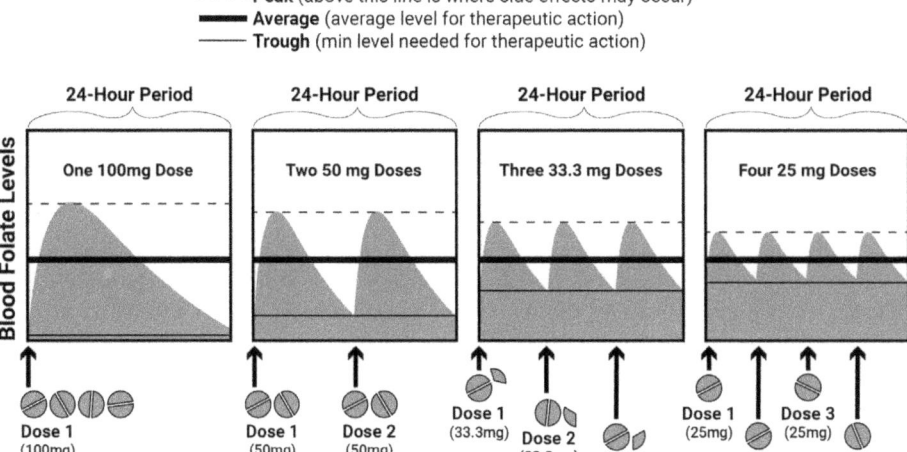

Figure 17.3 Different ways of dividing and dosing 100mg of leucovorin. Graphs depict blood levels at steady state.

Children who have comorbid conditions such as epilepsy who are taking certain anti-epileptic drugs (AEDs), and children who are taking folate-inhibitors such as methotrexate for cancer, arthritis, or other autoimmune conditions need to work closely with their physicians to understand possible drug interactions. While taking these other medications, the dosage, timing and administration method of their leucovorin treatment may need to be adjusted accordingly to ensure safety and effectiveness.

Unlike many medications used to treat acute illnesses, leucovorin is often taken for years when managing CFD. Depending on the underlying cause of the patient's CFD, the condition may be life-long. Given this, it is not uncommon for children who respond well to leucovorin to need dose adjustments several times throughout their treatment, particularly as their weight increases during periods of rapid growth, such as puberty. These adjustments ensure that the dosage remains effective in supporting the patient's folate needs as they develop.

Brands

Leucovorin is a generic drug produced by multiple manufacturers. However, not all brands of leucovorin are identical, and certain brands can even cause unwanted adverse effects in some patients. This variability is illustrated in several patient stories, where switching brands has led to different therapeutic outcomes or side effects.

Parent Story: Mysterious Regression

When we went to the pharmacy last month to pick up our leucovorin prescription, I noticed that the tablets looked different. They were the same size, but a different color and the letters on the pills were not the same as before. When I took a closer look, I found that the leucovorin tablets were from a different company than the ones we usually get. I didn't think much of this change until I realized that my son was falling asleep two hours after taking the medication.

Over the next several weeks, my son's speech started to regress. He had a difficult time expressing himself and he could not pronounce words well anymore. We then stopped giving him leucovorin. He was no longer tired, but his speech was still unintelligible.

The next month, I went back to the pharmacy and requested the original brand of leucovorin. After just the first dose of the original brand of leucovorin, his speech started to become clearer, and he eventually returned to his old self. The timing was too suspicious - I had to assume that there was something different about the other brand that did not allow leucovorin to work the same.

Parent Story: Leucovorin Suddenly Works

I had been giving my daughter leucovorin for years with a mild, but not impressive, effect on her development. One day the pharmacy changed the brand of leucovorin. Suddenly, within a few weeks, my daughter became energetic, had less brain fog and started speaking and communicating like she never had before.

I remembered that a few months back she also had transient improvements in speech. When I reviewed my prescriptions, I found that she was on this new brand during that time for only a month. She is now on the new brand with continual improvements. Her outcomes aligned with the switch of brands, making me believe that one brand was more effective than the other.

Coincidence or True Effect of Brands?

After noticing some negative effects following a brand switch, one parent reached out to an online group to see if other families had experienced similar sensitivities to leucovorin brands. Responses revealed that two specific brands frequently resulted in adverse effects, while three others were consistently well-tolerated and produced the desired therapeutic outcomes. The "bad" brands were associated with skill regression or ineffectiveness, whereas the "good" brands led to improvements in CFD symptoms.

Believing these observations were more than coincidental, I began investigating why leucovorin produced by different manufacturers could lead to such varied outcomes. My team identified two likely explanations: (1) variations in potency between brands or (2) differences in excipients (additives) used by each manufacturer, which may have adversely affected some patients. Excipients can include fillers, binders, dyes, preservatives, and other substances added for stability, taste, or manufacturability.

Different brands of leucovorin were analyzed for potency. To maintain objectivity, the pills were crushed so that the brands could not be identified. The analysis results showed that all samples contained 99% of the expected leucovorin dose, suggesting that potency was not the issue. This finding indicated that the variations in patient response were likely due to factors other than the active ingredient, prompting us to investigate other possibilities, such as differences in excipients among the brands.

Upon examining the two brands associated with adverse reactions, we found that one contained numerous undesirable excipients, while the other had the same excipients as the brands that did not cause issues. However, a parent contacted the manufacturer of this brand to inquire further about the additives and discovered that the tablets contained additional excipients not listed on the label. This was surprising, but we learned that drug companies can change a product's excipients without updating the label, provided that the excipients are on a list approved by the Food and Drug Administration (FDA).

This issue is not unique to leucovorin. Research indicates that excipients can contribute significantly to adverse effects. In fact, one study estimated that around 50% of adverse reactions associated with medications are due to these excipients rather than the active drug itself. [231]

Some patients with high sensitivities may not tolerate any of the commercial leucovorin brands. In such cases, a compounding pharmacy can create a custom formulation without any additives. Because I work with a population of children who often have unique metabolic issues, when introducing therapy for CFD, I sometimes recommend starting with compounded leucovorin. This approach minimizes the variability that commercial brands might introduce.

If the child responds well to the compounded leucovorin and the family later wishes to switch to a commercial version for cost savings or convenience, having an established baseline effect on a leucovorin formulation without excipients is beneficial for comparison. Should the child experience regression or adverse effects with the commercial version, the family can either return to the compounded formulation or work with their local pharmacy to try different generic brands.

Administration Method	Explanation
Oral (PO)	Administered by mouth, absorbed through the digestive system and processed by the liver. Available in tablets and compounded capsules or liquid. Convenient but slower onset due to metabolism.
Intravenous (IV)	Injected directly into a vein, providing rapid absorption and immediate effect. Usually administered by a medical professional in a hospital or clinic setting.
Subcutaneous (SC)	Injected into the fatty tissue just beneath the skin with a small syringe. For younger children, this is commonly injected into the buttocks. For adult children and adults, it can be injected into the back of the arm, thigh, or abdomen. Slower absorption than IV. Administered at home.
Intramuscular (IM)	Injected into muscle tissue, allowing for faster absorption than SC but slower than IV. Leucovorin is not typically administered by this method.
Intrathecal	Injected into the space surrounding the spinal cord and brain (CSF) for direct access to the central nervous system. Very uncommonly used. Always administered by a medical professional in a hospital setting.

Figure 17.4 - Different ways of administering leucovorin

Alternate Routes of Administration

For various reasons discussed later, the oral administration of leucovorin may not be optimal for certain patients. In such cases, leucovorin can be delivered through alternative routes. See Figure 17.4 for explanations of the different delivery methods. Next to oral leucovorin, the most common administration methods for CFD are subcutaneous, intravenous, and intramuscular in that order of prevalence. All three of these methods have been used in combination with chemotherapy with good tolerance.[232]

One study treating refractory CFD used intrathecal administration[233] (directly into the spinal fluid); however, this type of administration is very rare and must be conducted in a medical setting under careful supervision.

Intravenous (IV) Administration

For most CFD patients, IV administration is uncommon; however, it may be suitable for some situations. Most of what we know about IV administration of leucovorin comes from cancer studies. In oncology, leucovorin is commonly administered IV following methotrexate or 5-fluorouracil treatments in a hospital setting. When treating children for colorectal cancer with 5-fluorouracil, leucovorin is given at 200 mg/m^2 daily for 5 days (approximately 300 mg for the average child). For standard rescue from methotrexate, leucovorin is given at 10 mg/m^2 (approximate 15 mg for the average child) every 6 hours for 10 doses. In the case of impaired methotrexate elimination or overdose, it is given at 100 mg/m^2 every 3 hours (approximately 150 mg for the average child) until the methotrexate blood concentration is acceptable.

IV administration is preferred when immediate absorption and high bioavailability are needed, especially when a patient's condition or treatment plan requires a rapid and controlled delivery of the medication. Figure 17.5 shows the corresponding folate serum levels over time based on different methods of leucovorin administration.

In Chapter 7, I reviewed some cases of children with refractory epilepsy who did not respond to typical drugs, but did respond to leucovorin. In cases when a child is hospitalized with treatment-resistant epilepsy and CFD is confirmed or suspected, a trial of IV leucovorin may be warranted due to the serious risks associated with prolonged seizures.

IV administration might also be considered when patients are already receiving infusions for other reasons. If CFD is confirmed or suspected, and there are no concerns about drug interactions, trialing IV leucovorin can provide immediate feedback on its effectiveness. Some clinicians, including myself, have observed improvements in symptoms, such as cognitive function, academic performance, and the resolution of seizures and involuntary movements, when leucovorin was added to ongoing infusion treatments.

Several studies have used IV administration to treat severe cases of CFD with good,[234,235,236,237,238,239,240] minimal,[241] and unremarkable[242] success. Some studies report treating with daily IV leucovorin for a certain period of time and then switching to daily oral leucovorin, although some studies continue IV leucovorin on a regular basis. Studies have used 4-6 mg/kg/day daily, 12 mg/kg/day every other day, 100mg weekly, 300mg and 25mg/kg monthly. Overall, the IV dosing regimens for CFD are a lot less standardized compared to oral administration.

The limitations of IV administration are primarily due to leucovorin's calcium content. As previously described, leucovorin is formulated as a salt combining

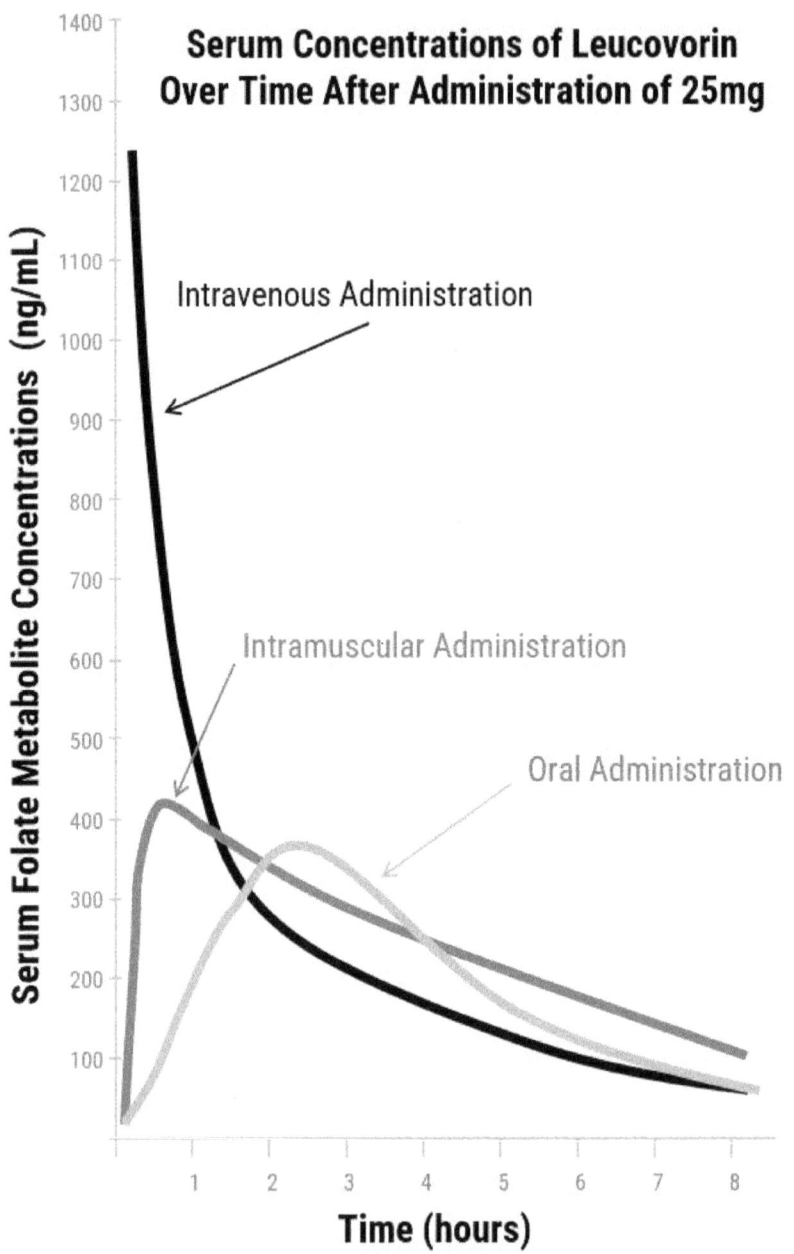

Based on Leucovorin Pharmacokinetics, Professional Service Lederle Laboratories, 1987.

Figure 17.5 Concentrations of leucovorin in the bloodstream over time based on different administration routes: oral, intravenous, and intramuscular. Adapted from data published in: Leucovorin Pharmacokinetics, Professional Service Lederle Laboratories, 1987.

folinic acid with calcium to enhance its stability and water solubility. Administering leucovorin intravenously carries the risk of calcium overload, which can lead to complications such as irregular heartbeats, kidney damage, or hypercalcemia (excess calcium in the blood). Additionally, administering more than 160 mg per minute can have serious consequences, and leucovorin may be incompatible with certain IV solutions.

Given these risks, it is crucial to consult an expert before considering IV administration. Since IV administration requires a medical professional to perform the procedure, it is generally less accessible than other routes of administration. However, IV remains an important option, especially for individuals with refractory epilepsy, where its rapid delivery and high bioavailability may provide significant therapeutic benefits.

Subcutaneous (SC) Administration

Leucovorin can also be given subcutaneously (SC)[243] into fatty tissue such as the buttocks, abdomen, thigh, or upper arm. Typically, this is done by parents at home using 3/8 to 5/8 inch, 25 to 30 gauge needles, which are very thin, similar to those used for insulin injections.

When given subcutaneously, leucovorin is sometimes combined with cobalamin (Vitamin B12). Many children with conditions such as anemia, gastrointestinal disorders, metabolic disorders, neurological disorders, or malabsorption issues require subcutaneous B12 injections. Children with autism spectrum disorder (ASD) often experience these comorbidities and frequently respond well to SC cobalamin, which is typically administered several times a week.[244]

Cobalamin contains a cobalt ion surrounded by a corrin ring. To make this base molecule more stable, it is commonly combined with a cyanide molecule or a methyl group, resulting in cyanocobalamin or methylcobalamin, respectively. Both forms are available as over-the-counter and prescription supplements. Since cyanocobalamin is synthetic and requires conversion to methylcobalamin to become bioactive, methylcobalamin is often preferred for children with metabolic issues.

An experienced compounding pharmacy can combine both methylcobalamin and leucovorin into a single SC injection, allowing children who need both treatments to receive only one shot instead of two. However, liquid methylcobalamin is a sensitive compound that can degrade when exposed to heat, light, or air. As a result, it typically requires special handling, including refrigeration and protection from light, to maintain its stability and effectiveness.

Many practitioners regularly use these combined injections for children with ASD who have biomarkers indicating a need for supplemental cobalamin. The combination of methylcobalamin and leucovorin appears to cause fewer adverse effects—such as hyperactivity and sleep disturbances—compared to cobalamin alone. Additionally, our recent case series suggested that this combination offers benefits for children with ASD and FRAAs, potentially enhancing therapeutic outcomes.[245] This delivery method has proven to be a beneficial alternative for some children who cannot tolerate oral leucovorin. While there are only preliminary results supporting this treatment approach, it appears to be a promising option for managing CFD and related conditions.

Intramuscular (IM) Administration

Leucovorin is also given on its own intramuscularly (IM)[246] for folate metabolism disorders. This is a much rarer form of administration, generally reserved for individuals who have folate absorption issues.

The absorption of dietary folate is facilitated by the proton-coupled folate transporter (PCFT) in the proximal intestine (as discussed in Chapter 2). Some children have a defect in the PCFT, which leads to a unique type of folate deficiency. For example, a 1-year-old child with hereditary malabsorption experienced low blood folate levels due to this defect. The depletion of folate in the blood led to secondary CFD, resulting in neurological symptoms.[247] Even with a very high oral leucovorin dose of 10 mg/kg/day, the child's CSF 5-MTHF concentration was only 12 nmol/L (normal levels for children under 2 years range from 81-184 nmol/L). After increasing the dose to 28 mg/kg/day, the CSF concentration only rose to 16 nmol/L.

It wasn't until the child received 2 mg/kg/day of IM injections for six weeks that the CSF concentration increased to 43 nmol/L. After six months of IM administration, the concentration approached normal values at 59 nmol/L. These CSF levels were only possible when the blood folate concentration reached 2042 nmol/L, hundreds of times higher than the typical range of 7-29 nmol/L. As the CSF folate levels normalized, the child's neurological symptoms resolved. In another case involving a child with epilepsy, a dosage of 4 mg/kg/day of IM leucovorin resulted in a significant reduction in seizures.[248]

Most patients with CFD will not require IM administration; however, severe cases with known absorption issues or rare forms of epilepsy may require this form of delivery. IM offers a more rapid concentration increase than oral leucovorin, and a slower decline concentration rate than IV.

Intrathecal Administration

Some medications are administered intrathecally, which means they are injected directly into the cerebrospinal fluid in the spinal canal. Due to the precision required and the potential risks involved, this type of administration is always performed by a trained healthcare professional.

Leucovorin, though commonly administered orally or intravenously, is rarely given intrathecally. In fact, its drug monograph—the official document providing detailed information about each medication—does not recommend intrathecal use. However, in some cases, this method has been utilized to treat CFD because intrathecal administration bypasses the blood-brain barrier.

As discussed in Chapter 4, mutations in the FOLR1 gene, which encodes the folate receptor alpha, can lead to severe cases of CFD by disrupting folate transport into the brain. One study treated seven patients with genetically confirmed abnormalities in the FOLR1 gene with intrathecal leucovorin. This method was chosen after failed results with oral treatment. Unlike all other administration techniques, intrathecal administration bypasses the blood-brain barrier, where FOLR1 mutations impede normal folate transport.

Intrathecal dosing ranged from 1-5 mg twice a month to 2-8 mg monthly. Three of the four symptomatic patients (75%) showed improvement, while one patient's condition worsened. Those who improved also showed improved myelination on MRI brain scans, which correlated with their clinical response.[249]

Use of 5-methyltetrahydrofolate (5-MTHF)

Chapter 3 explains how folinic acid is partially converted into 5-MTHF, which is another active form of folate. Since 5-MTHF generates a free methyl group, it plays a crucial role in fueling the methylation cycle, which is essential for numerous metabolic processes, including DNA synthesis and neurotransmitter production.

For these reasons, some clinicians prefer using 5-MTHF directly as a treatment. They argue that since 5-MTHF is the substrate for methionine synthase it should be as effective or even superior to leucovorin. By providing the body with the end product of folate metabolism, 5-MTHF bypasses potential genetic or enzymatic blockages in the folate cycle.

While this reasoning is understandable, there are still significant advantages to using leucovorin as the primary treatment for CFD. Firstly, leucovorin has been more extensively studied than 5-MTHF, so there is greater certainty regarding the appropriate dosages for treatment. Secondly, at least half of leucovorin is converted into 5-MTHF, providing the same benefit. Thirdly, leucovorin directly enhances the production of 10-formyl-tetrahydrofolate, the precursor to purines, which is essential for DNA and RNA synthesis as well as neurotransmitter and nitric oxide production.

That said, some patients may not tolerate leucovorin well. Individuals with MTHFR polymorphisms may have reduced enzyme functionality and a lower capacity to convert leucovorin into 5-MTHF efficiently. However, at the therapeutic doses used for CFD, this conversion still occurs, even when the enzyme operates at a reduced capacity.

In addition, much of the conversion from leucovorin to 5-MTHF occurs in the gut by the microbiome, so the capacity of the MTHFR is not a major issue. Patients with homozygous C667T MTHFR polymorphisms (two copies of C677T) or severe MTHFR mutations may benefit from additional 5-MTHF supplementation to ensure adequate levels without relying on MTHFR enzyme activity. Most forms of 5-MTHF are available over the counter, making them highly accessible, though product quality and potency can vary significantly by manufacturer.

Use of Deplin® to Treat CFD

I'm sometimes asked by clinicians and patients about using Deplin® to treat CFD. Deplin® is a brand name product that was developed for a specific group of individuals who are concurrently taking antidepressants for the management of psychiatric illnesses. It has not been studied as a treatment for CFD. While it contains similar folates as those used for CFD, patients and physicians should also be aware that it has other ingredients including milk,[250] which may cause issues for some patients with CFD (See Chapter 16).

Deplin® (generic name: L-methylfolate from Metafolin® and Algae-S powder Schizochytrium) is marketed as a targeted nutrition product for people with depression and schizophrenia, and it requires a prescription. It contains L-methylfolate, a reduced folate like leucovorin (folinic acid) and 5-MTHF. It is the precursor to folinic acid in the folate cycle. It is used for psychiatric illnesses because its conversion to 10-formyl-tetrahydrofolic acid can enhance neurotransmitter production.

While patients with CFD may find some symptom improvement with this product, the dosing, safety, side effects, and outcomes have not yet been investigated for this specific use. With all factors that go into choosing a treatment—safety, effectiveness, cost, accessibility, dosing, etc., I have yet to encounter a case of CFD that would point to the use of Deplin® over leucovorin.

What About Folic Acid?

As discussed in Chapter 2, folic acid (FA) is a synthetic compound and is not the appropriate treatment for CFD. For reasons detailed earlier, it is strongly advised to discontinue all forms of folic acid supplementation if diagnosed with CFD. The conversion of folic acid into its active folate form depends on the Dihydrofolate Reductase (DHFR) enzyme.

While DHFR polymorphisms are less studied than MTHFR polymorphisms, they are still believed to be fairly common, meaning many individuals may have a diminished ability to convert synthetic folic acid into a bioavailable form of folate.

Unmetabolized folic acid (UMFA) can interfere with folate metabolism, potentially worsening symptoms. FA is also thought to compete with folinic acid and 5-MTHF at folate transport sites. Specifically, FA may bind to FRα (folate receptor alpha), preventing 5-MTHF from binding effectively.

A study systematically examined this effect in two patients—one with Kearns-Sayre syndrome and another with a homozygous MTHFR C677T polymorphism.[251] Both patients had low 5-MTHF concentrations in the cerebrospinal fluid (CSF) and received three sequential treatments: high-dose FA alone, folinic acid combined with high-dose FA, folinic acid alone. The study found that CSF 5-MTHF levels did not improve until FA was discontinued and the patients were treated with folinic acid only. During high-dose FA treatment, FA levels in the CSF increased, but 5-MTHF levels remained low, suggesting that an elevated CSF concentration of UMFA may inhibit folate metabolism in the brain, making it the wrong treatment for CFD.

Adjunctive Treatments

When studying the effectiveness of certain medications, scientists often use genetically engineered mouse models to replicate the human condition being researched. To study CFD, mouse models have been developed without the folate receptor alpha (FRα)—the primary mechanism for transporting folate into the brain. These genetically modified mice provide a valuable animal model to investigate potential therapeutics and adjunctive treatments, which will be explored in this section.

Vitamin D and PQQ

Three studies have demonstrated that in mice lacking the FRα, the reduced folate carrier (RFC) can be enhanced by Vitamin D and pyrroloquinoline quinone (PQQ).[252,253,254] Recall from Chapter 4 that the RFC is an alternative pathway for folate to cross the blood-brain barrier.

Vitamin D has numerous health benefits and has been shown to improve symptoms in neurodevelopmental disorders. Maintaining adequate levels of Vitamin D is important in treating conditions like CFD where therapeutic effectiveness depends on the proper function of the RFC.

PQQ is a naturally occurring compound produced by bacteria, which aids in energy production from alcohol and sugars. Fruits and vegetables absorb PQQ from soil. Recent mouse studies suggest that PQQ may reverse inflammation, oxidative stress, and mitochondrial dysfunction in glial cells (neuronal support cells) caused by folate deficiency.[255] Additionally, PQQ has been proposed to enhance cerebral blood flow and improve sleep quality.

These initial studies indicate that using PQQ as an adjunct therapy alongside leucovorin could provide additional benefits. However, optimal dosing and the long-term effects of PQQ supplementation remain underexplored and require further investigation.

Cobalamin (Vitamin B12)

Folate supplementation can mask a cobalamin (Vitamin B12) deficiency, so it is crucial to assess cobalamin needs alongside the investigation of CFD. In cases of cobalamin deficiency, metabolic imbalances may result in a condition called "folate trapping." Normally, 5-MTHF donates a methyl group to convert homocysteine into methionine, a process catalyzed by the enzyme methionine synthase, which requires cobalamin as a cofactor (See Chapter 3). Methionine is critical for many metabolic processes, including the methylation cycle.

However, when cobalamin levels are insufficient, 5-MTHF accumulates and becomes "trapped," unable to participate in other folate-dependent processes such as nucleotide synthesis for DNA and RNA. This results in a functional folate deficiency, despite adequate folate levels in the body.

Since CFD primarily affects the brain, where biomarkers of cobalamin metabolism cannot be easily assessed, it is important to consider cobalamin supplementation alongside folate treatment. This ensures that the folate can be properly utilized in key biochemical pathways. Without sufficient cobalamin, the methylation cycle may stall, leading to symptoms resembling both folate and cobalamin deficiencies.

As discussed in earlier sections, cobalamin is commonly seen in the form of cyanocobalamin or methylcobalamin. Since cyanocobalamin is synthetic and requires conversion to be absorbed and utilized by the body, methylcobalamin (methyl B12) is the preferred choice for children with metabolic issues. Additionally, since the metabolism of cyanocobalamin produces cyanide as a byproduct, it is not recommended for individuals with impaired detoxification abilities (which are commonly seen in children with neurodevelopmental disorders).

L-Carnitine

L-carnitine is a naturally occurring amino acid derivative that helps transport long-chain fatty acids into the mitochondria, where they are oxidized and used to produce energy. L-carnitine is also important for removing unmetabolized molecules from the body. Such molecules can build up when metabolic systems are dysfunctional.

As mentioned in several cases, mitochondria are essential for the proper functioning of the folate transporter, to such an extent that dysfunctional mitochondria can actually cause CFD. Many neurological and neurodevelopmental disorders involve mitochondrial dysfunction, which may arise secondary to other pathophysiological processes such as inflammation or oxidative stress.

Given this, supporting mitochondrial health may enhance the effectiveness of leucovorin treatments. Many clinicians, including myself, have found that adding L-carnitine supplementation to the treatment regimen can significantly improve the response to leucovorin by supporting mitochondrial function.[256]

L-carnitine is vital for maintaining cellular energy levels, particularly in tissues that require high energy, such as muscles and the heart. While it can be obtained through dietary sources, individuals with metabolic disorders may have low levels of L-carnitine, which is why supplementation can help support mitochondrial function.

Lower doses of L-carnitine are available over-the-counter, while higher doses can be prescribed, often under the name of Carnitor or Levocarnitine. Most of the time, this medication is liquid and can be taken with food to reduce stomach upset.

Pyridoxine

Pyridoxine, also known as Vitamin B6, is a water-soluble vitamin essential for numerous biological functions in the nervous system. Pyridoxine plays a critical role in synthesizing neurotransmitters that regulate neural excitability. For this reason, low pyridoxine levels are closely linked to seizures and epliepsy. Pyridoxine-Dependent Epilepsy (PDE) is a rare genetic condition characterized by seizures that respond dramatically to pyridoxine supplementation.

As discussed in Chapter 7, folinic acid-responsive seizures have an overlap with PDE, leading to current guidelines recommending the use of leucovorin and pyridoxine together. This combination proved necessary for a boy with CFD who also had seizures, suggesting that the addition of pyridoxine may be essential for optimal treatment in some cases.[257] This highlights the importance of addressing both folate and pyridoxine pathways when managing patients with seizure disorders.

Milk-Free Diet

As discussed extensively in Chapter 16, as part of the treatment for CFD, I frequently recommend that my patients follow an animal milk-free diet if they have tested positive for FRAAs or are awaiting their FRAA test results. Studies have shown a link between animal milk consumption and elevated FRAA titers. In some cases, patients were able to lower their autoantibody levels by adhering to a milk-free diet for several months.[258]

Parents who are waiting for a specialist consultation to evaluate CFD may consider trying an animal milk-free diet, as it is a simple intervention that might alleviate symptoms and provide valuable insights. If the child shows improvement on the animal milk-free diet, this can be an effective, affordable, and medication-free treatment that not only addresses CFD but may also help with other inflammatory or gastrointestinal issues.

Since cow milk contains high levels of proteins like casein and whey—common triggers for sensitivity—dairy products that are higher in fat or have undergone processing that denatures proteins may be better tolerated. In some cases, I recommend a strict dairy-free approach, and if improvement is observed, I suggest gradually reintroducing less aggravating dairy products, such as yogurt and cheese, one at a time to test tolerability.

In conclusion, this chapter has summarized the most common primary and adjunct treatments for CFD; however, it is not an exhaustive overview of every therapeutic approach used in managing this complex condition. Patients with co-morbid disorders, such as epilepsy, ASD, and/or mitochondrial diseases, often require highly individualized treatment regimens that must be closely monitored and adjusted over time.

Chapter 19 provides a collection of Frequently Asked Questions (FAQs), many of which address specific treatment-related issues that may not have been fully explored in this chapter. This FAQ section serves as an additional resource for parents and clinicians seeking further guidance.

It is important to recognize that CFD impacts numerous aspects of a patient's life. While leucovorin remains a safe, effective, and generally well-tolerated medication, achieving optimal outcomes often involves addressing broader health factors as well. Prioritizing proper nutrition, healthy sleep patterns, fresh clean air, sunlight exposure, regular physical activity, and supportive therapies can significantly enhance overall health, quality of life, and treatment success for individuals with CFD and should always be encouraged.

CHAPTER 18
Following Outcomes

Often, it seems like we approach medical treatment with the expectation that every intervention will work for every patient. However, many people are surprised to learn that even medications proven in clinical trials don't help everyone. In fact, there's a metric in clinical trials called Number Needed to Treat (NNT). For some approved drugs, the NNT may be 6 or 8, meaning that 6 or 8 patients need to be treated for one to benefit.

When treating CFD, the success rate is high, and the NNT for leucovorin is lower than for many other medications. As explained in Chapter 5, our previous studies show that for patients who are positive for FRAAs, the NNT is about 1.8.[259] Even with these promising findings, not all patients respond to treatment. It is important to remember that CFD symptoms are often non-specific and overlap with many other conditions. Not everyone with suspected CFD will end up having the condition. Additionally, each patient has a unique genetic make-up and possible comorbidities that may impact how symptoms present and how they respond to medication. Even in confirmed or strongly suspected cases of CFD, leucovorin may not work for everyone. This underscores the importance of closely monitoring patients and providing tailored care to meet their unique needs.

In clinical practice, it's critical to evaluate whether a prescribed treatment is making a meaningful difference. If it's not, it's important to explore the reasons why and take appropriate action. This might mean adjusting the dosage or frequency of the medication or considering an alternative treatment that could be more effective. In Chapter 17, I discussed some variables that commonly require adjustment throughout the course of treating CFD, including different administration methods, dosing, timing, and conjunctive therapies such as methylcobalamin.

For over a decade, I have used quantitative questionnaires to track symptom changes in my patients and to assess the effectiveness of treatments. One of the first tools I developed, along with my colleague Dr. Dan Rossignol, was the Parent-Rated Autism Symptom Change (PRASC) Scale. We collaborated to use this questionnaire in our clinics so that we could gather combined data on treatment outcomes. This effort proved valuable when we discovered the effectiveness of leucovorin in treating children with ASD who tested positive for FRAAs. Our collaboration allowed us to demonstrate that leucovorin was superior to a waitlist control group, and we published these findings in our first paper on leucovorin.[260]

We use the PRASC scale to track any changes—positive or negative—after starting leucovorin or, in the case of the control group, during a period when no treatment changes were made. The simplicity of the scale allows parents to answer the questions quickly, without becoming fatigued or distracted. The PRASC uses a 7-point Likert scale, ranging from "much worse" to "much better," and focuses on symptoms associated with ASD, which are often the primary concerns during clinical visits.

Some children with folate issues do not have ASD, yet this tool is still useful to track progress of CFD symptoms, including seizures, motor function, and different areas of cognition such as speech and attention. There is also a free-form space to report any observed side effects. This straightforward questionnaire can be given to patients before they see the doctor, perhaps while they are in the waiting room, ensuring that any changes in symptoms are documented in their chart.

Although the PRASC is copyrighted, it is available for free to any clinician who wants to use it to track changes in their patients, allowing for more personalized, quantitative medicine.

As our understanding of CFD continues to grow, so too does our ability to change the lives of those affected by this complex condition. Promising research is ongoing, fueled by dedicated scientists, clinicians, families, and advocates committed to uncovering new therapies and deeper insights. You, as patients, parents, caregivers, and medical providers, are essential partners in this journey. Your support, whether through advocacy, participation in research, or spreading awareness, plays a crucial role in shaping future advancements. Above all, never lose hope. Remain optimistic, because with every new discovery, we move closer to enhancing the well-being, quality of life, and future possibilities for every individual living with CFD and neurodevelopmental disorders.

Parent Rated Autism Symptomatic Change Scale (PRASC)

	Change Since Baseline						
	Much Worse	Moderately Worse	Mildly Worse	No Change	Mildly Better	Moderately Better	Much Better
Receptive Language							
Expressive Language							
Verbal Communication							
Non-Verbal Communication							
Stereotyped Behavior							
Expressive Language							
Hyperactivity							
Mood							
Attention							
Aggression							
Fine Motor Skills							
Gross Motor Skills							
Seizures							
Side Effects Reported:							

© Richard E. Frye and Daniel A. Rossignol, 2010

Part V.

Frequently Asked Questions

This final part of the book will address many of the frequently asked questions (FAQs) received in conferences, online discussions, peer-to-peer reviews, and patient appointments.

I would like to take a moment to sincerely thank the parents, patients, and my fellow healthcare providers who continually bring thoughtful and insightful questions to our discussions. Your curiosity and commitment to patient care not only deepen my understanding of individual experiences but often inspire new avenues of research.

Many of the advancements in treatment have been driven by the important questions asked by parents. The collaboration between families and healthcare teams is invaluable, and I am deeply grateful for the role each of you plays in advancing our collective knowledge and improving patient care.

Thank you for being essential partners on this journey.

CHAPTER 19
Frequently Asked Questions (FAQs)

FAQs: Diagnosis

1. How can I test for cerebral folate abnormalities?

Currently, there is a commercial test called the Folate Receptor Autoantibody Test (FRAT), which detects the presence of antibodies against the folate receptor alpha (FRα). The FRAT can also identify if the patient has soluble folate binding protein (sFBP) in their blood, an abnormality that may have significant implications for treatment.

Physicians can order the FRAT test, which comes with a collection kit containing all the necessary supplies to return the samples to the laboratory. The test requires a blood sample. Since many commercial labs do not handle specialty tests, it is important for families to find a phlebotomy service that can perform the blood draw.

The samples can be returned in the same kit, which includes an ice pack to preserve the integrity of the test. Results may be available in a few weeks, though in some cases it may take a few months due to the laboratory's rigorous quality assurance procedures.

It is important to remember that FRAAs are just one potential contributor to CFD, so if CFD is suspected but the FRAT results are negative, a lumbar puncture, mitochondrial workup, or genetic testing may be appropriate next steps.

2. **To get accurate results for the FRAT test, should the child avoid any foods or supplements prior to testing, and if so, for how long?**

There are certain precautions to take before undergoing the FRAT test. As discussed in Chapter 16, Drs. Quadros and Ramaekers demonstrated that cow milk significantly raises FRAA levels and should be avoided in individuals who are FRAA positive. Other types of milk, such as goat milk, can also elevate antibody levels, while human milk appears to have lesser effects. Therefore, avoiding animal's milk is crucial before the FRAT test. While the effects of other dairy products are unknown, there is a possibility that they may also increase FRAA levels.

Additionally, we have found that folate can raise FRAA levels. We believe this occurs because folate competes with the antibodies at the receptor level. When more folate is present in the blood, it displaces the antibodies from the receptors resulting in an increase in antibodies circulating in the blood. Although this displacement can be helpful as a treatment by removing the antibodies from the folate receptors, it also causes the titers to rise. For this reason, it is important to stop taking folate supplements before performing the FRAT test.

The exact duration for avoiding these substances is unclear, but a period of three to five days prior to testing is likely sufficient. The half-life for most folate supplements is approximately 3-4 hours, although this can vary depending on the dosage and specific product. The reason for the longer waiting period is that folates are stored in the liver and released gradually, meaning it can take the body longer to eliminate excess folate. It is recommended to avoid folate for several days before the FRAT test to allow for this extended clearance time.

3. **What can one interpret from a high FRAT value (something over 3.0 OD) versus a low FRAT value (something below 0.5 OD)? Do these correlate with symptom severity?**

We recently correlated FRAA titers with symptoms and response to leucovorin and found a significant relationship between binding titers, symptom severity, and treatment outcomes. Higher binding titers were associated with more severe ASD symptoms and a greater improvement in symptoms when treated with leucovorin.[261] For very high titers, such as 3.0 OD, there was a notable reduction of eight to sixteen points on social responsiveness subscales.

In contrast, the changes were much milder for lower titers, such as 0.5 OD. This suggests that the level of FRAA binding titer can be an important indicator of both symptom severity and potential response to leucovorin treatment.

4. Is there a different diagnosis/prognosis for a child with positive Binding versus Blocking autoantibodies? What about for children with both?

Except for the study mentioned in the previous question, binding and blocking FRAA titers have not been extensively studied in detail. In most research, FRAAs are typically classified as either positive or negative. In our double-blind, placebo-controlled study, we also dichotomized the FRAAs into positive or negative categories.[262]

In that study, we found that being positive for either antibody was predictive of a positive response to treatment. Further research is needed to better understand the prognostic value of FRAAs, but it's likely that other factors—such as mitochondrial dysfunction and polymorphisms in key folate-related genes—also play a significant role in the response to leucovorin.

5. Can CFD be diagnosed from a FRAT alone, or do you need to do a lumbar puncture to confirm the diagnosis? Likewise, if you already did a LP, is there a point in doing the FRAT?

CFD is diagnosed by measuring 5-MTHF concentration in the cerebrospinal fluid (CSF), which requires a lumbar puncture (LP) for definitive confirmation. While the FRAT can help assess whether an LP is warranted, it is not the only factor contributing to CFD and should not be the sole consideration when deciding whether to proceed with the procedure.

In my opinion, an LP should be performed in conjunction with the FRAT and markers of mitochondrial function, as these factors are critical in understanding the underlying causes of CFD. Additionally, these markers could potentially be used to monitor the severity of the disease over time, reducing the need for repeated LPs.

If an LP has already confirmed CFD, a FRAT is not necessary for diagnosis but may still provide valuable insights for treatment. For example: High FRAA titers may indicate that a milk-free diet could be beneficial. A negative FRAT test suggests alternative causes of CFD, such as mitochondrial dysfunction, metabolic disease, or specific genetic mutations. Identifying these factors can help inform a long-term treatment plan and determine potential adjunct therapies to optimize patient outcomes.

6. What are normal values for the 5-MTHF levels in the CNS? Some say 40 nmol/L is normal while others say "normal" should be above 80 nmol/L - please explain.

The lower limit of normal for 5-MTHF in the CSF is 41 nmol/L. However, it's important to recognize that these normal ranges are based on healthy individuals and may not fully apply to children with neurodevelopmental disorders, particularly ASD. In these cases, metabolic systems are often in overdrive, requiring higher levels of certain vitamins and nutrients.

Rather than labeling this as a deficiency, we refer to it as an *insufficiency*, meaning there is an insufficient amount of cofactors and/or nutrients to support the heightened demands of these overactive metabolic processes. As a result, a 5-MTHF concentration that falls within the low-normal range might still be inadequate for certain individuals, even though it technically falls within normal limits.

7. How do folate levels in the blood factor into the diagnosis for CFD? What folate levels in serum are typically seen in children who have CFD?

CFD is characterized by below-normal concentrations of 5-MTHF in the cerbrospinal fluid (CSF), despite normal folate concentrations in the blood. This is because the disorder involves a disruption of folate transport from the bloodstream to the CSF. In contrast, individuals with low blood folate levels may experience neurological consequences due to a systemic folate deficiency, but these symptoms are not specific to the brain.

In children with neurodevelopmental disorders such as ASD, we often observe high blood folate concentrations. We believe this occurs because the folate is not reaching where it is needed most, particularly the brain. Instead, it remains in the bloodstream, indicating that folate is not being properly transported to the brain and other tissues, where it would normally support metabolic and neurological functions.

8. Is there an age where either the FRAT or a lumbar puncture to diagnose CFD becomes less reliable?

There does not seem to be a specific age where the FRAT or an LP is less reliable. CFD manifests itself slightly differently at different ages, but it has been diagnosed throughout the entire age range, from neonate to adult, with good reliability.

9. When would either a positive FRAT or a lumbar puncture warrant additional testing (such as a genetic work-up)? In general, what additional tests are recommended to monitor a patient with CFD?

CFD is often associated with mitochondrial dysfunction, so in addition to testing for FRAAs, screening for mitochondrial or other metabolic disorders should be considered. I typically recommend whole genome sequencing (WGS) for most of my patients to ensure that no additional disorders are overlooked.

FRAAs have also been linked to autoimmune conditions, such as juvenile rheumatoid arthritis. Therefore, if a patient presents with symptoms like joint pain or other signs of inflammation, it is important to conduct a thorough workup for autoimmune or immune-related abnormalities.

Further testing is necessary when a patient does not respond to treatment as expected. If a patient shows improvement with standard treatment, extensive additional testing may not be necessary. However, if progress is lacking, a deeper investigation is warranted to identify any underlying factors.

In general, I monitor patients based on their response to leucovorin. However, if a patient stops responding as anticipated, repeating the FRAT or performing a lumbar puncture may be needed to reassess the situation and adjust the treatment plan accordingly.

10. For primary physicians, what are the implications of CFD? Are there other health issues that should be monitored if the patient has CFD?

Once a patient is diagnosed with CFD, the most critical neurological concern is monitoring for seizures. Seizures associated with CFD can be particularly refractory and difficult to manage. They pose a significant risk because even a first seizure can lead to status epilepticus, a life-threatening condition where the seizure does not stop on its own.

Studies have shown that patients with CFD may experience elevated thyroid-stimulating hormone (TSH) levels despite normal thyroid function, making it important to monitor thyroid activity.

CFD presents differently depending on the patient's age. Young children with CFD should have regular vision and hearing evaluations. Studies suggest that teenagers who are FRAA-positive may be at risk for developing Pediatric Acute-onset Neuropsychiatric Syndrome (PANS), while CFD has been linked to schizophrenia in young adults and severe, refractory depression with suicidal ideation in adults.

Therefore, individuals with CFD should be closely monitored throughout life for these age-related comorbid conditions and any new or evolving symptoms.

The folate receptor alpha (FRα) which is problematic in CFD is also found in other organs, though the full implications of this are not yet known. Additionally, because FRα is present in the placenta, women of childbearing age need to be cautious during pregnancy to ensure that FRAAs are not inhibiting folate transport to the fetus, which could affect fetal development.

11. When, if ever, do you recommend repeating the FRAT or a lumbar puncture? For example, if both are negative, but CFD is suspected, should these tests be repeated?

Further testing is necessary in certain circumstances, particularly if the patient is not responding to treatment as expected or if there is a sudden worsening of symptoms. I typically repeat a FRAT when considering discontinuing leucovorin.

If the FRAT is negative and the LP is within expected normal ranges for the patient (see Chapter 15 for more details), it indicates that the patient likely does not have CFD, and alternative diagnoses should be explored. This ensures that the patient receives appropriate care based on their evolving condition.

12. Would any other tests help confirm or make one suspicious of CFD? For example, are ANA tests or other autoimmune panels generally positive when the child has CFD?

CFD can be caused by FRAAs, mitochondrial dysfunction, and rare genetic mutations, making it essential to test for these factors when diagnosing or suspecting CFD. In some cases, brain imaging may show changes in white matter on an MRI, and generalized slowing may appear on an EEG. However, these findings are nonspecific and do not definitively indicate CFD.

Traditional immunological tests are usually negative or only slightly abnormal in individuals with CFD. For example, an antinuclear antibody (ANA) test may occasionally show a low positive result.

While autoimmune disorders and inflammation can contribute to folate depletion, these factors are not specific to CFD. However, autoimmune inflammatory disorders have been associated with FRAAs. Therefore, if an individual with an inflammatory disorder experiences unexpected cognitive changes, CFD should be considered as a potential underlying cause.

13. Are there specific EEG or Brain MRI findings that are indicative of CFD? Are EEGs or MRI needed or helpful to diagnosis or monitoring the course of CFD?

EEGs and MRIs may be nonspecifically abnormal in patients with CFD. An EEG may show generalized slowing while a brain MRI may show delays in white matter development. These can be used to monitor improvements in individuals with CFD. An EEG may be particularly useful because it is non-invasive and does not require sedation.

14. Is there a difference between the diagnosis of Cerebral Folate Deficiency and Cerebral Folate Transport Deficiency?

The diagnosis of Cerebral folate transport deficiency (CFTD) has generally been applied to patients who have mutations in the FOLR1 gene, which encodes for FRα. As discussed in Chapter 9, patients with these rare genetic mutations may have trouble transporting folate into the brain.

CFD is defined by a below normal concentration of 5-MTHF in the CSF. A patient who has CFTD may also develop CFD when the deficiency in the transporter is severe enough that the 5-MTHF levels are below normal.

If there is a suspicion of CFDT, it is important to monitor for CFD as it may occur depending on the severity of the biological process that's causing the transporter deficiency.

15. How should CFD be coded to ensure that insurance will cover the necessary leucovorin treatment?

Cerebral Folate Deficiency is generally coded as ICD-10 G93.41, Metabolic Encephalopathy. If CFD is associated with underlying causes such as mitochondrial dysfunction, genetic conditions, or other neurological disorders, additional codes may be required to reflect these contributing factors.

16. Is CFD a diagnosis that lasts for life, or will the child outgrow it or later be "undiagnosed" with CFD?

In my experience, most children who respond to leucovorin, presumably due to CFD, require long-term treatment with the medication. While it is reassuring that folate is known to be safe for extended use, it remains important to regularly reevaluate patients for any new symptoms or potential adverse effects during prolonged treatment.

There have been several cases where children have shown normalization with leucovorin, and their repeat FRAT tests became negative. However, it is uncertain whether the FRAT will turn positive again in the future, so lifelong monitoring is necessary to watch for any recurrence of symptoms or changes in health status, particularly through periods of rapid change, like puberty.

In my clinical practice, I've observed that children with CFD who exhibit Autism Spectrum Disorder (ASD) symptoms and initially meet the diagnostic criteria for ASD sometimes experience sufficient symptom improvement to no longer meet the criteria for an ASD diagnosis.

FAQs: Treatment

17. What is the difference between folic acid and folinic acid (leucovorin)?

This is a very common question, and many people, even medical providers, often confuse folic acid with folinic acid. The key differences between folic acid and folinic acid (leucovorin) lie in their chemical structures, how the body processes them, and how they are used therapeutically. (See Chapter 3 for more details).

Folic acid (B9) is the synthetic form of folate and is not found in nature. It is used in commercial products because it is more stable than natural folates and is lower in cost. It is commonly used in prenatal vitamins, fortified foods (like cereals), and most folates supplements.

As a supplement, folic acid must be converted by the body into its active form, tetrahydrofolate (THF), through several enzymatic steps. While most people can easily convert folic acid to useable forms of folate, individuals with certain genetic polymorphisms in the DHFR gene may have trouble efficiently converting folic acid into its active form. In addition, the throughput of the DHFR enzyme is limited and it can become saturated when high doses of folic acid are consumed. In such cases, elevated unmetabolized folinic acid (UMFA) can occur, which can inhibit folate metabolism.

Folinic Acid, on the other hand, is a naturally occurring form of folate and doesn't require conversion by the DHFR enzyme. It bypasses several steps in the folate metabolism pathway and enters the folate pathway directly, making it optimal for people with metabolic or genetic issues.

Patients with CFD generally have problems transporting folate across their blood-brain barrier (BBB) because of a blocked or malfunctioning FRα. They rely on getting folate into their brains via the reduced folate carrier (RFC). Because leucovorin is a reduced form of folate, it is able to cross the BBB through the RFC. For this reason, folinic acid, rather than folic acid, is the standard treatment for CFD.

While folic acid is used for general supplementation, folinic acid is more often used to treat specific medical conditions. In addition to treating CFD, leucovorin is used in cancer treatments to rescue healthy cells from the damaging effects of methotrexate (a form of chemotherapy). Because it is harder and more expensive to make, folinic acid is often reserved for those with specific medical conditions and generally requires a prescription for higher doses.

18. What is the difference between folinic acid (leucovorin) and 5-MTHF for treating CFD?

Folinic acid and 5-MTHF are both active (reduced) forms of vitamin B9 (folate) and play important roles in various biological processes. These are two forms of reduced (active) folate in the folate cycle.

The choice to use either form depends on the underlying medical need. Leucovorin is often preferred in complex conditions, such as CFD or autoimmune-related folate transport issues, whereas 5-MTHF is typically used for more general metabolic folate supplementation. Below is a chart with a more detailed comparison, followed by explanations for typical usage:

	Leucovorin (Folinic Acid)	**5-MTHF**
Methylation Potential	Does not directly participate in methylation. Primarily acts as a coenzyme in reactions involved in nucleotide synthesis, DNA repair, and amino acid metabolism.	Directly involved in methylation by converting homocysteine to methionine in the methylation cycle. Methylation plays a crucial role in gene expression, neurotransmitter synthesis, detoxification, and many other processes.
Medical Uses	Commonly used in medicine. Rescues the toxic effects of certain drugs which inhibits folate metabolism. It can also be used in the treatment of certain anemias.	Often used in medicine and nutrition to address methylation imbalances or for those with severe MTHFR polymorphisms. 5-MTHF can help ensure an adequate supply of active folate for methylation processes.
Bioavailability	Readily absorbed with good bioavailability. Much is converted to 5-MTHF by the liver and gut microbiome when taken orally.	Well-absorbed and has good bioavailability. Can be readily used by cells.
Safety	Generally well-tolerated with low risk of toxicity. Can cause insomnia so needs to be given in the afternoon rather than evening for some.	Generally safe. However, high doses may lead to an overstimulation of the methylation cycle, which can cause anxiety, irritability, or insomnia.

	Leucovorin (Folinic Acid)	5-MTHF
When it's used	Often used when there's a problem with the body's ability to get a high enough concentration of folate into the central nervous system to support the brain's activities. This is common in conditions like CFD where patients have mitochondrial dysfunction and/or FRAAs that block the transport of folate into the brain. Leucovorin bypasses the conversion step required to turn folic acid into the active form of folate and provides a usable form that can be readily taken up by cells, including those in the nervous system.	5-MTHF is the bioactive form of folate and can be used directly by the body without needing to go through the conversion process. It is often used in patients who have severe MTHFR gene polymorphisms, which impairs the body's ability to convert leucovorin into 5-MTHF. It can also be used in general folate deficiencies where there are no FRAAs or autoimmune conditions.
Why it's chosen	Leucovorin is available in higher doses which are often needed for CFD and inflammatory or autoimmune conditions that affect folate transport. It is also chosen because of its well-known safety profile and dosing standards that have been established over decades of study. An additional benefit of treating CFD with leucovorin is that the costs are sometimes covered by insurance, providing some financial relief for patients who must incur the medical costs associated with this condition.	5-MTHF is often preferred for patients with genetic issues in folate metabolism or those who simply need supplementation of folate in its active form. It is also chosen because it is generally available without a prescription. 5-MTHF is a direct way to support folate pathways and is commonly used for neurological, psychiatric, or general metabolic needs. It is less preferred for treating a complex condition like CFD.
Typical dosage	Typically dosed in milligrams (mg) based on body weight for children and adults. Doses for those with FRAAs generally range from 0.5 to 2 mg/kg/day, depending on the patient's specific medical factors. The doses are often divided into two doses daily. For example, a child weighing 20 kg might receive between 10 to 40 mg per day, with half given in the morning, and half given in the afternoon. It is not uncommon for some children to require doses over 50 mg per day to achieve therapeutic results.	5-MTHF is generally available over-the-counter without a prescription. Common starting doses for individuals with severe MTHFR polymorphisms are about 1 mg to 5 mg daily. Higher doses, 7.5 mg to 15 mg per day, may be used for those with significant folate metabolism issues or psychiatric conditions, such as depression or anxiety, that are linked to folate deficiencies.

In summary, leucovorin (folinic acid) and 5-MTHF are both active forms of Vitamin B9, but they have different roles and applications. Leucovorin is primarily used to treat CFD, while 5-MTHF is commonly used to support methylation processes and address genetic variations. Folinic acid does not directly participate in methylation, while 5-MTHF is specifically involved in methylation reactions. Both forms have good bioavailability, but 5-MTHF carries a higher risk of overstimulation if taken in excessive doses.

Because 5-MTHF is available over-the-counter, some parents independently trial this supplement with their children before pursuing a formal medical evaluation and diagnostic workup for CFD. It's important to note, however, that folate supplementation may result in elevated folate levels in the CSF if a lumbar puncture is performed later, potentially affecting diagnostic accuracy. For this reason, parents should always consult a healthcare professional for personalized guidance regarding leucovorin (folinic acid) or 5-MTHF supplementation, appropriate dosing adjustments, and the management of potential side effects.

19. Why do some kids seem to do better with 5-MTHF than with leucovorin alone?

All controlled studies to date have used either leucovorin alone or in combination with a multivitamin. No studies have specifically examined 5-MTHF alone or compared leucovorin with 5-MTHF. Controlled clinical trials have demonstrated that leucovorin by itself is effective and does not result in increased side effects compared to placebo.

While some children might potentially benefit more from 5-MTHF, anecdotal reports lack the necessary controls to make accurate comparisons due to factors like genetics, concurrent medications, and differing symptoms. Leucovorin dosing is well-established from decades of clinical research and use, whereas the appropriate dosage for 5-MTHF is less well understood.

Another factor that complicates comparisons is the variability in preparation and additives in different products. For example, commercial leucovorin products may contain lactose and other additives, which can affect tolerance and efficacy in a subset of children, leading some patients to require a compounded formulation.

This variability is even greater with 5-MTHF. As a supplement, it is not as tightly regulated, making it difficult to know the precise composition of a particular product or whether observed effects are due to additives or other substances.

One of the advantages of folinic acid (leucovorin) is that at least half of it is converted to 5-MTHF when taken orally. This means that it provides two key folates—both of which play crucial roles in metabolism.

20. When/why do some children with CFD require injections or infusions? Would most children benefit from injections or infusions instead of pills?

Oral leucovorin has been highly effective for many of my patients with FRAAs and suspected CFD, and in these cases, alternative administration routes have not been necessary. However, injections or infusions of leucovorin may be more effective for individuals with severe transportation blocks that hinder folate from entering the nervous system.

In patients with severe symptoms, known genetic issues affecting folate transport, or low 5-MTHF levels confirmed through a lumbar puncture, injections or infusions should be considered. These methods result in higher peak concentrations in the blood, which can enhance folate transport into the nervous system. Chapter 17 provides guidance on specific situations, such as intractable seizures, where alternative administration routes may be necessary to address folate deficiencies.

Additionally, Dr. Quadros and his team recently demonstrated in an animal model that administering leucovorin by injection has a different effect compared to oral administration.[263] When taken orally, folinic acid is first processed in the liver before it enters the bloodstream. In contrast, injections appear to deliver leucovorin directly and rapidly to the brain.

This suggests that injections may be more effective at replenishing folate in the nervous system and supporting neurotransmitter production. As this exciting area of research continues to evolve, it has the potential to guide practitioners in selecting the most appropriate administration methods and dosing strategies for each specific case of CFD, allowing for more tailored and effective treatments.

21. Does the brand of leucovorin make a difference? Can you switch between brands easily?

Leucovorin is a generic drug produced by various companies, and while generic medications are required to be bioequivalent to their brand-name counterparts, two key factors can influence this equivalence. First, there is an acceptable range for the resulting blood levels of a generic drug, but in some cases, these levels can be significantly lower than those produced by another product with the same dose. This has been a concern with critical medications like antiepileptics, where individuals have experienced breakthrough seizures after switching to a different generic version that resulted in insufficient blood levels to control their condition. Second, different generics may contain different additives, which can affect how individuals respond to the medication. For example, many children with ASD are sensitive to certain additives, which can trigger allergic reactions or gastrointestinal distress.

Most commercial forms of leucovorin contain lactose as an additive. While the small amount of lactose is tolerated by most children, about 5% may not tolerate it well. In such cases, a compounded form of leucovorin without additives is recommended. Inactive ingredients can also affect the absorption of the medication. One study found that many medications contain so-called "inactive" ingredients that may actually cause adverse effects[264] suggesting that some reported side effects may stem from these additives rather than the active drug itself. Additionally, the composition of additives in generic products can be changed without notice and may not be reflected in the package insert.

Because of these variables, different generic forms of leucovorin may not be entirely equivalent. Therefore, if a generic brand is being used, it's important to track the specific brand that seems to work well for the patient to work with the pharmacy to continue that brand if possible. Likewise, if the patient has a suboptimal reponse to leucovorin, it may be worthwhile to try a different generic brand to see if symptoms improve.

22. If the parent cannot find a doctor to prescribe leucovorin, are there over-the-counter products they can start with, and what would the dosage be for those products?

Most over-the-counter (OTC) formulations of folinic acid range from 400 mcg to 800 mcg (mcg = microgram and mg = miligram; 1 mcg = 1/1000th of a mg). This means that each folinic acid pill is equivalent to only 0.4 mg to 0.8 mg of leucovorin. Given that the standard daily dose for leucovorin in treating conditions like CFD is around 50 mg, a person would need to take more than 62 OTC pills per day just to reach the recommended dose. This approach is not only costly but impractical, as it would expose the individual to an unnecessary amount of additives.

While other OTC reduced folate compounds are available, leucovorin is the preferred treatment for several important reasons. One major advantage is that leucovorin has been used in medicine for decades, so the proper dosing and potential side effects are well established. Moreover, the majority of studies on ASD and CFD have been conducted using leucovorin, making it the only compound for which management guidance is available for these conditions.

It is crucial that a medical professional experienced in treating folate disorders prescribes leucovorin. While the treatment may appear straightforward, there are many nuances in managing folate disorders, and individual responses to treatment can vary. Having leucovorin prescribed and monitored by a knowledgeable healthcare provider ensures the best chance of success and reduces the risk of unexpected reactions. Hopefully, as awareness of folate disorders grows, more healthcare professionals will recognize the importance of addressing these issues, particularly in children with neurodevelopmental disorders.

23. How long before one should expect some sign of improvement on leucovorin? At what point should you give up?

The length of time required to see improvement with leucovorin varies from child to child. Clinical trials have generally observed responses over a 3-month period, during which improvements in language and behavior have been noted, particularly in children who are FRAA positive. However, some children may respond more slowly. For instance, those with soluble folate binding proteins (sFBPs) often require higher doses of leucovorin and exhibit a more gradual response. Additionally, children with mitochondrial disorders or subclinical epilepsy may need adjunctive treatment for those conditions before leucovorin becomes effective.

When considering leucovorin treatment, it is important to evaluate the need for a lumbar puncture (LP) to guide therapy, particularly if additional medical conditions are expected to complicate treatment. An LP before treatment can provide a diagnosis and establish a baseline. If there is uncertainty about whether adequate concentrations of folate are reaching the brain during treatment, a repeat LP can help clarify this. That said, LPs are typically not favored in most cases, where an empirical trial of leucovorin can be attempted without invasive testing.

The decision to discontinue leucovorin treatment depends on the strength of the clinical suspicion for CFD prior to initiating therapy (See Chapter 15 for the criteria defining Definite, Probable, Possible, and Unlikely CFD diagnoses).

If a patient has undergone a LP revealing significantly low 5-MTHF levels in cerebrospinal fluid (CSF) but does not show clear improvement on leucovorin, the issue may lie in the dosage, administration method, or formulation rather than the efficacy of treatment itself. In such cases, it is reasonable to trial higher doses, injectable formulations, or different leucovorin brands for longer periods of time before discontinuing, provided the treatment remains well-tolerated. Conversely, if FRAA testing is negative, the LP results are normal or inconclusive, and the child's symptoms can be explained by other conditions, then CFD is unlikely to be the underlying cause. In such cases, continuing leucovorin treatment is less likely to provide meaningful benefits, and discontinuation may be appropriate.

For parents who trial OTC folinic acid and observe little to no improvement, it is likely that the dose is too low to be therapeutic if their child has CFD. Since proper dosing can vary significantly, working with a medical professional is essential to determine the appropriate dosage, formulation, and administration method.

24. What are the side effects of leucovorin?

For the most part, leucovorin is well tolerated. In our recent meta-analysis of studies on leucovorin for treating ASD, we found that around 10% of parents reported aggression, agitation, and/or insomnia, while about 5% reported headaches and/or tantrums when leucovorin was given alone. When leucovorin was administered as part of a multivitamin, typically at lower doses, only about 1% reported aggression, though 8% reported worsening behavior.

However, controlled clinical trials using leucovorin to treat folate abnormalities in ASD showed that adverse effects were no higher than with placebo, suggesting that many of these side effects might be related to typical ASD behavior variations rather than the medication itself.

In clinical practice, we have observed some consistent adverse effects that appear to be linked to leucovorin treatment in certain children. Approximately 10-20% of children experience excitement or hyperactivity within the first few weeks of treatment (See Chapter 5).

Fortunately, these symptoms usually resolve with continued use, and the child often improves beyond their pre-treatment state. Another adverse effect seen in about 5% of children is insomnia, which is typically managed by administering the second dose of leucovorin in the afternoon instead of the evening.

As explained in earlier chapters, folate is a water-soluble vitamin that is primarily excreted through urine. If side effects occur and discontinuation is necessary, folate typically clears from the body relatively quickly, minimizing the risk of prolonged adverse effects.

25. What is the best time of day to give injections?

Most children receiving injections of leucovorin also receive a combination shot that includes B12. Since both of these ingredients can be energizing, it's generally best to give the injection in the morning if possible.

However, for patients who are just starting with injections, the process can be challenging due to both the apprehension of the person administering the shot and the nervousness of the child. In these situations, I recommend waiting until after the child falls asleep to give the injection, as they are less likely to notice or feel it. The needles used are small and typically cause minimal discomfort. They do not seem to interfere with sleep when given in this manner.

In my experience, over time, children tend to become more comfortable with their injections, and some even begin to look forward to them, especially if they notice the energy boost that often follows the treatment.

26. Is it safe to combine leucovorin with ADHD drugs?

Absolutely. Leucovorin appears to help with ADHD symptoms. In addition, folate is important for making neurotransmitters in the brain such as dopamine and norepinephrine which are key for controlling hyperactivity and attention.

27. Why is leucovorin given in divided doses versus just once per day?

Administering medications multiple times a day can help maintain higher and more consistent blood levels. In some cases, to increase the blood levels of leucovorin, it may need to be given three or four times daily.

It's important to note that simply giving a higher dose of a medication doesn't always result in more absorption by the body, as the body can only absorb a limited amount at one time. Therefore, medications often need to be given more frequently to achieve and sustain higher levels in the body (See Chapter 17).

The dosing of leucovorin is highly individualized. Some children do well with a single morning dose, while others may require multiple doses throughout the day to maintain therapeutic levels. The optimal dosing schedule depends on the child's specific needs and response to treatment.

28. Is CFD treatment for life? When is it safe to stop treatment?

Many individuals with CFD, particularly those who are FRAA positive or have mitochondrial disorders, seem to require long-term leucovorin treatment. If there is uncertainty about whether leucovorin is still benefiting the patient, it is often gradually weaned off to assess whether it is making a significant difference in cognition or behavior.

In some instances, children have shown normalization in both behavior and cognition, and retesting the FRAT revealed that the autoantibodies were no longer present. In such cases, stopping leucovorin treatment may be considered.

29. How do you stop leucovorin? Must it be slowly weaned or can you quit suddenly? Are there risks during withdrawal?

Technically, leucovorin can be stopped at any time. However, regression is seen in many children in which it is stopped abruptly. Sometimes the effect of stopping leucovorin is not immediate but may occur over months, so it is important to monitor a child after leucovorin is stopped.

30. How do you know if you should try to increase the dose of leucovorin?

The decision to increase leucovorin depends on several factors. If a lumbar puncture (LP) has been performed and the 5-MTHF concentration has been measured, a repeat LP can assess whether leucovorin dosing has effectively raised the 5-MTHF levels.

In the absence of an LP, the patient can be monitored clinically to evaluate how much benefit they are receiving from leucovorin. If the expected improvements are not seen, the leucovorin dose can be increased to assess whether additional benefits result. If no benefits are observed with the higher dose, the dosage can always be reduced back to the original level.

Children taking leucovorin on a long-term basis may need several dose adjustments during their treatment. Since dosing is usually based on weight, the dose may need to be increased if the effects seem to be wearing off as the child grows. Additionally, children going through rapid changes during puberty may need higher doses.

In the absence of a LP, adjusting the dose and monitoring clinical changes typically provides flexibility to optimize treatment based on each individual's response.

31. Are there any pre-existing conditions where leucovorin would be harmful or not recommended for the patient?

In general, there are no specific conditions where leucovorin would be harmful. In rare instances, such as when it is given with certain medications like methotrexate or similar chemotherapies, the timing of leucovorin administration needs to be coordinated with the other drug to avoid interactions.

Leucovorin is a form of folate, which interacts with other vitamins. A severe deficiency in other vitamins, particularly vitamin B12, can lead to unwanted effects. Since folate requires other cofactors to function properly, it's important to ensure that the patient is taking a good multivitamin before starting leucovorin treatment.

FAQs: Other Questions

32. Are the symptoms of CFD typically progressive? Are there periods where they tend to get worse (like puberty)?

Some of the earliest cases of CFD reported in the literature involved infantile-onset CFD, where symptoms developed gradually over the first year of life. These children often had a progressive course, which unfolded over time and sometimes led to epilepsy, vision and hearing loss, and abnormal brain development. As our understanding of CFD has evolved, we now recognize that the severity of the condition depends on both the underlying cause and the age at which it develops. The absence of folate during critical periods of rapid development in childhood can lead to the accumulation of more severe symptoms if left untreated.

One of the most exciting aspects of CFD is that treatment with leucovorin has proven highly effective in preventing the worsening of symptoms in many patients, and in some cases, even reversing them. Many of the patient stories in this book describe how severe symptoms, such as vision loss, seizures, and movement disorders improved once the child started taking leucovorin.

When FRAAs are involved, symptoms are often linked to antibody titers, which can fluctuate over time. Regular reevaluation is crucial to ensure the condition is not worsening. If improvement is seen, further assessment can help determine if the biological process causing CFD has resolved. If the condition worsens, it may be necessary to try higher or more frequent doses of leucovorin or consider alternative routes of administration to optimize treatment.

33. Is there any relationship between CFD and abnormal endocrinology testing or children needing human growth hormones?

FRAA titers have been linked to atypical levels of thyroid-stimulating hormone (TSH) in the blood. It has been hypothesized that maternal FRAAs may bind to fetal thyroid tissue, potentially leading to abnormal thyroid development.

While correlations between CFD and/or FRAAs and other endocrine abnormalities have not been clearly established, it is important to recognize that the brain regulates hormone release. If areas of the brain are affected by abnormal 5-MTHF concentrations, hormone levels may also be impacted.

If you believe your child exhibits symptoms consistent with an endocrine disorder, it is important to inform your doctor to ensure a comprehensive evaluation, as these conditions may not be identified through standard CFD diagnostic testing. Additionally, if an endocrine abnormality is detected, targeted treatments beyond

CFD management will likely be necessary to address the underlying hormonal imbalance and optimize overall health.

34. Is there any relationship between CFD and Cerebral Creatine Deficiency or Methylmalonic Acidemia?

In many cases, the underlying cause of CFD is mitochondrial dysfunction. Mitochondrial dysfunction acts as a link between CFD and several metabolic disorders, such as cerebral creatine deficiency and methylmalonic acidemia. Both of these conditions result in impaired mitochondrial function. Patients with mitochondrial dysfunction often experience reduced energy production, which can affect the FRα.

Without sufficient energy, FRα is unable to effectively transport folate into the brain, ultimately leading to CFD. This connection highlights the importance of addressing mitochondrial issues in patients with CFD to ensure proper folate transport and brain function.

35. Is there any relationship between CFD and anemia?

Anemia is a medical condition in which the body lacks healthy red blood cells. Red blood cells contain hemoglobin, a protein that binds to oxygen and transports it throughout the body. When anemia occurs, there is a shortage of hemoglobin or red blood cells, resulting in symptoms such as fatigue, weakness, and shortness of breath.

Anemia can be caused by various factors, including iron deficiency, chronic disease, genetic disorders, and vitamin deficiencies. If the cause of anemia is unclear, it may be due to a folate deficiency. Unlike CFD, which is restricted to low folate levels in the central nervous system, anemia suggests low folate levels throughout the entire body (systemically).

Low folate concentrations in the blood can lead to both systemic anemia and neurological symptoms because the available folate is insufficient to meet the demands of the central nervous system. Systemic folate deficiency is treated differently from CFD and requires restoring folate levels in the body to address both anemia and neurological symptoms.

36. Is leucovorin typically covered by insurance? If not, are there any specific steps to help get it covered by insurance?

Whether leucovorin is covered by insurance depends on the specific insurance company and their policies. If coverage is denied, your doctor can submit a letter of medical necessity. This letter should reference clinical trials that support the use of leucovorin for conditions such as FRAAs, mitochondrial dysfunction, or low 5-MTHF concentrations in the CSF. This documentation can help strengthen the case for insurance coverage.

37. What genetic testing is typically recommended for children with CFD?

If no cause for CFD is identified, or if the condition does not respond to treatment, it is important to investigate the folate-related genes, especially FOLR1. Mutations or variations in these genes can impair folate transport and metabolism, which may explain the condition and help guide more effective treatment strategies.

While the presence of a FOLR1 mutation strongly supports a CFD diagnosis, analyzing this one gene will not correctly identify most CFD cases. Other factors, like FRAAs and mitochondrial dysfunction, are more common causes of CFD and should be considered in the diagnosis.

Comprehensive genetic testing, such as whole genome sequencing (WGS) or whole exome sequencing (WES), offers a broader understanding of a patient's genetics and how metabolic issues might contribute to CFD. For example, a patient with mitochondrial disease could develop secondary CFD, even if the gene mutations do not directly affect folate metabolism.

As these genetic technologies become more affordable and accessible, they provide a fuller picture of the factors contributing to a child's CFD diagnosis and should be considered as part of the initial evaluation.

38. There is literature about children with the FOLR1 mutation having CFD, but what does it mean if a child has an FOLR2 mutation?

Much of our understanding of folate receptors comes from cancer research. Folate receptors are commonly overexpressed in cancer cells. Many cancer treatments target these receptors to either block folate from entering diseased cells or to attach drugs to folate, using the receptors to deliver medication directly into the cancer cells. In contrast, research into folate metabolism issues, such as those affecting non-cancerous conditions, is less advanced.

What we do know is that there are three types of folate receptors, all encoded on the same region of chromosome 11. The folate receptor alpha (FRα) is encoded by the FOLR1 gene, the folate receptor beta (FRβ) is encoded by the FOLR2 gene, and the folate receptor gamma (FRγ) is encoded by the FOLR3 gene.

Each one is expressed on different tissues in the body. The FRα is very important for transport of folate into the central nervous system. The FRβ is found on several tissues, including placenta, spleen, bone marrow and thymus. It is also thought that FRβ is expressed in the choroid plexus of infants, but this expression is phased out by 4-6 months of age, at which point FRα becomes more prominent in transporting folate into the CNS.[265]

FRγ is primarily found in blood cells. While its exact role is less understood compared to FRα and FRβ, it is believed to be involved in immune responses and folate transport in specific blood cell types.

Mutations in FOLR1 can lead to CFD because defective FRα inhibits the transport of folate into the brain and CNS. A child with mutations in FOLR2 or FOLR3 may also have disorders related to folate metabolism, but since these receptors are mainly expressed in tissues outside the CNS, such mutations would likely lead to other folate-related issues rather than CFD.

39. Is there a relationship between a CASK gene mutation (like Rett's) and CFD?

Both Rett syndrome and calcium/calmodulin-dependent serine protein kinase (CASK) gene mutations are rare conditions, involving genes located on the X chromosome. They tend to affect females more than males. Most cases of Rett syndrome are caused by mutations in the MECP2 gene, which produces a protein essential for brain development and nerve function.

Like MECP2, CASK plays a critical role in brain development, as well as in cell signaling, neuron communication, and the formation of synapses (connections between neurons). Children with mutations in these genes may present with a range of neurological disorders.

CFD is often not tested in genetic cases because cognitive and behavioral symptoms are typically attributed to the underlying gene mutations. As a result, medical providers may not see a reason to order a lumbar puncture to evaluate for CFD. However, there is one documented case where a CASK gene mutation was associated with abnormal cerebrospinal fluid (CSF) chemistry.[266] As explained in Chapter 9, children with various genetic conditions may also have CFD. While some links between genetic mutations and CFD are known, others remain unclear. Regardless, if CFD is identified, it should be treated accordingly.

40. How do you know if the child also has a methylation problem? How does that factor into CFD treatment?

Methylation is a critical biochemical process that influences gene expression and detoxification. At the center of this process is S-adenosylmethionine (SAM), a key methyl donor involved in numerous biochemical reactions throughout the body. Currently, there is no reliable clinical test to directly measure SAM levels, but several indirect markers can help assess whether the methylation cycle is functioning optimally. Blood and urine tests commonly used to evaluate methylation status include:

- Genetic tests – MTHFR, MTR, MTRR, and others may have polymorphisms
- Homocysteine levels – Both elevated and lowered values can indicate that methylation is impaired
- SAM:SAH ratio – A high ratio suggests overactive methylation, while a low ratio indicates impaired methylation
- Methylmalonic acid (MMA) – Elevated levels may indicate a Vitamin B12 deficiency, which can disrupt methylation

If methylation abnormalities are detected, addressing these imbalances may be necessary before initiating treatment for CFD. Since methylation plays a foundational role in cellular function and detoxification, unresolved methylation issues may contribute to a poor response to treatment and should be optimized to support overall health.

41. What's the relationship between MTHFR mutations (C677 and A1298) and CFD, if any?

Many people, including medical professionals, often assume that CFD is caused by MTHFR polymorphisms or mutations; however, this is not the case. The MTHFR (Methylenetetrahydrofolate Reductase) gene plays a crucial role in converting 5-formyl-THF (folinic acid) into 5-MTHF, which is essential for methylation, SAM production, and homocysteine metabolism—all of which influence glutathione synthesis and overall cellular function.

Despite MTHFR's role in folate metabolism, there is no direct link between MTHFR polymorphisms and CFD. The C677T and A1298C polymorphisms are relatively common in the general population, with C677T found in approximately 30-40% of individuals and A1298C in 7-12%. As discussed in Chapter 2, polymorphisms represent minor genetic variations that can impact enzyme efficiency but do not typically result in severe dysfunction. In contrast, mutations are rare and more likely to cause significant impairments in gene function.

When true MTHFR mutations are present, the gene's function can be compromised, making it more difficult for the body to convert folinic acid into 5-MTHF. Among common polymorphisms, C677T is generally considered more significant than A1298C. A heterozygous (single copy) polymorphism is usually not a major concern, while homozygous (two copies) C677T polymorphisms are associated with reduced enzyme activity and abnormalities in homocysteine metabolism.

A key advantage of leucovorin in CFD treatment is that, when taken orally, a portion of it is naturally converted into 5-MTHF, bypassing the need for MTHFR enzyme activity. Since leucovorin enters the folate cycle just before MTHFR, and 5-MTHF enters just after MTHFR, the enzyme's function becomes irrelevant in the context of CFD treatment, making leucovorin an effective option for most people regardless of MTHFR status.

42. What percentage of CFD is caused by genetic mutations, versus folate receptor autoantibodies, versus mitochondrial dysfunction?

In a recent meta-analysis conducted by myself and Dr. Rossignol, we found that cerebral folate deficiency (CFD) was caused by folate receptor autoantibodies (FRAAs) in 83% of cases, mitochondrial dysfunction in 43% of cases, and genetic abnormalities in 14% of cases.[267] In some cases, multiple contributing factors were identified, with the most common combination being FRAAs and mitochondrial dysfunction.

43. If the child does not have FRAAs, but has CFD from mitochondrial dysfunction, how does that impact the course of treatment and/or expected recovery?

In cases where a child has CFD but does not test positive for folate receptor autoantibodies (FRAAs), the condition is most often associated with mitochondrial disease rather than mitochondrial dysfunction. Unlike mitochondrial dysfunction, mitochondrial disease is a more severe and systemic condition that requires a thorough evaluation to guide appropriate treatment.

Patients with mitochondrial disease and CFD often require significantly higher doses of leucovorin, typically in the range of 4-8 mg/kg/day, to achieve therapeutic benefits. However, due to the complexity of mitochondrial disorders and the potential for variability in response, it is crucial to consult an expert in mitochondrial medicine when considering treatment at these higher doses. Proper monitoring and individualized care are essential to ensure both safety and efficacy in these cases.

Most of these cases also require concurrent treatment of the mitochondrial disease with a "mitochondrial cocktail." This refers to a combination of supplements and vitamins used to support mitochondrial function, improve energy production, and reduce oxidative stress. Examples of components may include: Ubiquinol (CoQ10), L-Carnitine, Creatine, Vitamin B2, Vitamin C, and Magnesium.[268]

The exact combination and dosages in a mitochondrial cocktail are personalized based on the individual's condition and needs. Addressing mitochondrial energy production is a crucial aspect of treating CFD and must work in tandem with high-dose leucovorin for effective management.

44. What types of doctors typically treat CFD?

Traditionally neurologists and metabolic experts diagnose and treat CFD. However, there is growing awareness of CFD among integrative medicine doctors, who combine traditional Western medical practices with evidence-based complementary and alternative therapies.

Parents seeking a physician to explore a CFD diagnosis may want to begin with a MAPS doctor. These physicians have been trained by the Medical Academy of Pediatric Special Needs (MAPS) to treat children with complex medical conditions, especially those with autism spectrum disorder (ASD) and other neurodevelopmental disorders. MAPS doctors use a biomedical approach, focusing on the medical, biochemical, and environmental factors that contribute to a child's developmental and behavioral challenges.

Many MAPS doctors have received specialized training in treating conditions such as ASD, ADHD, PANS/PANDAS, mitochondrial dysfunction, CFD, and other metabolic disorders, making them well-equipped to help families navigate complex diagnoses like CFD.

45. Where could a doctor go to get training on CFD?

CFD was only defined as a medical condition in the last two decades. Many doctors who completed medical school prior to that time would not have learned about this condition in school.

CFD is now taught in neurology and metabolic residency. Doctors interested in learning more about Cerebral Folate Deficiency (CFD) and how to diagnose and treat it can pursue training through several avenues:

1. **MAPS (Medical Academy of Pediatric Special Needs) Training**
   - MAPS offers a specific biomedical approach to complex pediatric disorders, including ASD, ADHD, mitochondrial disorders, and CFD. Their training focuses on addressing the underlying medical, biochemical, and environmental causes of these conditions - website: www.medmaps.org

2. **Medical Conferences and Continuing Education**
   - Specialized Neurology and Metabolic Disorder Conferences: These conferences often have sessions on rare diseases like CFD, mitochondrial dysfunction, and metabolic disorders
   - Society for Inherited Metabolic Disorders (SIMD): This organization offers resources and conferences on metabolic diseases, including CFD
   - Child Neurology Society (CNS): Offers conferences and continuing education in pediatric neurology and metabolic disorders

3. **Metabolic Specialists and Geneticists**
   - Consulting with or shadowing metabolic specialists: Physicians can gain experience by collaborating with doctors who specialize in genetic and metabolic disorders, particularly those in large academic or research institutions
   - Training at genetic/metabolic centers: Many large hospitals have departments focused on metabolic disorders, where physicians can undergo specialized training or fellowships in conditions like CFD

4. **Fellowships in Pediatric Neurology and Metabolic Disorders**
   - Many teaching hospitals and academic institutions offer fellowships in pediatric neurology and metabolic genetics. These fellowships provide in-depth training in diagnosing and treating disorders like CFD, mitochondrial disease, and other rare metabolic conditions

5. **Online Courses and CME Programs**
   - UpToDate: Provides comprehensive, evidence-based content on CFD, metabolic diseases, and mitochondrial dysfunction, offering CME credits
   - Medscape: Offers courses and articles on CFD, ASD, and related neurodevelopmental and metabolic conditions
   - American Academy of Neurology (AAN): Provides educational resources on pediatric neurology and metabolic disorders
   - Coming Soon! The Metabolic Learning Resource will be offering modules featuring the contents of this book (www.metaboliclearn.com)

6. **Research Literature and Journals**
    - Reviewing CFD case studies and research: Physicians can read peer-reviewed articles on CFD in journals like Neurology, Journal of Inherited Metabolic Disease, and Pediatric Neurology to stay up-to-date with advances in diagnosis and treatment

CFD is an active area of research. My foundation, the Autism Discovery and Treatment Foundation (ADTF), is a 501(c)(3) non-profit organization dedicated to researching and discovering treatments for CFD, as well as other conditions affecting children with ASD and neurodevelopmental disorders. Our research projects and publications can be found on our website: www.autismdiscovery.org.

REFERENCES

Chapter 1. The Importance of Vitamins
1. Imai, S. & Guarente, L. NAD+ and sirtuins in aging and disease. Trends Cell Biol 24, 464-471 (2014).

Chapter 2. Folate: The Most Essential Vitamin
2. L, W. Nutrition Classics. British Medical Journal 1:1059–64, 1931. Treatment of "pernicious anaemia of pregnancy" and "tropical anaemia" with special reference to yeast extract as a curative agent. Nutrition Reviews 35, 149–151 (1978).
3. Mitchell HK, S.E., Williams RJ The concentration of "folic acid". J Am Chem Soc 63, 2284 (1941).
4. Angier, R.B., et al. Synthesis of a Compound Identical with the L. Casei Factor Isolated from Liver. Science 102, 227-228 (1945).
5. Farber, S. & Diamond, L.K. Temporary remissions in acute leukemia in children produced by folic acid antagonist, 4-aminopteroyl-glutamic acid. N Engl J Med 238, 787-793 (1948).
6. Prevention of neural tube defects: results of the Medical Research Council Vitamin Study. MRC Vitamin Study Research Group. Lancet 338, 131-137 (1991).
7. Prevention of neural tube defects: results of the Medical Research Council Vitamin Study. MRC Vitamin Study Research Group. Lancet 338, 131-137 (1991).
8. Bjork, M., et al. Association of Folic Acid Supplementation During Pregnancy With the Risk of Autistic Traits in Children Exposed to Antiepileptic Drugs In Utero. JAMA Neurol 75, 160-168 (2018).
9. Levine, S.Z., et al. Association of Maternal Use of Folic Acid and Multivitamin Supplements in the Periods Before and During Pregnancy With the Risk of Autism Spectrum Disorder in Offspring. JAMA Psychiatry 75, 176-184 (2018).
10. Ren, X., et al. Association of folate intake and plasma folate level with the risk of breast cancer: a dose-response meta-analysis of observational studies. Aging (Albany NY) 12, 21355-21375 (2020).
11. Lin, H.L., An, Q.Z., Wang, Q.Z. & Liu, C.X. Folate intake and pancreatic cancer risk: an overall and dose-response meta-analysis. Public Health 127, 607-613 (2013).
12. Zhao, Y., et al. Folate intake, serum folate levels and esophageal cancer risk: an overall and dose-response meta-analysis. Oncotarget 8, 10458-10469 (2017).
13. Wei, Y., et al. Serum total folate, 5-methyltetrahydrofolate and vitamin B12 concentrations on incident risk of lung cancer. Int J Cancer 152, 1095-1106 (2023).
14. Du, L., Wang, Y., Zhang, H., Zhang, H. & Gao, Y. Folate intake and the risk of endometrial cancer: A meta-analysis. Oncotarget 7, 85176-85184 (2016).
15. Moazzen, S., et al. Folic acid intake and folate status and colorectal cancer risk: A systematic review and meta-analysis. Clin Nutr 37, 1926-1934 (2018).
16. Browne HP, Shao Y, Lawley TD. Mother-infant transmission of human microbiota. Curr Opin Microbiol. 2022 Oct;69:102173. doi: 10.1016/j.mib.2022.102173. Epub 2022 Jul 1. PMID: 35785616.

17. Dunn, A.B., Jordan, S., Baker, B.J. & Carlson, N.S. The Maternal Infant Microbiome: Considerations for Labor and Birth. MCN Am J Matern Child Nurs 42, 318-325 (2017).
18. Slattery, J., MacFabe, D.F. & Frye, R.E. The Significance of the Enteric Microbiome on the Development of Childhood Disease: A Review of Prebiotic and Probiotic Therapies in Disorders of Childhood. Clin Med Insights Pediatr 10, 91-107 (2016).
19. Losurdo G, Caccavo NLB, Indellicati G, Celiberto F, Ierardi E, Barone M, DiLeo A. Effect of Long-Term Proton Pump Inhibitor Use on Blood Vitamins and Minerals: A Primary Care Setting Study. J Clin Med. 2023 Apr 17;12(8):2910. doi: 10.3390/jcm12082910. PMID: 37109245; PMCID: PMC10146626.
20. Bailey, S.W. & Ayling, J.E. The extremely slow and variable activity of dihydrofolate reductase in human liver and its implications for high folic acid intake. Proc Natl Acad Sci U S A 106, 15424-15429 (2009).

Chapter 3. Folate: The Workhorse Vitamin

21. Wright, A.J., Dainty, J.R. & Finglas, P.M. Folic acid metabolism in human subjects revisited: potential implications for proposed mandatory folic acid fortification in the UK. Br J Nutr 98, 667-675 (2007).
22. Kao, T.-T., et al. Characterization and Comparative Studies of Zebrafish and Human Recombinant Dihydrofolate Reductases—Inhibition by Folic Acid and Polyphenols. Drug Metabolism and Disposition 36, 508-516 (2008).
23. Heyden, K.E., Malysheva, O.V., MacFarlane, A.J., Brody, L.C. & Field, M.S. Excess Folic Acid Exposure Increases Uracil Misincorporation into DNA in a Tissue-Specific Manner in a Mouse Model of Reduced Methionine Synthase Expression. J Nutr (2024).
24. Troen, A.M., et al. Unmetabolized Folic Acid in Plasma Is Associated with Reduced Natural Killer Cell Cytotoxicity among Postmenopausal Women1. The Journal of Nutrition 136, 189-194 (2006).
25. Raghavan, R., et al. A prospective birth cohort study on cord blood folate subtypes and risk of autism spectrum disorder. Am J Clin Nutr 112, 1304-1317 (2020).
26. Whitrow, M.J., Moore, V.M., Rumbold, A.R. & Davies, M.J. Effect of supplemental folic acid in pregnancy on childhood asthma: a prospective birth cohort study. Am J Epidemiol 170, 1486-1493 (2009).
27. Krishnaveni, G.V., Veena, S.R., Karat, S.C., Yajnik, C.S. & Fall, C.H. Association between maternal folate concentrations during pregnancy and insulin resistance in Indian children. Diabetologia 57, 110-121 (2014).
28. Hoyo, C., et al. Methylation variation at IGF2 differentially methylated regions and maternal folic acid use before and during pregnancy. Epigenetics 6, 928-936 (2011).
29. Ondičová, M., et al. Folic acid intervention during pregnancy alters DNA methylation, affecting neural target genes through two distinct mechanisms. Clinical Epigenetics 14, 63 (2022).
30. Richmond, R.C., et al. The long-term impact of folic acid in pregnancy on offspring DNA methylation: follow-up of the Aberdeen Folic Acid Supplementation Trial (AFAST). International Journal of Epidemiology 47, 928-937 (2018).
31. Harlan De Crescenzo, A., et al. Deficient or Excess Folic Acid Supply During Pregnancy Alter Cortical Neurodevelopment in Mouse Offspring. Cereb Cortex 31, 635-649 (2021).
32. Henzel, K.S., Ryan, D.P., Schröder, S., Weiergräber, M. & Ehninger, D. High-dose maternal folic acid supplementation before conception impairs reversal learning in offspring mice. Sci Rep 7, 3098 (2017).

Chapter 4. Cerebral Folate Deficiency

33. Girotto, F., et al. High dose folic acid supplementation of rats alters synaptic transmission and seizure susceptibility in offspring. Scientific Reports 3, 1465 (2013).
34. Ramaekers, V.T., Häusler, M., Opladen, T., Heimann, G. & Blau, N. Psychomotor retardation, spastic paraplegia, cerebellar ataxia and dyskinesia associated with low 5-methyltetrahydrofolate in cerebrospinal fluid: a novel neurometabolic condition responding to folinic acid substitution. Neuropediatrics 33, 301-308 (2002).
35. Ramaekers, V.T. & Blau, N. Cerebral folate deficiency. Dev Med Child Neurol 46, 843-851 (2004).
36. Masingue, M., et al. Cerebral folate deficiency in adults: A heterogeneous potentially treatable condition. J Neurol Sci 396, 112-118 (2019).
37. Ramaekers, V.T., et al. Reduced folate transport to the CNS in female Rett patients. Neurology 61, 506-515 (2003).
38. Ramaekers, V.T., et al. Autoantibodies to folate receptors in the cerebral folate deficiency syndrome. N Engl J Med 352, 1985-1991 (2005).
39. Moretti, P., et al. Cerebral folate deficiency with developmental delay, autism, and response to folinic acid. Neurology 64, 1088-1090 (2005).
40. Ramaekers, V.T., Weis, J., Sequeira, J.M., Quadros, E.V. & Blau, N. Mitochondrial complex I encephalomyopathy and cerebral 5-methyltetrahydrofolate deficiency. Neuropediatrics 38, 184-187 (2007).
41. Alam, C., et al. Upregulation of reduced folate carrier by vitamin D enhances brain folate uptake in mice lacking folate receptor alpha. Proc Natl Acad Sci U S A 116, 17531-17540 (2019).
42. Naz, N., et al. Cerebral Folate Metabolism in Post-Mortem Alzheimer's Disease Tissues: A Small Cohort Study. Int J Mol Sci 24(2022).
43. Hughes, V. In Rare Cases, Scientist Link Autism to Folate Deficiency. in The Transmitter (2008).
44. Moretti, P., et al. Cerebral folate deficiency with developmental delay, autism, and response to folinic acid. Neurology 64, 1088-1090 (2005).
45. DeLuca, E. In Search of a Diagnosis: Cerebral Folate Deficiency. in Complex Child Magazine (2020).
46. News, A. Diagnosis Gets Girl, 5, Out of Wheelchair. in ABC News (2006).
47. Hyland, K., Shoffner, J. & Heales, S.J. Cerebral folate deficiency. J Inherit Metab Dis 33, 563-570 (2010).
48. Kovoor, P.A., Karim, S.M. & Marshall, J.L. Is levoleucovorin an alternative to racemic leucovorin? A literature review. Clin Colorectal Cancer 8, 200-206 (2009).
49. Campbell, I.M., et al. Novel 9q34.11 gene deletions encompassing combinations of four Mendelian disease genes: STXBP1, SPTAN1, ENG, and TOR1A. Genet Med 14, 868-876 (2012).
50. Brunetti, S., et al. Cerebral folate transporter deficiency syndrome in three siblings: Why genetic testing for developmental and epileptic encephalopathies should be performed early and include the FOLR1 gene. Am J Med Genet A 185, 2526-2531 (2021).
51. Dreha-Kulaczewski, S., et al. Folate receptor α deficiency - Myelin-sensitive MRI as a reliable biomarker to monitor the efficacy and long-term outcome of a new therapeutic approach. J Inherit Metab Dis 47, 387-403 (2024).
52. Ramaekers VT, Weis J, Sequeira JM, Quadros EV, Blau N. Mitochondrial complex I encephalomyopathy and cerebral 5-methyltetrahydrofolate deficiency. Neuropediatrics. 2007 Aug;38(4):184-7. doi: 10.1055/s-2007-991150. PMID: 18058625.

53. Shoffner, J., et al. CSF concentrations of 5-methyltetrahydrofolate in a cohort of young children with autism. Neurology 86, 2258-2263 (2016).
54. Ramaekers VT, Blau N. Cerebral folate deficiency. Dev Med Child Neurol. 2004 Dec;46(12):843-51. doi: 10.1017/s0012162204001471. PMID: 15581159.

Chapter 5. Autism Spectrum Disorder

55. Maenner, M.J., et al. Prevalence and Characteristics of Autism Spectrum Disorder Among Children Aged 8 Years - Autism and Developmental Disabilities Monitoring Network, 11 Sites, United States, 2020. MMWR Surveill Summ 72, 1-14 (2023).
56. Baio, J., et al. Prevalence of Autism Spectrum Disorder Among Children Aged 8 Years - Autism and Developmental Disabilities Monitoring Network, 11 Sites, United States, 2014. MMWR Surveill Summ 67, 1-23 (2018).
57. Cakir, J., Frye, R.E. & Walker, S.J. The lifetime social cost of autism: 1990–2029. Research in Autism Spectrum Disorders 72, 101502 (2020).
58. Baron-Cohen, S. Leo Kanner, Hans Asperger, and the discovery of autism. The Lancet 386, 1329-1330 (2015).
59. Tan, C., Frewer, V., Cox, G., Williams, K. & Ure, A. Prevalence and Age of Onset of Regression in Children with Autism Spectrum Disorder: A Systematic Review and Meta-analytical Update. Autism Res 14, 582-598 (2021).
60. Ramaekers VT, Blau N. Cerebral folate deficiency. Dev Med Child Neurol. 2004 Dec;46(12):843-51.
61. Ramaekers, V.T., et al. Autoantibodies to folate receptors in the cerebral folate deficiency syndrome. N Engl J Med 352, 1985-1991 (2005).
62. Moretti, P., et al. Cerebral folate deficiency with developmental delay, autism, and response to folinic acid. Neurology 64, 1088-1090 (2005).
63. Moretti, P., et al. Brief report: autistic symptoms, developmental regression, mental retardation, epilepsy, and dyskinesias in CNS folate deficiency. J Autism Dev Disord 38, 1170-1177 (2008).
64. Ramaekers, V.T., Blau, N., Sequeira, J.M., Nassogne, M.C. & Quadros, E.V. Folate receptor autoimmunity and cerebral folate deficiency in low-functioning autism with neurological deficits. Neuropediatrics 38, 276-281 (2007).
65. Frye, R.E., Sequeira, J.M., Quadros, E.V., James, S.J. & Rossignol, D.A. Cerebral folate receptor autoantibodies in autism spectrum disorder. Mol Psychiatry 18, 369-381 (2013).
66. Shoffner, J., et al. CSF concentrations of 5-methyltetrahydrofolate in a cohort of young children with autism. Neurology 86, 2258-2263 (2016).
67. Ramaekers, V.T., Sequeira, J.M., Thöny, B. & Quadros, E.V. Oxidative Stress, Folate Receptor Autoimmunity, and CSF Findings in Severe Infantile Autism. Autism Res Treat 2020, 9095284 (2020).
68. Rossignol, D.A. & Frye, R.E. Cerebral Folate Deficiency, Folate Receptor Alpha Autoantibodies and Leucovorin (Folinic Acid) Treatment in Autism Spectrum Disorders: A Systematic Review and Meta-Analysis. J Pers Med 11(2021).
69. Frye, R.E., Sequeira, J.M., Quadros, E.V., James, S.J. & Rossignol, D.A. Cerebral folate receptor autoantibodies in autism spectrum disorder. Mol Psychiatry 18, 369-381 (2013).
70. Rossignol, D.A. & Frye, R.E. Cerebral Folate Deficiency, Folate Receptor Alpha Autoantibodies and Leucovorin (Folinic Acid) Treatment in Autism Spectrum Disorders: A Systematic Review and Meta-Analysis. J Pers Med 11(2021).
71. Rossignol DA, Frye RE. Cerebral Folate Deficiency, Folate Receptor Alpha Autoantibodies

and Leucovorin (Folinic Acid) Treatment in Autism Spectrum Disorders: A Systematic Review and Meta-Analysis. J Pers Med. 2021 Nov 3;11(11):1141. doi: 10.3390/jpm11111141. Erratum in: J Pers Med. 2022 Apr 29;12(5):721. doi: 10.3390/jpm12050721. PMID: 34834493; PMCID: PMC8622150.

72. Rossignol, D.A. & Frye, R.E. Cerebral Folate Deficiency, Folate Receptor Alpha Autoantibodies and Leucovorin (Folinic Acid) Treatment in Autism Spectrum Disorders: A Systematic Review and Meta-Analysis. J Pers Med 11(2021).
73. Frye, R.E., et al. Folinic acid improves verbal communication in children with autism and language impairment: a randomized double-blind placebo-controlled trial. Mol Psychiatry 23, 247-256 (2018).
74. Renard, E., et al. Folinic acid improves the score of Autism in the EFFET placebo-controlled randomized trial. Biochimie 173, 57-61 (2020).
75. Panda, P.K., et al. Efficacy of oral folinic acid supplementation in children with autism spectrum disorder: a randomized double-blind, placebo-controlled trial. Eur J Pediatr (2024).
76. Frye, R.E., et al. The Soluble Folate Receptor in Autism Spectrum Disorder: Relation to Autism Severity and Leucovorin Treatment. J Pers Med 12(2022).
77. Frye, R.E., et al. Binding Folate Receptor Alpha Autoantibody Is a Biomarker for Leucovorin Treatment Response in Autism Spectrum Disorder. J Pers Med 14(2024).
78. Ramaekers, V.T., Sequeira, J.M., Blau, N. & Quadros, E.V. A milk-free diet downregulates folate receptor autoimmunity in cerebral folate deficiency syndrome. Dev Med Child Neurol 50, 346-352 (2008).
79. Frye, R.E., Donner, E., Golja, A. & Rooney, C.M. Folinic acid-responsive seizures presenting as breakthrough seizures in a 3-month-old boy. J Child Neurol 18, 562-569 (2003).
80. Frye, R.E., et al. Folinic acid improves verbal communication in children with autism and language impairment: a randomized double-blind placebo-controlled trial. Mol Psychiatry 23, 247-256 (2018).
81. Frye RE, Rossignol DA, Scahill L, McDougle CJ, Huberman H, Quadros EV. Treatment of Folate Metabolism Abnormalities in Autism Spectrum Disorder. Semin Pediatr Neurol. 2020 Oct;35:100835. doi: 10.1016/j.spen.2020.100835. Epub 2020 Jun 25. PMID: 32892962; PMCID: PMC7477301.
82. Frye, R.E., et al. The Soluble Folate Receptor in Autism Spectrum Disorder: Relation to Autism Severity and Leucovorin Treatment. J Pers Med 12(2022).
83. Ramaekers, V.T., Sequeira, J.M., Blau, N. & Quadros, E.V. A milk-free diet downregulates folate receptor autoimmunity in cerebral folate deficiency syndrome. Dev Med Child Neurol 50, 346-352 (2008).
84. Frye, R.E., et al. Treatment of Folate Metabolism Abnormalities in Autism Spectrum Disorder. Semin Pediatr Neurol 35, 100835 (2020).
85. Alam, C., et al. Upregulation of reduced folate carrier by vitamin D enhances brain folate uptake in mice lacking folate receptor alpha. Proc Natl Acad Sci U S A 116, 17531-17540 (2019).
86. Sangha, V., Aboulhassane, S., Qu, Q.R. & Bendayan, R. Protective effects of pyrroloquinoline quinone in brain folate deficiency. Fluids Barriers CNS 20, 84 (2023).
87. Alam, C., Hoque, M.T., Sangha, V. & Bendayan, R. Nuclear respiratory factor 1 (NRF-1) upregulates the expression and function of reduced folate carrier (RFC) at the blood-brain barrier. Faseb j 34, 10516-10530 (2020).

Chapter 6. Down Syndrome

88. Pogribna, M., et al. Homocysteine metabolism in children with Down syndrome: in vitro modulation. Am J Hum Genet 69, 88-95 (2001).
89. Ellis, J.M., et al. Supplementation with antioxidants and folinic acid for children with Down's syndrome: randomised controlled trial. BMJ 336, 594-597 (2008).
90. Blehaut, H., et al. Effect of leucovorin (folinic acid) on the developmental quotient of children with Down's syndrome (trisomy 21) and influence of thyroid status. PLoS One 5, e8394 (2010) .
91. Mircher, C., et al. Thyroid hormone and folinic acid in young children with Down syndrome: the phase 3 ACTHYF trial. Genet Med 22, 44-52 (2020).
92. Santoro, J.D., Filipink, R.A., Baumer, N.T., Bulova, P.D. & Handen, B.L. Down syndrome regression disorder: updates and therapeutic advances. Curr Opin Psychiatry 36, 96-103 (2023).
93. Rosso, M., et al. Down Syndrome Disintegrative Disorder: A Clinical Regression Syndrome of Increasing Importance. Pediatrics 145(2020).
94. Cardinale, K.M., et al. Immunotherapy in selected patients with Down syndrome disintegrative disorder. Dev Med Child Neurol 61, 847-851 (2019).
95. Ramaekers, V.T., et al. Folinic acid treatment for schizophrenia associated with folate receptor autoantibodies. Mol Genet Metab 113, 307-314 (2014).
96. Baumer, N.T., et al. Co-occurring conditions in Down syndrome: Findings from a clinical database. Am J Med Genet C Semin Med Genet 193, e32072 (2023).
97. Prajjwal, P., et al. Association of Alzheimer's dementia with oral bacteria, vitamin B12, folate, homocysteine levels, and insulin resistance along with its pathophysiology, genetics, imaging, and biomarkers. Dis Mon 69, 101546 (2023).
98. Naz, N., et al. Cerebral Folate Metabolism in Post-Mortem Alzheimer's Disease Tissues: A Small Cohort Study. Int J Mol Sci 24(2022).
99. Rossignol, D.A. & Frye, R.E. Cerebral Folate Deficiency, Folate Receptor Alpha Autoantibodies and Leucovorin (Folinic Acid) Treatment in Autism Spectrum Disorders: A Systematic Review and Meta-Analysis. J Pers Med 11(2021).
100. Reker, D., et al. "Inactive" ingredients in oral medications. Sci Transl Med 11(2019).
101. McKeown, D.A., et al. Olfactory function in young adolescents with Down's syndrome. J Neurol Neurosurg Psychiatry 61, 412-414 (1996).
102. Pogribna, M., et al. Homocysteine metabolism in children with Down syndrome: in vitro modulation. Am J Hum Genet 69, 88-95 (2001).
103. Frye, R.E., Sequeira, J.M., Quadros, E.V., James, S.J. & Rossignol, D.A. Cerebral folate receptor autoantibodies in autism spectrum disorder. Mol Psychiatry 18, 369-381 (2013).

Chapter 7. Epilepsy

104. Woody, R.C., Brewster, M.A. & Glasier, C. Progressive intracranial calcification in dihydropteridine reductase deficiency prior to folinic acid therapy. Neurology 39, 673-675 (1989).
105. Ventzke, A., et al. 'Malignant Phenylketonuria' (PKU) Due to Dihydropteridine Reductase (DHPR) Deficiency. Ir Med J 108, 312-314 (2015).
106. Ray, S., et al. Disorders of Tetrahydrobiopterin Metabolism: Experience from South India. Metab Brain Dis 37, 743-760 (2022).
107. Opladen, T., Hoffmann, G.F. & Blau, N. An international survey of patients with tetrahydrobiopterin deficiencies presenting with hyperphenylalaninaemia. J Inherit Metab Dis 35, 963-973 (2012).

108. Hyland, K., et al. Folinic acid responsive seizures: a new syndrome? J Inherit Metab Dis 18, 177-181 (1995).
109. Torres, O.A., Miller, V.S., Buist, N.M. & Hyland, K. Folinic acid-responsive neonatal seizures. J Child Neurol 14, 529-532 (1999).
110. Frye, R.E., Donner, E., Golja, A. & Rooney, C.M. Folinic acid-responsive seizures presenting as breakthrough seizures in a 3-month-old boy. J Child Neurol 18, 562-569 (2003).
111. Nicolai, J., van Kranen-Mastenbroek, V.H., Wevers, R.A., Hurkx, W.A. & Vles, J.S. Folinic acid-responsive seizures initially responsive to pyridoxine. Pediatr Neurol 34, 164-167 (2006).
112. Gallagher, R.C., et al. Folinic acid-responsive seizures are identical to pyridoxine-dependent epilepsy. Ann Neurol 65, 550-556 (2009).
113. Dill, P., et al. Pyridoxal phosphate-responsive seizures in a patient with cerebral folate deficiency (CFD) and congenital deafness with labyrinthine aplasia, microtia and microdontia (LAMM). Mol Genet Metab 104, 362-368 (2011).
114. Ramaekers, V.T., Häusler, M., Opladen, T., Heimann, G. & Blau, N. Psychomotor retardation, spastic paraplegia, cerebellar ataxia and dyskinesia associated with low 5-methyltetrahydrofolate in cerebrospinal fluid: a novel neurometabolic condition responding to folinic acid substitution. Neuropediatrics 33, 301-308 (2002).
115. Moretti, P., et al. Cerebral folate deficiency with developmental delay, autism, and response to folinic acid. Neurology 64, 1088-1090 (2005).
116. Sofer, Y., et al. Neurological manifestations of folate transport defect: case report and review of the literature. J Child Neurol 22, 783-786 (2007).
117. Ramaekers, V.T., Weis, J., Sequeira, J.M., Quadros, E.V. & Blau, N. Mitochondrial complex I encephalomyopathy and cerebral 5-methyltetrahydrofolate deficiency. Neuropediatrics 38, 184-187 (2007).
118. Thome, U., et al. Electrographic status epilepticus in sleep in an adult with cerebral folate deficiency. Neurol Clin Pract 6, e4-e7 (2016).
119. Rossignol, D.A. & Frye, R.E. Cerebral Folate Deficiency, Folate Receptor Alpha Autoantibodies and Leucovorin (Folinic Acid) Treatment in Autism Spectrum Disorders: A Systematic Review and Meta-Analysis. J Pers Med 11(2021).
120. Vidaurre, J. & Nunley, S. Atypical Presentation of a Progressive and Treatable Encephalopathy in an Older Child With Gelastic and Dacrystic Seizures. SemPediatr Neurol 26, 95-100 (2018).
121. Shein, S.L., Reynolds, T.Q., Gedela, S., Kochanek, P.M. & Bell, M.J. Therapeutic hypothermia for refractory status epilepticus in a child with malignant migrating partial seizures of infancy and SCN1A mutation: a case report. Ther Hypothermia Temp Manag 2, 144-149 (2012).
122. Girgis, M.Y., Mahfouz, E., Abdellatif, A., Taha, F. & ElNaggar, W. Cerebral Folate Transport Deficiency in 2 Cases with Intractable Myoclonic Epilepsy. J Epilepsy Res 14, 29-36 (2024).

Chapter 8. Neuroinflammation

123. Swedo, S. E., Leonard, H. L., Garvey, M., Mittleman, B., Allen, A. J., Perlmutter, S., Dow, S., Zamkoff, J., Dubbert, B. K., & Lougee, L. . Pediatric autoimmune neuropsychiatric disorders associated with streptococcal infections: Clinical description of the first 50 cases. The American Journal of Psychiatry, 155(2), 264–271. (1998).
124. Swedo, S.E., Leckman, J.F, & Rose, N.R. From Research Subgroup to Clinical Syndrome: Modifying the PANDAS Criteria to Describe PANS (Pediatric Acute-onset Neurophychiatric Syndrome). Pediatrics & Therapeutics, Vol 2, Iss 2, 113 (2012).
125. Jones, P., Lucock, M., Scarlett, C.J., Veysey, M. & Beckett, E.L. Folate and Inflammation – links

between folate and features of inflammatory conditions. Journal of Nutrition & Intermediary Metabolism 18, 100104 (2019).

126. Vaccaro, J.A., Qasem, A. & Naser, S.A. Folate and Vitamin B(12) Deficiency Exacerbate Inflammation during Mycobacterium avium paratuberculosis (MAP) Infection. Nutrients 15(2023).

127. Jones, P., Lucock, M., Scarlett, C.J., Veysey, M. & Beckett, E.L. Folate and Inflammation – links between folate and features of inflammatory conditions. Journal of Nutrition & Intermediary Metabolism 18, 100104 (2019).

128. Cheng, M., et al. Folic acid deficiency exacerbates the inflammatory response of astrocytes after ischemia-reperfusion by enhancing the interaction between IL-6 and JAK-1/pSTAT3. CNS Neurosci Ther 29, 1537-1546 (2023).

129. Cheng, M., et al. Folic acid deficiency enhanced microglial immune response via the Notch1/nuclear factor kappa B p65 pathway in hippocampus following rat brain I/R injury and BV2 cells. J Cell Mol Med 23, 4795-4807 (2019).

130. Shaikh, A. & Roy, H. Folate deprivation induced neuroinflammation impairs cognition. Neurosci Lett 807, 137264 (2023).

131. Mokgalaboni, K., Mashaba, G.R., Phoswa, W.N. & Lebelo, S.L. Folic acid supplementation on inflammation and homocysteine in type 2 diabetes mellitus: systematic review and meta-analysis of randomized controlled trials. Nutr Diabetes 14, 22 (2024).

132. Asbaghi, O., et al. Effects of Folic Acid Supplementation on Inflammatory Markers: A Grade-Assessed Systematic Review and Dose-Response Meta-Analysis of Randomized Controlled Trials. Nutrients 13(2021).

133. Ramaekers, V.T., et al. Folate receptor autoantibodies and spinal fluid 5-methyltetrahydrofolate deficiency in Rett syndrome. Neuropediatrics 38, 179-183 (2007).

134. Wells, L., O'Hara, N., Frye, R.E., Hullavard, N. & Smith, E. Folate Receptor Alpha Autoantibodies in the Pediatric Acute-Onset Neuropsychiatric Syndrome (PANS) and Pediatric Autoimmune Neuropsychiatric Disorders Associated with Streptococcal Infections (PANDAS) Population. J Pers Med 14(2024).

135. Mashayekhi, F. et al. Folate receptor alpha autoantibodies in the serum of patients with relapsing-remitting multiple sclerosis (RRMS). Clinical Neurology and Neruosurgery. 237 (2024).

136. Blau, N., et al. Cerebrospinal fluid pterins and folates in Aicardi-Goutières syndrome: a new phenotype. Neurology 61, 642-647 (2003).

137. Koenig, M.K., Perez, M., Rothenberg, S. & Butler, I.J. Juvenile onset central nervous system folate deficiency and rheumatoid arthritis. J Child Neurol 23, 106-107 (2008).

138. Frye, R.E., et al. Biomarkers of mitochondrial dysfunction in autism spectrum disorder: A systematic review and meta-analysis. Neurobiol Dis 197, 106520 (2024).

Chapter 9. Genetics

139. Ramaekers, V.T., et al. Reduced folate transport to the CNS in female Rett patients. Neurology 61, 506-515 (2003).

140. Ormazabal, A., Artuch, R., Vilaseca, M.A., Aracil, A. & Pineda, M. Cerebrospinal fluid concentrations of folate, biogenic amines and pterins in Rett syndrome: treatment with folinic acid. Neuropediatrics 36, 380-385 (2005).

141. Neul, J.L., et al. Spinal fluid 5-methyltetrahydrofolate levels are normal in Rett syndrome. Neurology 64, 2151-2152 (2005).

142. Ramaekers, V.T., et al. Folate receptor autoantibodies and spinal fluid 5-methyltetrahydrofolate deficiency in Rett syndrome. Neuropediatrics 38, 179-183 (2007).

143. Temudo, T., et al. Evaluation of CSF neurotransmitters and folate in 25 patients with Rett disorder and effects of treatment. Brain Dev 31, 46-51 (2009).
144. U.S. Food and Drug Administration. Food standards: Amendment of standards of identity for enriched grain products to require addition of folic acid (Docket No. 91N-100S). Federal Register, 61(44), 8781-8797 (1996).
145. Tso, W.W., Kwong, A.K., Fung, C.W. & Wong, V.C. Folinic acid responsive epilepsy in Ohtahara syndrome caused by STXBP1 mutation. Pediatr Neurol 50, 177-180 (2014).
146. Wang, Q., et al. The first Chinese case report of hereditary folate malabsorption with a novel mutation on SLC46A1. Brain Dev 37, 163-167 (2015).
147. Ahmad, I., Mukhtar, G., Iqbal, J. & Ali, S.W. Hereditary folate malabsorption with extensive intracranial calcification. Indian Pediatr 52, 67-68 (2015).
148. Torres, A., et al. CSF 5-Methyltetrahydrofolate Serial Monitoring to Guide Treatment of Congenital Folate Malabsorption Due to Proton-Coupled Folate Transporter (PCFT) Deficiency. JIMD Rep 24, 91-96 (2015).
149. D'Aco, K.E., et al. Severe 5,10-methylenetetrahydrofolate reductase deficiency and two MTHFR variants in an adolescent with progressive myoclonic epilepsy. Pediatr Neurol 51, 266-270 (2014).
150. Garcia-Cazorla, A., et al. Mitochondrial diseases associated with cerebral folate deficiency. Neurology 70, 1360-1362 (2008).
151. Lob, K., Sawka, D.M., Gaitanis, J.N., Liu, J.S. & Nie, D.A. Genetic Diagnostic Yield in Autism Spectrum Disorder (ASD) and Epilepsy Phenotypes in Children with Genetically Defined ASD. J Autism Dev Disord (2024).
152. Pérez-Dueñas B, Ormazábal A, Toma C, Torrico B, Cormand B, Serrano M, Sierra C, De Grandis E, Marfa MP, García-Cazorla A, Campistol J, Pascual JM, Artuch R. Cerebral folate deficiency syndromes in childhood: clinical, analytical, and etiologic aspects. Arch Neurol 68(5):615-21. (2011)

Chapter 10. So What About Vaccines?

153. Postma, J.K., et al. The diagnostic yield of genetic and metabolic investigations in syndromic and nonsyndromic patients with autism spectrum disorder, global developmental delay, or intellectual disability from a dedicated neurodevelopmental disorders genetics clinic. Am J Med Genet A, e63791 (2024).
154. Kuo, S.S., et al. Developmental Variability in Autism Across 17 000 Autistic Individuals and 4000 Siblings Without an Autism Diagnosis: Comparisons by Cohort, Intellectual Disability, Genetic Etiology, and Age at Diagnosis. JAMA Pediatr 176, 915-923 (2022).
155. Pode-Shakked, B., et al. A single center experience with publicly funded clinical exome sequencing for neurodevelopmental disorders or multiple congenital anomalies. Sci Rep 11, 19099 (2021).
156. Burger, B.J., et al. Autistic Siblings with Novel Mutations in Two Different Genes: Insight for Genetic Workups of Autistic Siblings and Connection to Mitochondrial Dysfunction. Frontiers in Pediatrics 5(2017).
157. Bar, O., Vahey, E., Mintz, M., Frye, R.E. & Boles, R.G. Reanalysis of Trio Whole-Genome Sequencing Data Doubles the Yield in Autism Spectrum Disorder: De Novo Variants Present in Half. Int J Mol Sci 25(2024).
158. Chaste, P. & Leboyer, M. Autism risk factors: genes, environment, and gene-environment interactions. Dialogues Clin Neurosci 14, 281-292 (2012).

159. Fan, H.C., Yang, M.T., Lin, L.C., Chiang, K.L. & Chen, C.M. Clinical and Genetic Features of Dravet Syndrome: A Prime Example of the Role of Precision Medicine in Genetic Epilepsy. Int J Mol Sci 25(2023).
160. Shoffner, J., et al. Fever plus mitochondrial disease could be risk factors for autistic regression. J Child Neurol 25, 429-434 (2010).
161. Klein, N.P., et al. Measles-mumps-rubella-varicella combination vaccine and the risk of febrile seizures. Pediatrics 126, e1-8 (2010).
162. Diseases, N.C.f.I.a.R. MMR & Varicella Vaccines or MMRV Vaccine: Discussing Options with Parents. (2021).
163. Wakefield, A.J., et al. Ileal-lymphoid-nodular hyperplasia, non-specific colitis, and pervasive developmental disorder in children. Lancet 351, 637-641 (1998).
164. Retraction--Ileal-lymphoid-nodular hyperplasia, non-specific colitis, and pervasive developmental disorder in children. Lancet 375, 445 (2010).
165. Motta M, Stecula D (2021) Quantifying the effect of Wakefield et al. on skepticism about MMR vaccine safety in the U.S. PLoS ONE 16(8): e0256395. (1998).
166. Gulle, B.T., Yassibas, U. & Sarigedik, E. Vaccine Hesitancy in the Autism Spectrum Disorder Context: Parental Vaccine Decision-Making and Coping with Stress Strategies. J Autism Dev Disord (2024).
167. Urion, D.K. Compassion as a Subversive Activity: Illness, Community, and the Gospel of Mark. Cowley Publications. (2006).

Chapter 11. Psychiatric Conditions

168. Wells, L., O'Hara, N., Frye, R.E., Hullavard, N. & Smith, E. Folate Receptor Alpha Autoantibodies in the Pediatric Acute-Onset Neuropsychiatric Syndrome (PANS) and Pediatric Autoimmune Neuropsychiatric Disorders Associated with Streptococcal Infections (PANDAS) Population. J Pers Med 14(2024).
169. Pan, L.A., et al. Metabolomic disorders: confirmed presence of potentially treatable abnormalities in patients with treatment refractory depression and suicidal behavior. Psychol Med 53, 6046-6054 (2023).
170. Godfrey, P.S., et al. Enhancement of recovery from psychiatric illness by methylfolate. Lancet 336, 392-395 (1990)   .
171. Papakostas, G.I., et al. L-methylfolate as adjunctive therapy for SSRI-resistant major depression: results of two randomized, double-blind, parallel-sequential trials. Am J Psychiatry 169, 1267-1274 (2012).
172. Papakostas, G.I., et al. Effect of adjunctive L-methylfolate 15 mg among inadequate responders to SSRIs in depressed patients who were stratified by biomarker levels and genotype: results from a randomized clinical trial. J Clin Psychiatry 75, 855-863 (2014).
173. Zajecka, J.M., et al. Long-term efficacy, safety, and tolerability of L-methylfolate calcium 15 mg as adjunctive therapy with selective serotonin reuptake inhibitors: a 12-month, open-label study following a placebo-controlled acute study. J Clin Psychiatry 77, 654-660 (2016).
174. Nierenberg, A.A., et al. L-Methylfolate For Bipolar I depressive episodes: An open trial proof-of-concept registry. J Affect Disord 207, 429-433 (2017).
175. Ramaekers, V.T., et al. Folinic acid treatment for schizophrenia associated with folate receptor autoantibodies. Mol Genet Metab 113, 307-314 (2014).
176. Roffman, J.L., et al. Randomized multicenter investigation of folate plus vitamin B12 supplementation in schizophrenia. JAMA Psychiatry 70, 481-489 (2013).

177. Roffman, J.L., et al. Biochemical, physiological and clinical effects of l-methylfolate in schizophrenia: a randomized controlled trial. Mol Psychiatry 23, 316-322 (2018).
178. Loria-Kohen, V., et al. A pilot study of folic acid supplementation for improving homocysteine levels, cognitive and depressive status in eating disorders. Nutr Hosp 28, 807-815 (2013).

Chapter 12. Cognitive Disorders of Older Age

179. Cooper, C., Sommerlad, A., Lyketsos, C.G. & Livingston, G. Modifiable predictors of dementia in mild cognitive impairment: a systematic review and meta-analysis. Am J Psychiatry 172, 323-334 (2015).
180. Rotstein, A., Kodesh, A., Goldberg, Y., Reichenberg, A. & Levine, S.Z. Serum folate deficiency and the risks of dementia and all-cause mortality: a national study of old age. Evid Based Ment Health 25, 63-68 (2022).
181. Kishida, R., et al. Serum folate and risk of disabling dementia: a community-based nested case-control study. Nutr Neurosci 27, 470-476 (2024).
182. Wang, Z., Zhu, W., Xing, Y., Jia, J. & Tang, Y. B vitamins and prevention of cognitive decline and incident dementia: a systematic review and meta-analysis. Nutr Rev 80, 931-949 (2022).
183. Ramos, M.I., et al. Low folate status is associated with impaired cognitive function and dementia in the Sacramento Area Latino Study on Aging. Am J Clin Nutr 82, 1346-1352 (2005).
184. Agnew-Blais, J.C., et al. Folate, vitamin B-6, and vitamin B-12 intake and mild cognitive impairment and probable dementia in the Women's Health Initiative Memory Study. J Acad Nutr Diet 115, 231-241 (2015).
185. Kim, J.M., et al. Changes in folate, vitamin B12 and homocysteine associated with incident dementia. J Neurol Neurosurg Psychiatry 79, 864-868 (2008).
186. Tu, M.C., Chung, H.W., Hsu, Y.H., Yang, J.J. & Wu, W.C. Neurovascular Correlates of Cobalamin, Folate, and Homocysteine in Dementia. J Alzheimers Dis 96, 1329-1338 (2023).
187. Chen, H., et al. Folic Acid Supplementation Mitigates Alzheimer's Disease by Reducing Inflammation: A Randomized Controlled Trial. Mediators Inflamm 2016, 5912146 (2016).

Chapter 13. Who Should Be Tested?

188. Girgis, M.Y., Mahfouz, E., Abdellatif, A., Taha, F. & ElNaggar, W. Cerebral Folate Transport Deficiency in 2 Cases with Intractable Myoclonic Epilepsy. J Epilepsy Res 14, 29-36 (2024).
189. Ramaekers, V.T., Häusler, M., Opladen, T., Heimann, G. & Blau, N. Psychomotor retardation, spastic paraplegia, cerebellar ataxia and dyskinesia associated with low 5-methyltetrahydrofolate in cerebrospinal fluid: a novel neurometabolic condition responding to folinic acid substitution. Neuropediatrics 33, 301-308 (2002).
190. Mafi, S., et al. Pharmacoresistant Epilepsy in Childhood: Think of the Cerebral Folate Deficiency, a Treatable Disease. Brain Sci 10(2020).
191. Frye, R.E., Sequeira, J.M., Quadros, E.V., James, S.J. & Rossignol, D.A. Cerebral folate receptor autoantibodies in autism spectrum disorder. Mol Psychiatry 18, 369-381 (2013).
192. Wells, L., O'Hara, N., Frye, R.E., Hullavard, N. & Smith, E. Folate Receptor Alpha Autoantibodies in the Pediatric Acute-Onset Neuropsychiatric Syndrome (PANS) and Pediatric Autoimmune Neuropsychiatric Disorders Associated with Streptococcal Infections (PANDAS) Population. J Pers Med 14(2024).
193. Leuzzi, V., Mastrangelo, M., Celato, A., Carducci, C. & Carducci, C. A new form of cerebral folate deficiency with severe self-injurious behaviour. Acta Paediatr 101, e482-483 (2012).

194. Ramaekers, V.T., et al. Folinic acid treatment for schizophrenia associated with folate receptor autoantibodies. Mol Genet Metab 113, 307-314 (2014).
195. Ho, A., Michelson, D., Aaen, G. & Ashwal, S. Cerebral folate deficiency presenting as adolescent catatonic schizophrenia: a case report. J Child Neurol 25, 898-900 (2010).
196. Pan, L.A., et al. Metabolomic disorders: confirmed presence of potentially treatable abnormalities in patients with treatment refractory depression and suicidal behavior. Psychol Med 53, 6046-6054 (2023).
197. Pan, L.A., et al. Metabolomic disorders: confirmed presence of potentially treatable abnormalities in patients with treatment refractory depression and suicidal behavior. Psychol Med 53, 6046-6054 (2023).
198. Ikeda, L., Capel, A.V., Doddaballapur, D. & Miyan, J. Accumulation of Cerebrospinal Fluid, Ventricular Enlargement, and Cerebral Folate Metabolic Errors Unify a Diverse Group of Neuropsychiatric Conditions Affecting Adult Neocortical Functions. Int J Mol Sci 25(2024).

Chapter 14. Symptoms of CFD

199. Thome, U., et al. Electrographic status epilepticus in sleep in an adult with cerebral folate deficiency. Neurol Clin Pract 6, e4-e7 (2016).
200. Ikeda, L., Capel, A.V., Doddaballapur, D. & Miyan, J. Accumulation of Cerebrospinal Fluid, Ventricular Enlargement, and Cerebral Folate Metabolic Errors Unify a Diverse Group of Neuropsychiatric Conditions Affecting Adult Neocortical Functions. Int J Mol Sci 25(2024).

Chapter 15. Diagnosing CFD

201. Frye, R.E., Sequeira, J.M., Quadros, E.V., James, S.J. & Rossignol, D.A. Cerebral folate receptor autoantibodies in autism spectrum disorder. Mol Psychiatry 18, 369-381 (2013).
202. Frye, R.E., et al. Binding Folate Receptor Alpha Autoantibody Is a Biomarker for Leucovorin Treatment Response in Autism Spectrum Disorder. J Pers Med 14(2024).
203. Frye, R.E., et al. Folinic acid improves verbal communication in children with autism and language impairment: a randomized double-blind placebo-controlled trial. Mol Psychiatry 23, 247-256 (2018).
204. Frye, R.E., et al. The Soluble Folate Receptor in Autism Spectrum Disorder: Relation to Autism Severity and Leucovorin Treatment. J Pers Med 12(2022).
205. Frye RE, McCarty PJ, Werner BA, Scheck AC, Collins HL, Adelman SJ, Rossignol DA, Quadros EV. Binding Folate Receptor Alpha Autoantibody Is a Biomarker for Leucovorin Treatment Response in Autism Spectrum Disorder. J Pers Med. Jan 1;14(1):62. (2024).
206. Frye, R.E., et al. Biomarkers of mitochondrial dysfunction in autism spectrum disorder: A systematic review and meta-analysis. Neurobiol Dis 197, 106520 (2024).
207. Dreha-Kulaczewski, S., et al. Folate receptor α deficiency - Myelin-sensitive MRI as a reliable biomarker to monitor the efficacy and long-term outcome of a new therapeutic approach. J Inherit Metab Dis 47, 387-403 (2024).
208. Masingue, M., et al. Cerebral folate deficiency in adults: A heterogeneous potentially treatable condition. J Neurol Sci 396, 112-118 (2019).
209. Liang, H., Chen, Z., Mo, C. & Tang, G. Synthesis and Preclinical Evaluation of [(18)F]AlF-NOTA-Asp(2)-PEG(2)-Folate as a Novel Folate-Receptor-Targeted Tracer for PET Imaging. J Labelled Comp Radiopharm 67, 334-340 (2024).

Chapter 16. Milk and CFD

210. U.S. Department of Agriculture and U.S. Department of Health and Human Services. Dietary Guidelines for Americans, 2020-2025. 9th Edition. (2020).
211. Ghozy S., et al. Association of breastfeeding status with risk of ASD: A systematic review, dose-response analysis and meta-analysis. Asian J Psychiatr. 48:101916. (2020).
212. Ballard O, Morrow AL. Human milk composition: nutrients and bioactive factors. Pediatr Clin North Am. 60(1):49-74. (2013).
213. Kent JC, et al. Volume and frequency of breastfeedings and fat content of breast milk throughout the day. Pediatrics. 117(3):e387–395. 2005-1417. (2006).
214. Wilkin, S., Ventresca Miller, A., Fernandes, R. et al. Dairying enabled Early Bronze Age Yamnaya steppe expansions. Nature 598, 629–633 (2021).
215. Bleasdale, M., Richter, K.K., Janzen, A. et al. Ancient proteins provide evidence of dairy consumption in eastern Africa. Nat Commun 12, 632 (2021).
216. Wal, J.M. Cow's Milk Allergens. Allergy Vol 53, Issue 11, p 1013 (1998).
217. Wunsch, N.G. Revenue of milk alternatives worldwide in 2024, by region. (2024).
218. Davoodi, S.H., et al. Health-Related Aspects of Milk Proteins. Iran J Pharm Res 15, 573-591 (2016).
219. Park,YW, Editor. Bioactive Components in Milk and Dairy Products. Wiley-Blackwell. (2009).
220. Singh, P. et al., Antiviral Properties of Milk Proteins and Peptides Against SARS-COV-2: A Review. Journal of Func Foods. Vol 117 (2024).
221. Hurley WL, Theil PK. Perspectives on immunoglobulins in colostrum and milk. Nutrients. 3(4):442-74. (2011).
222. Hansen SI, Holm J, Lyngbye J. Cooperative binding of folate to a protein isolated from cow's whey. Biochim Biophys Acta. 535(2):309-18. (1978).
223. Salter, D.N. et al., The Preparation and Properties of Folate-Binding Protein from Cow's Milk. The Biochemical Journal. Vol 193, Issue 2, 469-476. (1981)
224. Nixon PF, Jones M, Winzor DJ. Quantitative description of the interaction between folate and the folate-binding protein from cow's milk. Biochem J. 15;382 (2004).
225. Sahoo BR, et al., Structural and dynamic investigation of bovine folate receptor alpha (FOLR1), and role of ultra-high temperature processing on conformational and thermodynamic characteristics of FOLR1-folate complex. Colloids Surf B Biointerfaces. 121:307-18. (2014).
226. Vanze, J.D., et al., Nanocarrier centered therapeutic approaches: Recent developments with insight towards the future in the management of lung cancer. Journal of Drug Delivery Science and Technology. Volume 60 (2020).
227. Brigle, KE et al., Characterization of Two cDNAs Encoding Folate-binding Proteins from L1210 Murine Leukemia Cells. Journal of Biological Chemistry. Vol 266, No. 26. pp 17243-17249 (1991).
228. Ramaekers, V.T., Sequeira, J.M., Blau, N. & Quadros, E.V. A milk-free diet downregulates folate receptor autoimmunity in cerebral folate deficiency syndrome. Dev Med Child Neurol 50, 346-352 (2008).
229. Bobrowski-Khoury N, Ramaekers VT, Sequeira JM, Quadros EV. Folate Receptor Alpha Autoantibodies in Autism Spectrum Disorders: Diagnosis, Treatment and Prevention. J Pers Med. 11(8):710. (2021).
230. Zhang, X., et al. Milk consumption and multiple health outcomes: umbrella review of systematic reviews and meta-analyses in humans. Nutr Metab (Lond) 18, 7 (2021).

Chapter 17. Treating CFD

231. Reker, D., et al. "Inactive" ingredients in oral medications. Sci Transl Med 11(2019).
232. Sanguinetti, J.M., et al. Patient Safety and Satisfaction in Home Chemotherapy. Home Healthc Now 39, 139-144 (2021).
233. Dreha-Kulaczewski, S., et al. Folate receptor α deficiency - Myelin-sensitive MRI as a reliable biomarker to monitor the efficacy and long-term outcome of a new therapeutic approach. J Inherit Metab Dis 47, 387-403 (2024).
234. Vidaurre, J. & Nunley, S. Atypical Presentation of a Progressive and Treatable Encephalopathy in an Older Child With Gelastic and Dacrystic Seizures. Sem Pediatr Neurol 26, 95-100 (2018).
235. Mafi, S., et al. Pharmacoresistant Epilepsy in Childhood: Think of the Cerebral Folate Deficiency, a Treatable Disease. Brain Sci 10(2020).
236. Susgun, S., et al. Reanalysis of exome sequencing data reveals a treatable neurometabolic origin in two previously undiagnosed siblings with neurodev disorder. Neurol Sci 44, (2023).
237. Jaafar, F. & Obeid, M. Successful Treatment of Cerebral Folate Transporter Deficiency With Intravenous Folinic Acid. Pediatr Neurol 135, 22-24 (2022).
238. Zhang, C., et al. First case report of cerebral folate deficiency caused by a novel mutation of FOLR1 gene in a Chinese patient. BMC Med Genet 21, 235 (2020).
239. Kobayashi, Y., et al. Severe leukoencephalopathy with cortical involvement and peripheral neuropathy due to FOLR1 deficiency. Brain Dev 39, 266-270 (2017).
240. Delmelle, F., Thöny, B., Clapuyt, P., Blau, N. & Nassogne, M.C. Neurological improvement following intravenous high-dose folinic acid for cerebral folate transporter deficiency caused by FOLR-1 mutation. Eur J Paediatr Neurol 20, 709-713 (2016).
241. Kanmaz, S., et al. Cerebral folate transporter deficiency: a potentially treatable neurometabolic disorder. Acta Neurol Belg 123, 121-127 (2023).
242. Brunetti, S., et al. Cerebral folate transporter deficiency syndrome in three siblings: Why genetic testing for developmental and epileptic encephalopathies should be performed early and include the FOLR1 gene. Am J Med Genet A 185, 2526-2531 (2021).
243. Frye, R.E., et al. Binding Folate Receptor Alpha Autoantibody Is a Biomarker for Leucovorin Treatment Response in Autism Spectrum Disorder. J Pers Med 14(2024).
244. Rossignol, D.A. & Frye, R.E. The Effectiveness of Cobalamin (B12) Treatment for Autism Spectrum Disorder: A Systematic Review and Meta-Analysis. J Pers Med 11(2021).
245. Frye, R.E., et al. Binding Folate Receptor Alpha Autoantibody Is a Biomarker for Leucovorin Treatment Response in Autism Spectrum Disorder. J Pers Med 14(2024).
246. Lubout, C.M.A., et al. Successful Treatment of Hereditary Folate Malabsorption With Intramuscular Folinic Acid. Pediatr Neurol 102, 62-66 (2020).
247. Akiyama, T., et al. Folic acid inhibits 5-methyltetrahydrofolate transport across the blood-cerebrospinal fluid barrier: Clinical biochemical data from two cases. JIMD Rep 63, 529-535 (2022).
248. Delmelle, F., Thöny, B., Clapuyt, P., Blau, N. & Nassogne, M.C. Neurological improvement following intravenous high-dose folinic acid for cerebral folate transporter deficiency caused by FOLR-1 mutation. Eur J Paediatr Neurol 20, 709-713 (2016).
249. Dreha-Kulaczewski, S., et al. Folate receptor α deficiency - Myelin-sensitive MRI as a reliable biomarker to monitor the efficacy and long-term outcome of a new therapeutic approach. J Inherit Metab Dis 47, 387-403 (2024).
250. DEPLIN [package insert]. Shreveport, LA: Alfasigma USA, Inc. (2024).
251. Akiyama, T., et al. Folic acid inhibits 5-methyltetrahydrofolate transport across the blood-cerebrospinal fluid barrier: Clinical biochemical data from two cases. JIMD Rep 63, 529-535 (2022).

252. Alam, C., et al. Upregulation of reduced folate carrier by vitamin D enhances brain folate uptake in mice lacking folate receptor alpha. Proc Natl Acad Sci U S A 116, 17531-17540 (2019).
253. Alam, C., Hoque, M.T., Sangha, V. & Bendayan, R. Nuclear respiratory factor 1 (NRF-1) upregulates the expression and function of reduced folate carrier (RFC) at the blood-brain barrier. Faseb j 34, 10516-10530 (2020).
254. Sangha, V., Aboulhassane, S., Qu, Q.R. & Bendayan, R. Protective effects of pyrroloquinoline quinone in brain folate deficiency. Fluids Barriers CNS 20, 84 (2023).
255. Sangha, V., Aboulhassane, S., Qu, Q.R. & Bendayan, R. Protective effects of pyrroloquinoline quinone in brain folate deficiency. Fluids Barriers CNS 20, 84 (2023).
256. Rossignol, D.A. & Frye, R.E. Cerebral Folate Deficiency, Folate Receptor Alpha Autoantibodies and Leucovorin (Folinic Acid) Treatment in Autism Spectrum Disorders: A Systematic Review and Meta-Analysis. J Pers Med 11(2021).
257. Dill, P., et al. Pyridoxal phosphate-responsive seizures in a patient with cerebral folate deficiency (CFD) and congenital deafness with labyrinthine aplasia, microtia and microdontia (LAMM). Mol Genet Metab 104, 362-368 (2011).
258. Ramaekers, V.T., Sequeira, J.M., Blau, N. & Quadros, E.V. A milk-free diet downregulates folate receptor autoimmunity in CFD syndrome. Dev Med Child Neurol 50, 346-352 (2008).

Chapter 18. Following Outcomes

259. Frye, R.E., et al. Folinic acid improves verbal communication in children with autism and language impairment: a randomized double-blind placebo-controlled trial. Mol Psychiatry 23, 247-256 (2018).
260. Frye, R.E., Sequeira, J.M., Quadros, E.V., James, S.J. & Rossignol, D.A. Cerebral folate receptor autoantibodies in autism spectrum disorder. Mol Psychiatry 18, 369-381 (2013).

Chapter 19. Frequently Asked Questions (FAQs)

261. Frye, R.E., et al. Binding Folate Receptor Alpha Autoantibody Is a Biomarker for Leucovorin Treatment Response in Autism Spectrum Disorder. J Pers Med 14(2024).
262. Frye, R.E., et al. Folinic acid improves verbal communication in children with autism and language impairment: a randomized double-blind placebo-controlled trial. Mol Psychiatry 23, 247-256 (2018).
263. Bobrowski-Khoury, N., Sequeira, J.M. & Quadros, E.V. Brain Uptake of Folate Forms in the Presence of Folate Receptor Alpha Antibodies in Young Rats: Folate and Antibody Distribution. Nutrients 15(2023).
264. Reker, D., et al. "Inactive" ingredients in oral medications. Sci Transl Med 11(2019).
265. Ramaekers, V.T., et al. Genetic assessment and folate receptor autoantibodies in infantile-onset cerebral folate deficiency (CFD) syndrome. Mol Genet Metab 124, 87-93 (2018).
266. Delhey, L.M., et al. The Effect of Mitochondrial Supplements on Mitochondrial Activity in Children with Autism Spectrum Disorder. J Clin Med 6(2017).
267. Rossignol, D.A. & Frye, R.E. Cerebral Folate Deficiency, Folate Receptor Alpha Autoantibodies and Leucovorin (Folinic Acid) Treatment in Autism Spectrum Disorders: A Systematic Review and Meta-Analysis. J Pers Med 11(2021).
268. Frye, R.E., et al. Biomarkers of mitochondrial dysfunction in autism spectrum disorder: A systematic review and meta-analysis. Neurobiol Dis 197, 106520 (2024).

Images and Illustrations

Figure 1.1 - Image credit: Anderson, SA
Figure 1.2 - Image credit: Anderson, SA
Figure 1.3 - Image credit: Anderson, SA
Figure 1.4 - Created in BioRender. Frye, R. (2025) https://BioRender.com/a35j525
Figure 1.5 - Image credit: Anderson, SA
Figure 1.6 - Image credit: Anderson, SA
Figure 1.7 - Image credit: Anderson, SA
Figure 1.8 - Components from BioRender. Frye, R. (2025) https://BioRender.com/c53l047
Figure 1.9 - Components from BioRender. Frye, R. (2025) https://BioRender.com/c53l047
Figure 2.2 - Image credit: Anderson, SA
Figure 2.4 - Image credit: Anderson, SA
Figure 2.5 - Image credit: Anderson, SA
Figure 2.7 - Image credit: Anderson, SA
Figure 2.8 - Image credit: Anderson, SA
Figure 2.9 - Image credit: Anderson, SA
Figure 3.1 - Image credit: Anderson, SA
Figure 3.2 - Created in BioRender. Frye, R. (2025) https://BioRender.com/t59m209
Figure 3.3 - Image credit: Anderson, SA
Figure 3.4 - Image credit: Anderson, SA
Figure 3.6 - Image credit: Anderson, SA
Figure 3.7 - Image credit: Anderson, SA
Figure 3.8 - Image credit: Anderson, SA
Figure 4.3 - Image credit: Anderson, SA
Figure 4.4 - Image credit: Anderson, SA
Figure 7.1 - Created in BioRender. Frye, R. (2025) https://BioRender.com/y03j698
Figure 7.2 - Created in BioRender. Frye, R. (2025) https://BioRender.com/t31s471
Figure 7.3 - Created in BioRender. Frye, R. (2025) https://BioRender.com/k57f479
Figure 7.4 - Created in BioRender. Frye, R. (2025) https://BioRender.com/x17c263
Figure 7.5 - Created in BioRender. Frye, R. (2025) https://BioRender.com/q66n273
Figure 7.6 - Created in BioRender. Frye, R. (2025) https://BioRender.com/i47x069
Figure 7.7 - Created in BioRender. Frye, R. (2025) https://BioRender.com/r62l585
Figure 8.1 - Created in BioRender. Frye, R. (2025) https://BioRender.com/e33y557
Figure 8.2 - Created in BioRender. Frye, R. (2025) https://BioRender.com/o15i159
Figure 8.3 - Created in BioRender. Frye, R. (2025) https://BioRender.com/c92u516
Figure 9.1 - Created in BioRender. Frye, R. (2025) https://BioRender.com/b76d269
Figure 9.2 - Created in BioRender. Frye, R. (2025) https://BioRender.com/x87u855
Figure 14.2 - Created in BioRender. Frye, R. (2025) https://BioRender.com/g05n888
Figure 14.3 - Created in BioRender. Frye, R. (2025) https://BioRender.com/a05l652
Figure 14.4 - Image credit: Anderson, SA
Figure 14.5 - Photos licensed from 123RF
Figure 17.1 - Image credit: Anderson, SA
Figure 17.3 - Image credit: Anderson, SA

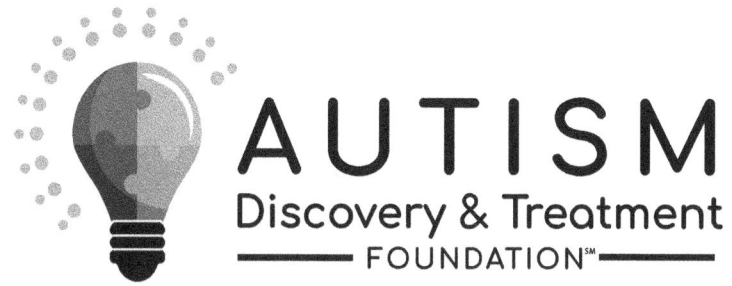

www.autismdiscovery.org

The Autism Discovery & Treatment Foundation

The Autism Discovery and Treatment Foundation (ADTF) is a 501(c)(3) nonprofit organization committed to enhancing the lives of individuals and families affected by autism and other neurodevelopmental disorders.

Founded by physicians dedicated to advancing our understanding of these complex conditions, ADTF focuses on identifying treatable biological mechanisms and developing practical, safe treatments.

By conducting cutting-edge research, particularly in areas like cerebral folate deficiency and mitochondrial dysfunction, the foundation strives to translate laboratory discoveries into effective clinical interventions, moving treatments from laboratories to lives.

ADTF's mission encompasses improving diagnostic accuracy, developing evidence-based clinical practices, and educating both the medical community and the public about new developments in autism research and treatment.

Please scan this QR code to learn about specific ongoing projects.

Want to Learn More?

The Metabolic Learning Resource, LLC will be launching a new online learning series in late 2025. Some modules are designed for clinicians, while others are tailored for families. These modules will provide in-depth exploration of the topics discussed in this book—particularly folate metabolism—as well as related subjects, such as the role of mitochondrial dysfunction in neurodevelopmental disorders.

As part of the series, Dr. Frye will host online Q&A sessions and offer clinical case reviews to support continued learning and engagement.

If you're interested in staying informed, please scan the QR code below to join our mailing list and let us know what topics and learning formats most interest you. You'll be notified as new resources become available.

Or visit www.metaboliclearn.com

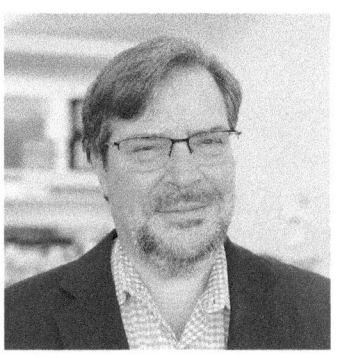

ABOUT THE AUTHOR

Dr. Richard E. Frye, MD, PhD, is a distinguished child neurologist and renowned research scientist specializing in neurodevelopmental and neurometabolic disorders, with a primary focus on autism spectrum disorder (ASD).

A leading voice in the ASD field, Dr. Frye's groundbreaking research has significantly advanced the understanding of the mechanisms underlying neurodevelopmental disorders and potential therapeutic strategies. His expertise encompasses mitochondrial dysfunction, folate metabolism defects, and the intricate interplay between the gut microbiome and brain function, which are critical areas of emerging ASD research.

Dr. Frye earned his MD and PhD in Physiology and Biophysics from Georgetown University and holds a Master's in Biomedical Science and Biostatistics from Drexel University. His extensive postgraduate training includes a Pediatrics residency at the University of Miami, a Child Neurology residency, and a Behavioral Neurology and Learning Disabilities fellowship at Harvard University/Children's Hospital Boston, as well as a Psychology fellowship at Boston University. He is board-certified in Pediatrics and in Neurology with Special Competence in Child Neurology.

With over 300 peer-reviewed publications and book chapters, Dr. Frye's work is widely cited and continues to shape the future of ASD research. He serves on several editorial boards, contributing his expertise to advance the field.

Currently, Dr. Frye serves as President and Chief Scientific Officer of the Autism Discovery and Treatment Foundation, Chief Medical Officer of the Neurological Health Foundation, Director of Research and Neurologist at the Rossignol Medical Center, and Principal Investigator at the Southwest Autism Research and Resource Center.

www.ingramcontent.com/pod-product-compliance
Lightning Source LLC
Chambersburg PA
CBHW052027030426
42337CB00027B/4899